# The Barefaced Doctor

## A mischievous medical companion

### Michael O'Donnell

I have lived open and barefaced... I will not die in a disguise.

*Roger Lestrange (1616 – 1704) Journalist and pamphleteer.*

Matador
9 Priory Business Park,
Wistow Road, Kibworth Beauchamp,
Leicestershire. LE8 0RX
Tel: (+44) 116 279 2299
Fax: (+44) 116 279 2277
Email: books@troubador.co.uk
Web: www.troubador.co.uk/matador

ISBN  978 1780884 264

British Library Cataloguing in Publication Data.
A catalogue record for this book is available from the British Library.

Typeset by Troubador Publishing Ltd, Leicester, UK

**Matador** is an imprint of Troubador Publishing Ltd

Printed and bound in the UK by TJ International, Padstow, Cornwall

Dedicated with respect and affection to those whose words are regular reminders that medicine remains an intellectually rigorous, humanitarian profession and who have over the years supplied me with anecdotal evidence of the uncertainties, paradoxes, life-affirming surprises, and black comedy that make practising medicine so rewarding.

Some are still with us. Some are not.
Others are I know not where.
But their words endure.

They include: Tim Albert, Marcia Angell, Peter Arnold, Richard Asher, Roger Bannister, Michael Baum, Austin Bradford Hill, Colin Brewer, Rob Buckman, Kenneth Calman, Mel Calman, Marie Campkin, Iain Chalmers, Anthony Clare, Archie Cochrane, David Colquhoun, Bev Daily, David Delvin, Bernard Dixon, Richard Doll, Christine Doyle, Annabel Ferriman, Faith Fitzgerald, Ben Goldacre, Raymond Greene, Phil Hammond, Ruth Holland, Antony Jay, Fred Kavalier, Geoffrey Keynes, Richard Leech, Richard Lehmann, Domhnall Macauley, Mary McCartney, Harvey Marcovitch, Francis Matthews, Peter Moloney, Larry Morton, Peter Medawar, George Mikes, Henry Miller, Jonathan Miller, John Mortimer, Frank Muir, Denis Norden, James O'Donnell, Gordon Ostlere (Richard Gordon), Sidney Joseph Perelman, James Penston, Robert Platt, Alison Pollock, Roy Porter, Michael Rawlins, Clare Rayner, Robert Robinson, Karl Sabbagh, Anne Savage, Sam Shuster, Bill Silverman, Petr Skrabanek, Richard Smith, Des Spence, Robin Steel, Raymond Tallis, Laurie Taylor, Lewis Thomas, Nick Timmins, Julian Tudor Hart, Paul Vaughan, Geoff Watts, Katherine Whitehorn, John Rowan Wilson, David Wood, David Wooton and the many others quoted in these pages.

# A

## Aaronical

High-priestly, pontifical role some doctors would like their profession to assume. Acceptable only if pronounced 'ironical'.

When I'm a patient I don't want a doctor with priestly aspirations but a skilled, kind, and intelligent sceptic who, in the words of the medical writer Donald Gould, "advises, persuades, supports, but never usurps".

If 21st century doctors are determined to have a fictional character as a role model, I suggest they eschew the wholly unsuitable Hippocrates (qv) and create one who approaches the Gould ideal, a unisex version of the loyal and dependable Reginald Jeeves.

## Abbreviation

Language that has replaced Latin (qv) as the vehicle for cabalistic medical utterance.

According to Dr Phil Hammond a patient will hear a junior doctor describe her to his boss as: "Mrs Simpson oriented times three, PERLA, cranials II to XII intact, LFs clear, JVP not displaced, Heart Sounds I plus II plus nil, Abdo NAD, TPCSR in RUL equals LUL equals RLL equals LLL."

All it means is that Mrs Simpson is fit to go home but, says Hammond, "If you can say it with a straight face, and know where the hospital laundry is, you can impersonate a doctor for life."

## Abnormal

Anything a doctor encounters for the first time.

## Absolute risk

Statistical term for the real risk we run, or can avoid, by changing our behaviour. This is the risk we need to know to make sensible decisions about our health but not the risk most often promulgated by the media.

In the age of cut-price journalism, too many 'health reports' and 'health scares' are based not on research data but on press releases. And too many press releases are written by people who hope to frighten us into changing our behaviour in a way that will profit them. Usually the profit is financial but sometimes it is just a bolstering of zealotry in those who believe they know what is good for us.

Even the *British Medical Journal (BMJ)*, which expects clinical trial reports to state absolute risks, can be complicit with deceivers. In May 2011 its news section, echoing national newspapers which relied on the same press release, published the results of an international study under a headline that suggested a pill could halve a particular risk. A reader, Dr John Doherty, pointed out the results could have been headlined: *International study shows that 94 per cent get no benefit and 58 per cent suffer side effects.*

That's a measure of the way data can be manipulated to impress people untrained or too bored to analyse statistics. The commonest trick is to quote relative rather than absolute risk. Suppose, for instance, we all run a risk of two in a thousand of getting a certain disease. That is our absolute risk. If a new treatment cuts that risk in half, it reduces the relative risk by 50 per cent but the absolute risk – our 'real' risk – only from two in a thousand to one in a thousand... a less impressive achievement.

In November 2011, another *BMJ* article claimed that research suggested that preventive 'treatment' could achieve a 10 per cent reduction in the risk of a specific cancer. A reader, Professor Florent Richy of Liege, pointed out that the data showed a 10 per cent reduction only of the relative risk; the reduction of the absolute risk was around 0.05 per cent.

In his book *stats.con* James Penston, a UK physician who has done much to clear muddled medical thinking about statistics, suggests that investigators quote relative risks because the inflated figures make their work look more significant. Others use them to promote their products, persuading doctors "to prescribe treatment, health service managers to pay for drugs, and patients to accept medication." (See Smoothsayer.)

## Academic values

Conditioned responses of those who live in Academe.

Unusually for her generation, Baroness Warnock had five children while she was still a young don. One morning in the early 1950s she met the aged Jocelyn Toynbee, then Professor of Roman History at Cambridge. Warnock was wheeling a pram containing two young children. A third toddled alongside. Toynbee peered into the pram and asked: "These all your children? Any of them any good?"

## Accent control centre

Group of cells in the cerebral cortex that ensures we speak foreign languages with the intonation of our own.

One man with a well tuned centre was General Charles de Gaulle who managed to speak English with an intonation that left no one in doubt of his distaste at having to use the language. Only once did he over-ride his central control. He and his wife were guests at a ceremony honouring British doctors who had helped the French Resistance during the war. Before the ceremony began, the wife of the president of one of our Royal Colleges sought to generate conversation by asking Madame de Gaulle what were her hopes for the future. To the consternation of the medical dignitaries (qv) she replied: "A penis." Her husband immediately intervened to explain: "In English, it is pronounced 'appiness'."

## Acceptable excuse

Essential semantic tool for NHS spin doctors. To gain acceptance an excuse needs to be couched in the language of Management.

Asked to explain a grave error, a Surrey hospital spokesman replied: "We regret that due to an oversight in the planning process, the service did not operate."

'An oversight in the planning process' approaches perfection. Error is freed from any taint of human culpability and becomes an unfortunate bug in the managerial software. And if you follow up the phrase, as the spokesman did, by reassuring critics that next time you will give "very careful consideration to the problem", you create the impression of concerned response without having to do anything.

Anyone seeking to couch an excuse in the language of the recipient should follow the example of Frank Muir and Denis Norden. When they were writing *Take it from Here*, the innovative post-war programme that severed radio comedy's last links with the Music Hall, the BBC accounts department sent them a cheque for an extra programme they had not written. A month later it wrote demanding its money back. After a pause to allow for due deliberation, Frank and Denis replied: "We regret we do not have the machinery for returning cheques."

The language and the tone of voice were so well-judged they heard nothing more.

## Acceptable gift
A definition that can pose tricky ethical decisions.

A consultant physician, asked to provide a 'second opinion', visited a patient in a high rise block in Liverpool. The patient was a member of a large family and, as the doctor was leaving, the family matriarch thanked him profusely for his kindness and, as a token of gratitude, handed him a box of eggs.

"Nice and fresh," she said. "And we'd like you to have them."

A glance out the window confirmed he was in a concrete ghetto with not a blade of grass in sight.

"Don't tell me you keep chickens up here," he said.

"Oh no, doctor. My daughter works in the hospital canteen."

## Accident prevention
Source of thoughtful advice from those at risk of paying compensation.

Warning on packet of Clotted Cream Rice: *IMPORTANT. Take care. Product will be hot after heating.*

Warning alongside a picture of a smiling baby on bottle of Teething Syrup: *May cause drowsiness. If affected, do not drive or operate machinery. Avoid Alcohol.*

Notice on top of television set in a Belgrade hotel bedroom: *If set breaks, inform manager. Do not interfere with yourself.*

## Acronyming

Game that medical institutions play with enthusiasm. Hospitals burdened with long names often translate them into Upper Case Abbreviation.

Characteristic examples are the LRI (Leicester Royal Infirmary) and UCH (University College Hospital). Sometimes abbreviation offers an harmonious acronym. MASH (Mobile Army Surgical Hospital) was so harmonious it served successfully as title of a best selling book and an award winning film.

This sort of harmony appeals to medical institutions when they choose to re-name themselves. The acronym NATASHA brings a hint of Eastern romance to the National Truss and Surgical Appliance Society unlike the original title bestowed by its founder William Pitt in 1772: An Institute for Relief of the Ruptured Poor.

A desperate search for harmony can, however, tempt new organisations to choose titles with an ear rather than a brain for meaning. I noticed the danger with the coming of ASH (Action on Smoking and Health) which seemed to overstrain syntax to achieve acronymity. Its creation caused the tobacco lobby to fight back, dare I say equally woodenly, with FOREST (Freedom Organisation for the Right To Enjoy Smoking Tobacco).

Harmony can also cause disharmony. I doubt the South Carolina Organisation of Ophthalmological Practitioners was pleased when its acronym SCOOP was hijacked by a New York City campaign to prevent dogs defecating in the streets. In New York the initials stand not for all that's best in southern ophthalmology but for Stop Crapping On Our Pavements.

## Acts of God

Delicious moments of retribution occasionally revealed unto doctors.

From the annals of the accident and emergency department at the Bristol Royal Infirmary: A driving examiner testing a moped driver, used one of the traditional procedures. "Drive round the block," he said. "When you re-appear in this street, I will step off the pavement and raise my hand to signal you to make an emergency stop." The moped driver disappeared, and when he came belting back around the corner, the examiner stepped from the pavement. It was the wrong moped.

## Acupuncture

Ancient Oriental treatment sometimes, thanks to its ritual, more effective than other placebos. Banned by the Chinese in 1929 but resuscitated in 1949 when the pragmatic Chairman Mao saw ancient Chinese medicine as a way to provide health care for a vast rural population in a country where the few doctors trained in Western medicine worked in cities.

When Nixon's visit to Beijing opened up China to the West, acupuncture, with its manikins, Qi channels, golden needles, and evocation of the mysterious Orient, seemed custom-tailored for seekers after alternative healing. The fervour which helped it conquer the West was generated predictably in California.

One evening in 1976 I called on my friend Ralph Schafferzick, in his office at St Michael's Hospital in San Francisco. His grin was so broad that instead of saying "Hello" I said, "Share the joke."

"I've just seen a woman from Chinatown. Her symptoms aren't serious but irksome and they don't respond to any treatment. When, as a last resort, I suggested we might try acupuncture she got very angry: 'Acupuncture very good for Americans visiting China,' she said. 'No good for Chinese woman living in San Francisco'."

## Address

Versatile verb that NHS managers filched from politicians. As in: "We are constantly addressing this important issue."

Conveys impression of asking or answering a question, or even doing both, while actually doing neither.

A survey of press releases issued by hospitals in 2006, revealed that by far the commonest subject being addressed was an 'agenda.' The next most common was 'ongoing problems.'

## Added value

What customers, once known as patients, really want from the NHS.

With the coming of the internal market (qv) a few enlightened individuals spotted the opportunities. One such visionary, Dr Mark Baker, chief executive of the Bradford Hospital Trust, told a conference of health service managers that the benchmark for judging NHS performance should be success in marketing clinical services to 'customers' rather than the ability to cure them. He exhorted his listeners to "hail successful selling staff as the heroes of the organisation." Other staff should look to their laurels and ensure that customers got more 'value' while in contact with the service.

Hospitals responded eagerly to the inspirational appeal of the visionaries. One of their first moves was to 'outsource' unglamorous services that made no contribution to 'sales', such as hospital cleaning.

Soon they were able to offer added value to their customers: patients admitted with just one illness were given a second one free, most commonly MRSA.

## Ad hominem
Time-honoured way to dismiss the arguments of someone on a lower branch of medicine's hierarchic tree.

Medicine's caste system provides a rich vocabulary of labels for 'upstarts' with unacceptable views. Most were forged and tested in the days of empire when everyone was expected to know his or her place. Traditional labels, all of them heard by me on GMC premises, include:

The Bit-of Group: *Bit of a show-off. Bit of a swat. Bit of an oik. Bit full of him/herself.*
The Too Group: *Too clever by half. Too big for his boots. A little too ambitious for my taste.*
The No-gentleman-no-lady Group: *No concept of decent behaviour. Can't stand that whine in her voice. One of the brown rice and sandals brigade.*
And, of course, the ultimate dismissal: *Unsound*

These phrases are most effective when used at a dinner table, a college reception, or a social gathering where they can float, in half-whisper, from the corner of a mouth into a receptive ear.

## Advice
Nostrum that has inherited the attributes of an old-style bottle of medicine: easy to dispense, difficult to swallow.

As a student I watched a young orthopaedic surgeon called Pickering-Pick give a butcher with a damaged shoulder not just advice but a detailed demonstration of how he should swing his cleaver. The patient was so impressed he couldn't bring himself to confess he worked in the accounts department.

Clare Rayner admitted that some advice she offered as an agony aunt could have been better expressed. One young couple had got themselves into such an emotional tangle the husband became impotent. The Rayner reply started: "There is one thing you must get straight between you... "

I once provoked a group of GPs into discussing the least helpful advice they could give to a patient. The most unhelpful phrases, we agreed, were those that sound good but lack precision: "Take it easy for a day or two", "Go on a light diet", or "Drink more fluid" ('more' is undefinitive and what else is there to drink other than fluid?).

Equally detested was advice impossible to follow: "Avoid stress", or the much more dangerous "Pull yourself together", usually addressed to those who'd lost their capacity to do just that.

I voted for "Don't worry", not just because it's advice impossible to follow but because a surgeon had recently told me, "Don't you worry, old chap, leave it all to me" and I would never leave anything to anyone who called me 'old chap'.

Nietzsche was probably right when he suggested that those who give advice to ill people acquire a feeling of superiority over them, whether the advice is taken or rejected. That was why, he suggested, susceptible and proud invalids hated their advisers even more than their illness.

## Aetiological blindness
The leading cause of muddled thinking about health and medicine.

> *"Heart disease (including heart attacks) was the leading cause of death for both sexes in England and Wales."*
> National statistics published by UK government.

> *"UN warns HIV/Aids leading cause of death in women."*
> BBC news website, 3 March 2010.

*"Tuberculous is the leading cause of death among curable infectious diseases."*

Health protection agency, July 2011.

None of these statements intend to mislead. Yet all are untrue. The leading cause of death remains what it always has been – birth.

I'm not being pedantic. Everyone involved in the 'healthcare business' needs a regular reminder of the implications of its ultimate achievement. Two of the most significant are:

1. The finest of medicine's technical triumphs are still just make-do-and-mend.
2. People who seek our help need more than just technical support along the route to the inevitable.

My experience in general practice taught me that an essential quality in a 'good GP' – by which I mean one I would like to look after my family or me – is an understanding that all patients suffer from the same incurable disease. Dealing with mortality is a more practical proposition than trying to instil an ill-defined entity called health.

The best doctors, whatever their specialty, help patients cope with the implications of their incurable disease and encourage them, during the course of it, to achieve some sort of harmony with the world around them. They learn to treat mortality not as an enemy to be fought on every front but as an awkward ally who has occasionally to be appeased.

## Affirmative action

The role of a yes man. Prudent activity for ambitious young medical persons.

When Dr John D Watt, of Kansas State University subjected bank employees to a personality test designed to measure sycophancy, he discovered that 'yes men' were more likely to be promoted, earn the approval of their superiors, and receive positive assessment reports. Juniors who indulged in high levels of ingratiating behaviour won high marks for co-operation, competence, motivation, promotion potential, and overall performance. Dr Watt found no difference between men and women in their willingness or ability to ingratiate.

Bankers, it seemed, had caught up with a truth already known to generations of junior doctors. Sucking up to the boss is good for you.

A senior World Health Organisation doctor visiting health workers in Malaysia in the 1990s concluded his homily with a joke. The interpreter translated it and everyone burst into laughter. Later, the visitor asked the interpreter how difficult it had been to translate the joke into local vernacular. 'I didn't think everyone would get the point, sir, so I said: "The doctor has just told a joke. Everyone will laugh".'

## Allergy
Useful and sometimes profitable diagnosis when all else has failed.

Dr Rob Buckman pointed out that a skin allergy is called eczema if it occurs on elbows, ears, or knees but dermatitis if it occurs on a private patient. Hence the riddle I once heard in a Californian hospital.

Q: What's the difference between an itch and an allergy?

A: About 200 dollars

Fear of allergy, and knowledge of ways to avoid it, is highest among the rich, particularly those who live in North America. When the incorrigible Sam Shuster, former professor of dermatology at the University of Newcastle-upon-Tyne, discussed the bizarre allergies diagnosed so readily and so profitably, he often showed his audience a funeral announcement culled from a US newspaper. The last sentence read: *No flowers please because of the deceased's allergies*.

## Almost a gentleman
Title the music hall comedian Billy Bennett bestowed on himself and which well-bred Victorian ladies bestowed on physicians and surgeons.

Doctors who whinge that our profession has lost its status should consider the opinion of Anthony Trollope's Miss Marrable, who appears in *The Vicar of Bullhampton* and "whom nobody could doubt was a lady; she looked it every inch."

*She had an idea that the son of a gentleman, if he intended to maintain his rank as a gentleman, should earn his income as a clergyman, or as a barrister, or as a soldier, or as a sailor. Those were the professions intended for gentlemen. She would not absolutely say that a physician was not a gentleman, or even a surgeon; but she would never allow to physic the same absolute privileges which, in her eyes, belonged to law and church.*

## Ambiguity

The well honed medical art of implying more than you actually say.

Often deployed in the writing of testimonials. In the 1960s Noel Glover, a surgeon at Guy's Hospital, wrote of one of his trainees: "You will be lucky to get this man to work for you."

The prospective employers of a junior orthopaedic surgeon received one that claimed: "He conceals his true character beneath a civilised veneer that is soluble in alcohol."

In another part of the forest, John Rowan Wilson, the surgeon turned novelist who died tragically young in the 1970s, was a regular recipient of unsolicited manuscripts from doctors who fancied they could emulate A J Cronin or Richard Gordon. Most of the texts were so long that if he read them he would have little time for anything else. John always replied politely: "Thank you for sending me your book. I shall lose no time in reading it."

## Ambivalence

Ingredient of even the most clearly defined dramatic gesture.

Evidence suggests, for instance, that many teenagers who make a 'suicide bid' by taking an overdose don't want to kill themselves but want to escape from distress they find unbearable. They seek not death but oblivion.

Their state of mind was illustrated by a youth who threw himself off the Brooklyn Bridge. He dithered so long before jumping that the river police had time to send a launch to the bridge. When he eventually jumped, the police launch sped towards him. A policeman threw him a rope and told him to grab it.

"Leave me alone," said the youth. "I want to die."

The New York cop drew his gun and pointed at the youth.

"Grab that rope," he said.

The youth obeyed immediately and was dragged aboard.

## Analgesic explanation.
One that in the words of the late Sir Peter Medawar, "dulls the ache of incomprehension without removing the cause".

> In the summer of 1981 William Bennett of Sheerness discovered he was pregnant. At the age of seventy-nine, he found it a bit tiresome but this was his thirtieth pregnancy and he had learned to put up with it. Whenever one of his four daughters became pregnant, Mr Bennett's abdomen began to swell and stayed swollen until his grandchild was delivered. Said his GP, "He hadn't swelled up when his wife was pregnant but never missed out on any of his twenty-six grandchildren and came out in sympathy with each of his four great grandchildren."

Medical textbooks call Mr Bennett's condition couvade but that is a label, not an explanation; medical dictionaries define it as a custom among primitive peoples by which a husband 'feigns illness' during his wife's pregnancy; medical journals have reported a few cases similar to Mr Bennett's but no medical texts give a convincing explanation of what was going on in his abdomen.

> One of my patients when I was a GP occasionally got a rash on her left hand. It always started under her wedding ring, usually as a small red patch which faded after a few weeks but it sometimes spread as a raw and peeling rash over her whole hand. Tests revealed no allergy to the metal of her ring. And when she didn't wear the ring, she still got the rash, starting at the point where the ring would have been.
> As often happens when doctors are baffled, the patient came up with the answer. She noticed the rash came only when her husband was due to fly abroad on business. She herself was terrified of flying and her family had once had to cancel a holiday after they'd arrived at the airport because she could not get on the plane. Her discovery of the link with her anxiety did not cure the rash but gave it a

name. Dermatologists recognise 'wedding ring dermatitis' as a rare affliction which sometimes occurs when a marriage is about to break up.

These days, most of us are prepared to accept that anxiety can cause headaches, indigestion, diarrhoea, or even rashes, but still think it odd when the rash is linked to a ring that is only a symbol. Such links, and Mr Bennett's 'pregnancy', so disturb some people they prefer to create a magical explanation which does not conflict with their idea of rigid 'natural laws'.

Some doctors suppress their unease over conditions like Mr Bennett's by calling them psychosomatic. Yet 'psychosomatic', like 'couvade' and 'wedding ring dermatitis' is an analgesic explanation. A barefaced doctor is happy to confess, "I see it happen but I don't know why... well, not yet."

## Anatomize

Making adroit use of anatomical knowledge to enhance a word picture, often to convey the grandeur of physical achievement.

The best examples are not extraneous images grafted on to an event but become part of the event itself. As in that offered by a stage hand who, in his youth, had stood in the wings of a Dublin theatre and heard the great John McCormick singing Mozart.

When a reporter asked him to describe the golden voice he said: "It may have sounded effortless out front, but when McCormick hit that top C, you couldn't have got a tram ticket between the cheeks of his arse."

## Animatism

The attribution of human emotions to inanimate objects. Occurs occasionally in schizophrenic patients and angry surgeons, more often in shopkeepers.

A *Times* reader described how his local DIY store had a notice explaining it no longer stocked one model of lawnmower because it was de-ranged. Another reader reported that notices around the Elephant and Castle claimed that local parking meters were alarmed. He wondered if they'd heard about the de-ranged lawnmowers.

A Lancashire surgeon found his hospital parking space blocked by a small car. He parked in a gap alongside and left a note, scrawled in angry block capitals, under the intruder's windscreen wiper: BLUE CAR. THIS IS A PRIVATE SPACE. DO NOT PARK HERE. When he returned he found the space empty and a reply under his own wiper. In tiny handwriting it said: *Please don't shout. I'm very sorry. Blue car.*

## Anonymity

Advantage bestowed by clothing worn in operating theatres.

In the 1950s the oldest medical student at St Thomas' was 'Pop' Manley, a retired Indian judge who'd taken up medicine in his sixties to become a missionary and was so deaf that rumour claimed he didn't pass his finals till he got a case that didn't require him to hear anything through a stethoscope.

When he made his first appearance in the theatre, his cap and mask obscured his grey hair and facial wrinkles and he stood quietly by while a pompous young surgeon lectured his new students on surgical etiquette and hinted how lucky they were to be apprenticed to a genius such as himself.

As he finished talking and raised his scalpel, one of his new students stepped forward and said: "Now, young man, perhaps you could tell us exactly what you're trying to do."

## APA

Acute penis awareness. Condition that afflicts men examined by women doctors.

And not just the men. Dr Susan Bewley described the culture shock she suffered in her first week working in a clinic for sexually transmitted infections where forty to fifty men dropped their trousers in front of her every day. Travelling home on the underground she half expected any man facing her to expose himself.

In her clinic, APA often induced shyness. One man said, "I couldn't possibly show you the offending part." She told him to look out of the window and pretend he was somewhere else. Others seemed all too eager to drop their trousers, unzipping their flies and whipping out the damaged organ as they strode into the consulting room. Discomfited by the lack of formality Dr Bewley would cry: "Hang on. Tell me your name first."

## Arcanian

Approved language for discourse between politicians, health department officials, health administrators, NHS managers, and all interdisciplinary in-depth strategic thinkers seeking to roll out a raft of innovative healthcare frameworks.

Advanced form of Decorated Municipal Gothic (qv), the language developed by management consultants and other spin doctors who need impressive words to hide the threadbare nature of the thought, if any, that lies behind the words.

Michael Leapman described it as "verbal detritus bred from the half-digested nostrums of the business schools and the self-important hype of the public relations industry." Simon Hoggart suggested it reflects "the desperate desire among people with just a little bit of power over our lives to turn the simplest human activity… into something vague, intangible, and pompous."

Administrators may find it less painful to refer to 'resource constraints' than to 'shortage of cash' but that's no excuse for forcing GPs to grope their way through plans "to provide a multi-agency preventative and problem solving approach for elderly care in the community." I suspect the authors mean 'care of old people' rather than 'elderly care' – an altogether different notion – but once you immerse yourself in sentences of that density, your brain grows dead to the actual meaning of the words.

Arcanians would, I suspect, prefer to address us in German, a language in which they could condense long composite phrases into a single noun. In evidence I offer a health authority memo that extols "a package of lifestyle associated health promotion initiatives." Package is clearly the word of the moment and nasty outbreaks of it have now been reported from most corners of the kingdom. The source of the epidemic in medicine was an Arcanian in the Department of Health who exhorted hospitals to offer their patients "consumer led packages", a phrase which conjures a vision of customers walking out of department stores with their parcels trotting behind them on a lead.

Sadly, its not only the managers who need to watch their language. I've seen otherwise intelligent doctors fall hopelessly in love with Arcanian and, like many who embark on passionate affairs in middle life, they quickly lose all sense of reason and discretion. As in this memorandum sent to all consultants at Addenbrooke's Hospital, Cambridge, and signed, may the Gods forgive him, by the Medical Director:

*You need to be aware that effective 9.00 am on 13th December, the Executive Board has agreed that a 'ring-fence' shall apply to the bed envelope of each general management grouping across the hospital. Thus the intention is that the Medical grouping and the Surgical grouping will consume their own smoke in meeting bed requirements.*

I was sent a copy by a Cambridge physician who wondered through which orifice he was expected to consume his smoke.

Arcanian has also polluted language and thought in academe. In 2011 Gary Kaye of Leeds pulled off a double whammy in a letter to the *Guardian* which, in two sentences, illustrates both the academic usefulness and the non-academic danger of the language.

*Media studies is often called a 'Mickey Mouse' subject, but I can say that the only time I reference Mickey Mouse is when teaching Jean Baudrillard's theory of the Disneyfication of the media world, related to his ideas of simulacra and simulacrum, with particular reference to the hegemonic model of conglomerate media ownership. Not such a soft subject after all, but one attacked with all the academic rigour it deserves.*

Not only does he suggest that 'academic rigour' is merely a matter of describing things in Arcanian, he tempts us to translate it into English. And, when we do, we discover his subject could be on the softish side. Nice one, Gary.

## Arcanian: recent advances
Unfortunately Arcanian is a living language and acquires regular accretions. Recent additions to its vocabulary include:

### Drill down into
Search desperately through complex data for any snippet you can use to your political or financial advantage.
### Empowerment
Word doctors use to persuade those who care about these

things that they involve others in implementing decisions they have already made.

### The patient journey
An unwell person sitting in a series of unfamiliar and vaguely threatening places wondering what's going to happen next.

### Narrative
All purpose noun. When used to describe a patient's history, a hospital building programme, a laundry list, indeed anything, adds a whiff of modernity.

### New era
Ill-defined period during which something exciting is predicted to happen but rarely does. In medicine, hijacked by politicians and journalists who expect us to welcome at least one a year.

### Pathway
1. A road to nowhere. Sometimes endowed with surrealistic properties. An enthusiast for the proposed 2012 NHS reforms described them on the radio as, "A pathway that manages to stretch the envelope without splitting it." Less a pathway, then, than a condom stretcher.
2. Euphemism for a track down which doctors usher patients on the way to their death, including those who've said emphatically they don't want to go that way.

### Road Map
A plan that isn't a plan, an agenda that isn't an agenda, a timetable that isn't a timetable… yet needs a name that infers that those who produced it have achieved something.

## Armorial bearings
Essential, if expensive, tackle for any thrusting young specialty. (See Mace.)

Soon after the inauguration of The Faculty of Accident and Emergency Medicine, its council decided it would like an armigerous logo to adorn its headed notepaper and its president's badge. The faculty's Registrar John Thurston was instructed to approach the College of Arms. After much rumination Portcullis, *aka* Pursuivant of Arms, was graciously pleased to present letters-patent to the president bearing the seals of the Kings of Arms: Garter, Clarenceux, and Norroy and Ulster.

The process cost about £6,000 but think of the consolation those letters-patent will bring to any unfortunate soul caught up in an accident or emergency.

## Aromatic nostalgia

A quirk of memory used by psychiatrists to lead the bewildered by their noses along the road to reality.

When Dorothy Brearley, aged ninety-two, becomes confused, she takes a quick sniff from a little brown bottle and her mind becomes clear. "Ah, yes," she says, "Monday was always washday." The genie in the bottle is an odiferous mixture designed to emulate the smell of soap suds, a boiling copper, and the wet wood of scrubbing board and mangle rollers. Her doctor prescribed it to help her clear occasional bouts of mild confusion.

Washday, according to the magazine *Health and Ageing,* is one of 130 Nostalgic Aromas produced by Dale Air Products of Blackpool for doctors who use reminiscence therapy to help elderly patients. Other aromas include First World War Christmas cake, a school cloakroom on a wet morning, and an old-fashioned corner shop. The company is particularly strong on persistent odours: a smoky mill town, steam trains, and Wolverhampton.

Reminiscence therapists claim the most effective smells are those that evoke memories of the Second World War particularly the Women's Voluntary Service Tea Wagon Aroma, provided by the Eden Camp museum near Malton in Yorkshire.

## Arts, The

The only database available to doctors trying to understand the perplexing emotions that can turn the same disease into a different illness in different individuals. (See Chekov.)

Doctors trained to diagnose and treat disease sometimes find it hard to cope with the individuality of illness. To treat it successfully they need to enhance their medical experience with the experience of others who contribute to our understanding of the world in which we struggle to survive.

Luckily help is at hand. Just as the knowledge doctors acquire from observing and investigating their patients can enhance their knowledge of disease, so the understanding they may absorb from literature, or any of the arts, can enhance their perception of the nature of illness. As E M Forster wrote in Howard's End:

*One death may explain itself, but it throws no light upon another: the groping inquiry must begin anew. Preachers or scientists may generalise, but we know that no generality is possible about those whom we love; not one heaven awaits them, not even one oblivion. Aunt Juley, incapable of tragedy, slipped out of life with odd little laughs and apologies for having stopped in it so long.*

The arts don't just help us understand the world beyond our experience, they also help us understand ourselves, our motives, and our attitudes. A lifetime of doctor-watching has convinced me that empathy and understanding – or, as the jargonists prefer, 'successful communication' – are as dependent on doctors' knowledge of themselves as on their knowledge of their patients.

The American physician Faith T Fitzgerald sees other advantages for doctors.

*The point is not, of course, that knowledge of literature, history, music, art, or other non-medical scientific subjects makes one a better diagnostician (although this may be true) or a better therapist (although that is almost certainly true), but that the possession by the doctor of the background necessary to explore these areas with patients vastly enriches the relationship, and generates those moments in the doctor's life that flavour memories ever after.*

## Asterisk

Prophylactic measure taken by printers to prevent allergic reaction in readers sensitive to smut (qv).

Sometimes a source of confusion. I once wrote a letter to the editor of the *Independent*:

*Dear Sir, You report that a journalist was criticised for using the word c\*\*\* on television but, thanks to your euphemistic use of asterisks, we don't know if the word he used was c\*\*\* or c\*\*\*."*

The paper published the letter but didn't answer the question.

## Astrology

Form of soothsaying once used in medicine. (Galileo taught astrology to medical students in Padua.)

Abandoned by doctors when they learned, also from Galileo, how to subject philosophical explanations to experimental testing. Now regarded as a science only by those who worship the irrational. Worshippers have included national newspapers, the BBC, and the old Abbey National Building Society.

In 1985 Dr Shawn Carlson of the University of California published the results of two exhaustive investigations of astrological interpretations. After three years of inquiry, he concluded:

*Despite the fact that we worked with some of the best astrologers... despite the fact they approved of the design of the experiment and predicted 50 per cent as the minimum effect they would expect to see, astrology failed to perform at a level better than chance. Tested, using double-blind methods, the astrologers' predictions proved to be wrong.*

Yet...

In 1985, despite Carlson's findings, BBC's *Breakfast Time* continued to field a resident astrologer every day, predicting the future with a dogmatic certainty that the resident doctor, restricted to one appearance a week and tethered by reason, could never hope to match. (The astrologer left in 1986 but only because he got a better offer from ITV.) Yet, when it came to the weather forecast, both BBC and ITV relied on meteorologists. They didn't get a presenter to disembowel an animal and give us a read of the entrails. Nor an old salt to have a feel of his seaweed.

In 1995, the Abbey National Building Society offered its customers a booklet *Your Astrological Guide to a Secure Future,* advising them how to find wise investments through the stars.

In January 2000, Jonathan Cainer, the *Daily Mail*'s appropriately billed 'star astrologer' announced he was turning down the *Mail*'s £1 million a year and defecting to the *Daily Express*.

James Randi, a magician who turns his hand to investigating paranormal happenings, conducted an experiment during an American television programme. He asked an audience of about thirty adults to give him their birth dates, then left the room to feed the data into a computer programmed to print individual natal charts. When he returned he handed a print-out to each participant. After they'd studied them, he asked any who thought the chart described them well to raise their hands. Most of the hands went up. He then invited them to pass their chart to the person on their right. As they read their neighbours' charts they began to giggle and soon the giggles grew into concerted laughter. He'd given the same chart to everyone.

## Audiogenic confusion
Common interpretative dysfunction.

A medical student doing a holiday job as a porter at a Teaching Hospital NHS Trust was asked to deliver a package to a Mr Ernest Sexhauer. Not knowing where to find him, he rang a woman telephonist at the largest hospital. "Do you have a Sexhauer there?" he asked.
"No," she said. "We don't even have a ten minute coffee break."

Dr Alan Greenwood was puzzled when a woman patient in his Warminster surgery told him, "I'm much better since going back on the Vegivan, doctor." He searched diligently through the index of drugs for what he guessed must be a combination of Veganin and Ativan. But in vain. Later in the week she waved to him from the driver's seat of her mobile greengrocer's shop.

One case reported to me is so neat I fear it may be apocryphal. Its only authentication, and my excuse for including it, is that I heard it from John Mortimer whose least believable tales about lawyers often turned out to be true.

> One Monday morning m'learned friends assembled in the High Court to hear the verdict in a complicated commercial case. The judge entered, settled behind the bench, and then confessed with some embarrassment that he had written his lengthy judgement over the weekend but had foolishly left it at his country home. He therefore feared he could not deliver it until the next day.
> A helpful junior counsel got to his feet with a suggestion.
> "Fax it up, my lord," he said.
> "Yes," said the judge wearily, "I suppose it does."

## Audiogenic dysarthria

Interpretative dysfunction similar to audiogenic confusion. Sufferers think the message they're pronouncing is the one their listeners are receiving.

The disorder most commonly afflicts radio and television commentators. The boxer Alan Minter claimed on television, "There have been injuries and deaths in boxing but none of them serious." And an Australian newsreader won immortality with, "In Taree today, a woman was bitten on the funnel by a finger-web spider."

In Britain, television newsman Jon Snow reported two cases: a commentator in Horseguards' Parade who praised the Queen's Royal Arse Artillery and a newsreader who converted World Cup Soccer into an unmistakably lewd event.

The most interesting cases are those in which the words remain unchanged but the meaning gets adjusted twixt utterance and reception. At the end of the 1977 Boat Race, Harry Carpenter exclaimed: "Ah, isn't that nice? The wife of the Cambridge president is kissing the cox of the Oxford crew."

## Aura

Nebulous mélange of authority, humility, kindliness, and preparedness to listen which, when possessed by doctors, inspires the loyalty of patients.

It's power became the driving force in the story of Freddie

Brant. In the 1950s Freddie worked as a laboratory technician for Dr. Reid L. Brown of Chattanooga where he learned something of the science of medicine and a lot about the behaviour of doctors. When he left, he took copies of Dr Brown's diplomas, assumed his boss's identity, and worked for three years in a State Hospital in Texas. In the 1960s, he became 'town doctor' in the Texas village of Groveton where he established a thriving practice and became a popular figure. His success grew not just from his engaging personality and his willingness to devote time to listening to his patients; he was respected for the way in which he referred all potentially serious cases to doctors in nearby towns, a move seen by his patients as a sign of commendable humility.

Yet, though careful about protecting his patients, he was careless about protecting himself. He ordered his practice drugs from the wholesaler who supplied the real Dr Brown and one day a clerk discovered she was processing orders from the same doctor practising in two different states. The wholesaler called the police who, after an investigation, charged Freddie with forgery and fraud.

The people of Groveton reacted angrily, directing their anger not at Freddie but at the authorities who sought to deprive them of their doctor. They inundated newspapers with testimonials to his skill. A local farmer wrote: *My wife has been sick for fourteen years. We've been to doctors in Lufkin, Crockett and Trinity, and he did her more good than any of 'em. She was all drawed up, bent over, you ought to have seen her. He's brought her up and now she's milking cows and everything.* When Freddie was taken to court, the people of Groveton stood by their man. A grand jury refused to prosecute him and, when the trial was moved to another county, the case ended with a hung jury, eight members voting for acquittal.

One newspaper suggested Groveton people should have known Freddie wasn't a doctor because he did so many non-doctorly things. He made house calls for only five dollars and charged only three dollars for an office visit; he approved of Medicare, fiercely condemned by the American Medical Association as 'socialised medicine'; he would drive for miles to visit a patient, often without fee if the patient were poor; and his handwriting was legible.

Though acquitted by the court, Freddie decided to leave Texas. Today, of course, he could have set up as an 'alternative practitioner' and stayed on as the hero of Groveton and the people's choice of doctor. But he was too decent a man to play that game.

## Authority

Postgraduate qualification acquired with little expenditure of effort.

Time was when its acquisition demanded self denial. Young doctors had to work long hours on low pay, show undue deference to persons who wielded power, spend a lot of time in libraries memorising minutiae they would never need, and pass postgraduate exams notorious for high fees and high failure rates.

In the age of Celebrity you don't need hard-won letters after your name to achieve authority, you just need to be dubbed an 'expert' (qv). A man recently introduced on TV as "nutrition expert" turned out to be the proprietor of a health food shop, and a doctor who gave us the benefit of his opinion on the *Daily Mail*'s editorial page was described as "GP and sexual health expert", a description that begged more questions than it answered. (I'm surprised the Mail didn't go for the *BMJ* correspondent who, on the eve of the London Olympics, described himself as "GP and London Sexual Health Champion for NHS London.")

On the evening of June 3, 2011, when people were worried by reports that a previously unknown strain of E coli was causing deaths across Europe, *Channel 4 News* wheeled on an 'expert' to explain the significance of the reports and give authoritative answers to questions that worried the punters. An internationally respected epidemiologist? A Nobel prize winning bacteriologist? Er no... a celebrity chef who could tell us only what he, and we, had already read in newspapers, heard on the radio, or seen on television.

Not any celebrity chef, mark you. A year before, food inspectors rated hygiene in his gastro-pub as "poor" with "standards generally low." He also created a recipe which the watchdog Food Commission nominated as one of the unhealthiest dessert recipes of all time, and in 2008 had recommended, in *Healthy and Organic Living* magazine, the poisonous plant hebane as a "tasty addition to salads."

But you had to hand it to him. Although he told us nothing we didn't already know, he did so with great authority.

## Autoerotic
Medical jargon for the goings-on in J G Ballard's novel (and film) *Crash*.

A nasty consequence of auto-erotism appeared in the programme at Burton Postgraduate Medical Centre, a session entitled "Diagnosis of Volvovaginitis."

## Autonomic dyslexia
Communication disorder that leads people to choose words that impose their own meaning on a sentence.

> From a hospital newsletter: *Sister Shirley competes for the Nurse of the Year title. She says: "The hospital's ambulance men entered me without my knowing."*

> Avon Health Authority organised a unique training programme for practice nurses: *The ins and outs of sex.*
> (The chosen venue was the Bristol Society for the Blind.)

> Michael Reid a Lytham GP attending a course at Lancaster University found a sign in the gentlemen's lavatory: *Fire Alarm Testing. Every Wednesday at 11.00 a.m. No need to evacuate.*

## Autonomy
A right that patients sometimes have to establish for themselves,

> An incident reported in the *Lancet* during the Second World War:
> When a school doctor arrived to examine a group of evacuees who'd arrived at a rural retreat, he saw that two of them, though dressed differently, looked identical.
> "Aha," he said with a patronising smile, "I see we have twins."
> One of the boys stared silently at the ground. The other looked the doctor in the eye. "We are *not* twins," he said contemptuously.

"Enough of that, young man," said the doctor, unaccustomed to being answered back by ragamuffins.

He brusquely ordered the boys to sit on a school bench while he leafed through their documents. He looked up triumphantly. "You're as like as two peas," he said. "You have the same address, the same birthday, and the same father and mother. You *are* twins."

"No we are *not*," said the stubborn boy.

"Then what the hell are you?" asked the doctor.

"We're all that's left of triplets."

From *The Evening Standard:*
In court Poddy, dressed in black rubber frogman's suit and wearing two pheasant feathers in his hair, said: "It's not me on trial today, but the mentality of the court."

## Awareness

Cognitive state alleged to be induced by a day, a week, a month – or, in extreme cases, a year – devoted to reminding us of those little things we're assumed to have forgotten.

In the late 20th century people proclaimed their awareness with badges in their lapels, bracelets on their wrists, or bumper stickers on their cars. Supporters of National Incontinence Awareness Week wore a badge wittily depicting a sweet pea and Hampshire GPs were invited to join a Condom Awareness Scheme with the promise that training sessions would be "kept small and filled on a first come first served basis".

By the time we strode into the new millennium, competition for our awareness had grown frenetic. *Health Events 2001*, a poster published by Health Promotion England (*sic*), is crammed with significant events: National Tampon Week, National Breastfeeding Awareness Week, Illicit Drug Trafficking Day, Twin, Triplets & More Week, Arthritis Education Week, Bug Busting Day, and British Cardiac Patients Association Awareness Day, which might have got more attention had it slid more easily across the tongue.

There were a couple of puzzling items. Why did we need a Europe Against Cancer Week; had there been an outbreak of Europe For Cancer rallies that needed rebuttal? And why was February 14th no longer dedicated to St Valentine Awareness but to National Impotence Day? I detect a whiff of what advertising persons call 'creativity'.

When I first saw the Health Events poster I was saddened that no month, nor week, nor even day was devoted to just gadding around feeling healthy. I decided to organise a Healthy Unawareness Month but once I turned my mind to the daily mundanities of life the idea slipped off my awareness screen.

# B

## Bad form

Serious breach of etiquette in modern general practice

Harassed by the multitasking demanded at the end of a surgery, a Glasgow GP Dr Margaret McCartney hunted for a referral form to get immediate home care for a patient. She completed it laboriously by hand and faxed it off. There then followed a protracted and, for her, tedious discussion with the receivers of the fax who refused to accept the referral because she had applied on "the wrong form." Eventually they faxed the right one to her surgery but the patient waiting to learn what fate had in store had to endure a long distressing delay.

Spurred by this incident Dr McCartney, her GP partner, and the practice secretary searched the premises to track down the forms GPs were expected to keep in stock and to use. They found sixty-eight varieties – each demanding roughly the same information but in a different format decreed by its progenitor. Most had to be completed by hand and GPs were expected to fill pre-defined boxes that didn't take account of patients' individual needs. Some might be needed only once or twice a year but referrals made on the wrong form could be rejected. In short, the forms were a barrier rather than an aid to the passage of information.

After careful assessment of the needs of the fillers and receivers, Dr McCartney announced in the *BMJ* that she and her colleagues had designed a universal form – "a blank sheet of paper on which we can write a letter of referral."

Which was of course what GPs used for generations before "the process of referral" was modernised, re-engineered, refurbished – call it what you will – in the name of improving efficiency, streamlining the patient journey, enhancing the patient experience etcetera, etcetera…

## Bad old days

Unenlightened times when 'community' was used more often as a noun than as an adjective, and GPs indulged in quaint practices such as visiting the sick.

From a medical careers booklet published by the *Lancet* in 1972:

*I work in a colliery practice – an industrial village with only one doctor and about 2000 patients. Not one is a stranger; they are not only patients, but fellow citizens. From many direct and indirect contacts, many non-medical, through shared activities, schools, shops and gossip, I have come to understand how ignorant I would be if I knew them only as a doctor sees them when they were ill. It is a compact world, in which integrity and a sense of proportion are more easily retained than in cities, provided that one accepts the multiple faces one must wear in an intimate communal life. There is immense friendliness, much bravery and generosity, a good deal of petty meanness, treachery and servile cowardice – but never indifference.*

## Ballroom dancing

Ritualised sexual foreplay now repackaged as a competitive sport and proclaimed to be healthy.

It was a sad day when the BBC announced that its new programme *Strictly Come Dancing* would "revitalise" ballroom dancing by "enhancing its healthy athletic quality." Is it really healthy? The very name 'fox-trot' conjures up a vision not of health but of suave Reynard gliding across the floor with the latest chicken he hopes to steer to his lair.

In its last few years, before it was expunged from the schedules, even the original *Come Dancing* programme had already become too flashy for *aficionados* like me. The rot set in when the men dancing 'South American' discarded their white tie and tails and the women were allowed to flaunt their knickers.

I have a fond hope that in a few thousand years when an archaeologist digs down to our layer in the silt, the only relic he'll find of 20th century Britain will be a videotape of *Come Dancing* in its original uncorrupted form with quantity surveyors from Penge clad in traditional dress – white tie, tails, white gloves, and key chain dangling from trouser pocket – clicking their patent leathers to the tempestuous music of Spain.

## Barometer

Useful instrument for measuring a student's aptitude for a medical education.

Medical schools try to pick students they can train to be good doctors but admit it's a difficult job. Help could be at hand from Copenhagen where the physics section of the pre-medical exam included the question: *Describe how to determine the height of a skyscraper with a barometer.*

One student wrote: *Tie a long piece of string to the neck of the barometer then lower it from the roof to the ground. The length of the string plus the length of the barometer will equal the height of the building.*

An unimaginative examiner failed the student who appealed against the decision and was invited to a *viva voce* conducted by an independent arbiter. The arbiter asked the same question but demanded an answer that revealed some knowledge of physics.

The student offered several:

*Take the barometer onto the roof, drop it over the edge, and measure the time it takes to reach the ground. The height of the building can be calculated from the formula $H = 1/2gt^2$ … height equals half times gravity time squared.*

*Measure the height of the barometer then set it on end and measure the length of its shadow. Next measure the length of the skyscraper's shadow and simple proportional arithmetic will provide the height.*

*A more elegant method would be to tie a short piece of string to the barometer and swing it as a pendulum at ground level and then on the roof. The height could be calculated by the difference in the gravitational restoring force.*

*If you want to be boring and orthodox, you could use the barometer to measure air pressure on the roof, compare it with air pressure on the ground, and convert the difference in millibars into metres.*

*But because I believe doctors should be encouraged to be imaginative, I would knock on the janitor's door and say: "I'll give you this nice new barometer, if you tell me the height of this building."*

The arbiter awarded him a pass: this student had the makings of a first rate doctor.

## Barrett manoeuvre

Psychotherapeutic technique designed for harassed motorists condemned to drive in cities.

One evening in the summer of 1950 Norman Barrett, chest surgeon at St Thomas' Hospital, London, left the hospital for home, driving the second-hand Rolls Royce that was then the prescribed car for teaching hospital consultants.

As he turned into Lambeth Palace Road, weary after a long operating list, he failed to pay due care and attention and cut straight across the bows of a taxi. The taxi driver managed to avoid contact thanks only to outstanding virtuosity at the wheel; Barrett drove on serenely as if nothing had happened. Three hundred yards down the road at Lambeth Bridge the traffic lights were at red and, when Barrett stopped, the taxi-driver drew alongside, flung down his window and subjected the weary surgeon to a full half-minute's worth of obscenity.

Barrett remained unmoved. When his tormenter paused for breath, he slowly wound down the window of the Rolls and said: "Don't worry, my man. You'll soon get used to driving in London."

Devotees of the Barrett Manoeuvre claim it never fails to induce contentment. It is guaranteed to revive the spirits of the weariest driver and when used as seemingly impromptu repartee can inspire the admiration of boyfriends or girlfriends, even of a wife or husband.

## Bedblockers

Sick and infirm patients who need care and attention which doesn't make use of the expensive capital equipment in which the hospital has invested.

Modern administrators, who prefer patients in whom 'outcome' is easier to measure, regard them as tedious creatures who clutter up well-managed institutions.

## Bedside manner

Medical salesmanship. There are three traditional approaches.

1. Charm or sympathy 'switched on' as a deliberate technique rather than generated by empathy. Sometimes called the 'game-show host' approach. Not particularly reassuring to patients. (See Communication skills.)

2. Impressive self confidence born of ignorance and lack of insight. Most common in those who specialise in diseases of the rich. Highly reassuring to patients, even those of some intelligence. In a stage direction in *The Doctor's Dilemma*, Bernard Shaw describes how the bombastic Sir Ralph Bloomfield Bonnington cheers, reassures and heals his patients because anxiety and disease are incompatible with his commanding presence. "Even broken bones, it is said, have been known to unite at the sound of his voice."

3. A quiet and caring air that gives every patient the impression that they are the only person on the doctors mind. Can be the most reassuring manner of all. In the 1930s and 40s, a GP in Cork, who was always referred to as Doctor Carney, as if Doctor were his first name, would say to the relatives of a sick man: "We'll be a little bit worried about him for the next twenty-four hours," a remark which earns full marks for artistic impression. It leaves the relatives with an image of the kindly doctor going about his business the next day with part of his mind constantly concerned about the health of their loved one. And whatever the outcome, the doctor will appear to have anticipated it. If the patient takes a turn for the worse, the relatives will say to themselves: "The doctor gave us a hint of what might happen but was kind enough to break it gently." If the patient recovers, as patients have a tendency to do despite the most rigorous of treatment, the doctor's 24 hours of concern is, in some mysterious way, seen to have played a part in the miraculous recovery. I suspect the technique had been handed down to Dr Carney by his GP father, and goodness knows how many generations of Carneys it passed through before it reached him.

## Belief

The mother of all placebos.

Every day patients ask doctors if they believe – not have they examined the evidence but do they believe – in acupuncture, homeopathy, the anti-arthritic properties of copper bracelets, or a future for Aston Villa. (Do they ever, I wonder, question their doctors' faith in less substantial propositions such as the nobility of Lord Archer or the existence of northbound trains on the Bakerloo line?)

Only the question about Aston Villa is acceptable. Football long ago ceased to be a game and became a source of doctrinal dispute based on an unquestioning belief in the power of good and evil. When the lads do well, it is because they believe in themselves. When they do badly, it is the work of the devil. In the words of the liturgy, the score, the referee's decision, or the referee himself was diabolical.

We forget at our peril the power of irrational belief or, as some prefer it, faith. We will never get rid of quackery, just as we will never learn from history, while the human instinct rates faith higher than reason.

When I was young and foolish I used to think that, as our society grew more scientifically literate, we would see a decline in superstition, maybe even a decline in the sort of quackery that exploits the fears and expectations of the sick. Now that I am old and foolish I accept the proposition Naguib Mahfouz puts into the mouth of a character in *The Cairo Trilogy*: "Belief is a matter of willing, not of knowing." The crevasse that lies twixt willing and knowing will, I fear, prevent us from ever achieving medical consensus on contentious issues such as abortion, assisted dying, even family planning. Adam and Eve were, after all, kicked out of Eden for daring to eat the fruit of the Tree of Knowledge.

I also accept – reluctantly – that quackery will always flourish, inside and outside the medical profession, and I should have paid more attention to the diagnosis made by Lady Mary Wortley Montague 200 years ago: "There is a fund of credulity in mankind that must be employed somewhere."

## Bereavement counselling

An art too often inspired by pity rather than understanding. Best left to those who have themselves been bereaved.

When my wife and younger daughter, both of whom I loved dearly, died suddenly and unexpectedly in the space of two years, I drew comfort from friends and acquaintances who behaved like the inadequate human beings we all are and spoke in stumbling phrases while their eyes radiated love. They knew, as I knew, that they had no magic potion to prescribe. I drew less comfort from the well-practised words of the trained professionals, medical, religious, and bureaucratic.

Once the immediate outpouring of kindness and sympathy from family and friends receded, I discovered I was an asylum seeker in an unfamiliar country. I was also a target for would-be counsellors who told me they knew how I must feel which was more than I knew myself. Understanding came only from friends who were similarly adrift.

One old friend Francis Matthews, whose wife Angela had died five years before, taught me how, when the waves of memory came rolling in unbidden, as they inevitably do, I could actually enjoy them, in a bittersweet way, by turning them into feelings of gratitude for the joyful, mischievous, heart-warming and occasionally heart rending times I'd shared with my wife and daughter.

Katherine Whitehorn wrote about the nuances of guilt and doubt, and the moments of ambivalence, that are part of grief. Honest as always, she described her guilt over the joy she felt when she realised her husband Gavin's death meant she at last had enough wardrobe space to hang her clothes without crushing them.

A neighbour, whose wife had died not long before, advised me not to waste time trying to return to 'the real world' but to accept that the old 'real world' had gone and been replaced by one in which two people who had been at the heart of the old one no longer existed.

Sue, widow of my friend Tony Rawlinson, reassured me that I was not the only person to learn that the platitude 'time heals' is a myth. Like me she had discovered that nothing makes things easier. Time just gives us space to adjust to things being different. The pain never goes.

In the immediate aftermath of death I got most help by remembering a nine-year-old girl whom I met when I was a young GP and tried, oh so ineptly, to console a few days after her mother died. As I stumbled and stuttered, she suddenly piped up: "People don't disappear when they die, you know. They're still here. It's just that we can't see them anymore." Sentimental maybe, and verging on the mawkish, but it expressed a truth I recognised when I needed it.

None of my would-be counsellors thought to mention it.

## Biological hazard

Domestic animal, usually a dog, that provokes a medical encounter of the third kind.

A community psychiatric nurse, making a home visit in Swansea, was followed into the patient's room by a large Alsatian dog that stretched out in front of the fire. In the middle of the interview, which lasted about an hour, the dog suddenly vomited over the hearthrug. The patient ignored it and kept on talking so the nurse thought it best not to comment. As she left at the end of the visit, the patient asked: "Aren't you going to take your dog with you?"

A young surgeon at St Thomas' Hospital, London, applied for a job at the Stanford Medical Center in California. He was invited to fly out for an interview and, desperately keen to get the job, was determined to stay on his best behaviour. On his first day he had an informal meeting with his prospective employer and, after it, the kindly Stanford surgeon offered him a lift back to his hotel. As they approached the car the young surgeon noticed that the front seat was occupied by a huge Great Dane and the back seat was crowded with his host's small grandchildren. He was about to sit in front but, after a close look at the dog, changed his mind and climbed in with the children. He'd no sooner cleared a space for himself when one of the children bit him.

## Blairite vision

View of the world inspired by a blend of hope and uplifting rhetoric unsustained by evidence or contact with reality. Named after Britain's first celebrity prime minister whose rhetoric uplifted his country into the beckoning promise of the 21st century before downlifting it into a catastrophic war.

Medical usage was exemplified by Michael Varnam, a Nottingham GP, when he wrote in the *BMJ*:

*We can all expect to die with dignity having a wide range of medical, social and spiritual needs met by enhanced Primary Care Teams appropriately prepared and effectively working together with the family and friends of the Patient.*

In just one sentence he captures the Blairite essentials: the omniscient confidence, "We can all expect", the high sounding yet empty phrases "wide range", "enhanced teams", "spiritual needs", "appropriately prepared", and the determined denial of reality.

I've no wish to be cruel to Dr Varnam but these days I have more contact with the reality than I would choose. I am angered by what I see when I visit octogenarian contemporaries in the hospitals or 'homes' to which they have been committed to endure the last weeks of their lives. Too many are subjected to a form of institutional neglect born of staff shortages and the desperate employment of untrained or ill-trained staff to whom notions of palliative care, or even of empathy, are as foreign as the English language.

I regard the development of the hospice (qv) movement as one of the great triumphs of 20th century medicine but we must not let proud declarations, seasoned with weasel words, blind us to what is happening in too many under-resourced public institutions and too many exploitive private ones.

To be fair, most Blairite statements about medicine come not from well-meaning GPs like Dr Varnam, whose aspirations are commendable, but from those who spend too little time in hospital outpatients or GP consulting rooms and too much time at meetings or conferences. There they absorb buzz words and jargon, the latest fashions in medical educationalism (qv), and other intellectual accoutrements which a *BMJ* editor, Domhnall Macauley, described as "a crib list for interviewees for GP teaching posts." He pointed out that the real test comes "when this comfortable world of the medical conference meets the queue of misery at a Monday morning surgery."

## Blame

Something someone has to shoulder after any mishap.

Declining faith in the existence of God prevents misfortune from being attributed to His will. Increasing faith in the benevolence of all things natural – from natural foods to natural medicines – inhibits people from acknowledging the existence of natural catastrophes. They turn a blind eye to the fact that most of us die from natural causes and apply the notion of bad luck only to picking the wrong numbers in the Lottery.

This communal delusion encourages litigation against any organisation that might deliver a jackpot. A woman from Memphis, Tennessee, sued a local pharmacist for $500,000 because she became pregnant after using a contraceptive jelly. She had spread the jelly on toast and eaten it. She told a newspaper reporter: "Who has time to sit around reading directions these days, especially when you're sexually aroused?"

More dangerously it engenders an intellectual state close to stagnation. The need for us to make errors is memorably stated by Lewis Thomas, American physician and essayist, in *The Medusa and the Snail.*

*Mistakes are at the very base of human thought, embedded there, feeding the structure like root nodules. If we were not provided with the knack of being wrong, we could never get anything useful done.*

*We think our way along by choosing between right and wrong alternatives, and the wrong choices have to be made as frequently as the right ones. We get along in life this way. We are built to make mistakes, coded for error.*

*We learn, as we say, by 'trial and error'… The old phrase puts it that way because that is, in real life, the way it is done.*

## Blonde

Sultry siren in a Top Doc Sex Shock.

When sociologists working for the Medical Research Council surveyed newspaper coverage of GMC disciplinary hearings they found that the tabloids nearly always described the 'other woman' as a blonde. During the hearing, the wronged wife was dark haired and "prim and proper." After the hearing, if the doctor was found not guilty, she was "devoted and loving"; if he was struck-off she was "loyal" or "standing by her man."

The relationship between 'blonde' and hair colour seemed arbitrary. One blonde in the *Daily Express* and *Daily Mail* was a brunette in the *News Of The World*. A blonde in the *Daily Mirror* was auburn-haired in the *Daily Mail*.

## Blood cholesterol
Biochemical measurement which some men, many of them American, treat as a golfer treats his handicap: working on it, taking pride in its reduction, and introducing it, none too artfully, into conversation.

## BMA Annual Representative Meeting
Premier event in the calendar of *Genus Medicopoliticus*. The names and the 'great issues of the moment' alter down the years but the ambience, the rhetoric and the posturing remain much the same.

When I was the editor of *World Medicine* I attended most of the self-styled 'great debates' but remember little of them now. What linger are the memories of off-stage incidents.

Like the representative who stood on the steps outside the hall at Hull – or was it Nottingham? – enjoying a few lungfuls of fresh air.

Somebody asked him: "Who's speaking in there now?"

"Dr Knowitall."

"What's he talking about?"

"I don't know. He didn't say."

And the time in Harrogate – or was it Eastbourne? – when another Dr Knowitall was at the rostrum.

A representative walked into the hall and exclaimed: "Good God, hasn't he finished yet?"

"He finished some time ago," said another, "but he hasn't stopped talking yet."

## BMA Speak
Coded language BMA politicians use at their Annual Representative Meeting.

In 1973 the *Lancet* published a brief guide. I'm told it is still a useful phrasebook.

**This is surely a matter of principle.**
This involves money.
**This is a matter of high principle.**
This involves a lot of money.
**Our general practice colleagues.**
That blackguard of a GP whose name I can never remember.
**Our valued delegate from the junior staff.**
That sickening young upstart whose name I have carefully noted.
**I am sorry to have to challenge the accuracy of para 147 of the Minutes.**
Para 147 is an accurate account of the committee once again failing to appreciate my point of view.
**A valuable and stimulating contribution which we might perhaps sometime take the opportunity of debating.**
A matter of principle.
**An interesting but wholly unrealistic concept, I'm afraid.**
A matter of high principle.

## Book learning
Essential ingredient of medical education.

A US medical student at a West Coast University won the year's top prize for outstanding achievement in her MD examination. On graduation day the prizes were presented at one of those ceremonies we know from the movies, where gowned and mortar boarded neo-graduates sit with their families on rows of white chairs set upon sunlit college lawns.

The chief guest was the editor of a leading medical text book. When, in an impressive ceremony amplified for all to hear, he handed over the top prize he asked the recipient rather archly which two books had helped her most as a student.

Without a blink she replied: "My mother's cook book and my father's cheque book."

## Bowels, pride in control over
Defining attribute of an Englishman. Few doctors have escaped the proud Englishman who, no matter how depressed he may

seem during a consultation, responds to the diffident inquiry "Bowels?" with a triumphant smile and a defiant: "Regular as clockwork, Doc."

Until the Second World War, the English bowel culture was dominantly a middle-class phenomenon. But after the war, it spread rapidly through the ranks, carried by returning soldiers who'd been brainwashed by officers like Apthorpe in Evelyn Waugh's *Men at Arms* who never advanced nor retreated without his personal thunder-box.

I suspect this bit of 'Englishness' originated in the public schools. Every morning at my prep school, all the boys had to pass in line before the matron who barked at each: "Been?" Those foolish enough to answer "No" were dosed with a foul tasting draught guaranteed to blast away the most intransigent of constipation.

Even those who were streetwise and responded, "Yes, matron" got to know the taste of the stuff because it was her universal panacea. Anyone confined to the infirmary, be it with a sore throat, German measles, or a sprained ankle, had to consume a morning dose. My class was blessed with a boy who didn't seem to mind the taste and would swallow anyone's draught on the payment of two sweets. One morning, during the great chicken pox epidemic, he actually consumed nine doses. His name was Gordon Reece. In later life he became a 'political strategist' to Margaret Thatcher and was credited with 'softening' her image. He clearly had the stomach for the job.

When it comes to bowels, Englishwomen tend to show concern rather than pride. A character in Alan Bennett's screenplay for *A Private Function* says, "My wife has two topics of conversation: the Royal Family and her bowels." And when Dr Kerr Donald, a retired GP, spent a holiday in a Scottish guest house, the guests who had assembled for dinner on the first evening were introduced to Auntie, a demure eighty-year-old former nurse. The hostess explained that Auntie would say grace. All bowed their heads reverently and the silence was broken by a clear authoritative voice: "O Lord. What we are about to receive, may it pass through us peacefully."

## Boxing

For years the British Boxing Board of Control maintained this was a dangerous sport for women who might damage their breasts but a healthy one for men who could damage only their brains.

## Breakdown in communication

Traditional excuse for ineptitude, incompetence, or laziness. Imported into the NHS from the corporate world.

Like its synonym, much favoured by politicians, 'failing to get the message across', it implies that people reject the message because they don't understand it not because they understand it all too well.

For fifty years I've earned my living as what some would call a 'communicator' though we who practice the craft rarely use that title. Getting people to understand what you mean is a relatively simple process. Calling it 'communication' suggests it is a specialised activity with complex techniques to be learned and a new academic discipline to be mastered, rather than a matter of taking an interest in people other than yourself, growing sensitive to their emotions and reactions, and being aware of how what you do and say appears to them.

The understanding needed to develop those qualities is, I submit, more likely to be absorbed from novels, films, and plays than from textbooks on communication skills.

One advantage of novels is that they are likely to be better written and easier to read than the textbooks. One of my most used lecture slides is a photograph of four people asleep in a lecture theatre while their teacher trundles his lecture along its predetermined groove. His subject is projected on the screen behind him: *Improving your communication skills.*

## Breakthrough

Dramatic breach of the frontiers of science reported in a medical journal.

Investigators at the Hospital del Salvador, Santiago, Chile, reported in the *BMJ* that when fifty-four healthy people had one hand immersed in warm water, the skin of thirty-eight wrinkled and that of sixteen did not. After due consideration they concluded this was "probably within the bounds of normal biological variation."

Three psychologists at the University of Wisconsin – Dennis Middlemist, Eric Knowles, and Charles Mather – investigated events at a men's public lavatory equipped with three urinals, to each of which they had attached a flowmeter. Keeping secret watch through a periscope, they discovered that micturition varied in speed, volume, and length of time according to whether one, two, or all three urinals were occupied.

After their groundbreaking investigation, *Handedness and longevity: archival study of cricketers,* J P Aggleton et al. were able to report in the *BMJ* that "Left handedness is not, in general, associated with an increase in mortality."

A team of six researchers at the Shisedo Research Center in Yokohama published *An Elucidation of Chemical Compounds Responsible for Foot Malodour.* Their breakthrough discovery was that people who think they have smelly feet do, and those who don't, don't.

## British cold, The
Jewel in the crown of the island race. (See Runny Nose.)

Few Britons with a cold have a virus infection. The British Cold is one of those maladies countries invent to provide their citizens with an acceptable excuse when they feel below par. The French have *crise de foie*, the Germans *Herzinsuffizienz*, and Americans a spectacular selection of allergies. The British cold, sometime referred to as 'a chill', is a malady not just for winter but for all seasons. Our Summer Cold is one of the season's great traditions, along with Wimbledon, Ascot, and Trooping the Colour..

Britons don't even talk about their colds as if they were an illness. "Got a bit of cold," they say. They'd never say that about a real illness, "Got a bit of brain tumour." And, unlike a real illness, a British Cold provokes little sympathy. If you mention your affliction, people respond by talking about their own. "Got that cold have you? Mine started with a sore throat." "Had it a week have you? Mine lasted three and I still haven't thrown it off." That's another sign it's not pathological. A cold is something you can throw off. People never talk of throwing off a myocardial infarction.

For some the British Cold is a source of consolation, for others a source of pride. Only a few see it as an opportunity. A *Punch* cartoon showed a woman in the salon of a grand couturier trying on fur coat while her husband bleated alongside: "For goodness sake Barbara, there are other ways of fighting a cold."

## Bulletinitis

Mild disorientation possibly induced by ionic radiation from BBC microphones. Afflicted speakers fail to distinguish between sports and medical bulletins.

A chronic sufferer was the endearing John Savage on BBC radio news. His case history included: "Yorkshire 232 all out, Hutton ill. I'm sorry. Hutton one hundred and eleven", and, "Ray Illingworth has relieved himself at the Pavilion end" .

## Bullish

The Irish attitude to matters medical. *The Oxford English Dictionary* claims, mistakenly, that the Irish bull involves "a ludicrous inconsistency unperceived by the speaker." In truth it involves a ludicrous consistency unperceived by non-Irish listeners such as Oxford English Dictionary editors.

Jim Kelly, a Mayo GP, was called to the house of a man who'd suffered a fatal heart attack during the night. As Jim expressed his condolences, the grieving widow sought to console herself. "You know doctor," she said, "isn't it a great way to go. In your sleep. He doesn't know he's dead yet."
After a moment of reflection, she added: "When he wakes in the morning and finds he is, the shock will kill him."

When Scottish GP Willie Angus was a medical student he took another student with him on the pillion of his motor bike on a holiday in Connemara. In the pre-helmet era they both wore flat caps. During one expedition, Willie's passenger tapped him on the shoulder and told him his cap had blown off. They rode back and found a man staring intently at something in the road. As they approached, he looked up.

"Is that your cap?" he asked.

"Yes, it is."

"Jasus, weren't you lucky your head wasn't in it?"

Some years ago, for reasons that would seem logical only to a television producer, I was filming an interview with a distinguished English medical scientist in a village in County Kerry. On our first morning I watched in wonder in the village shop while my interviewee asked if they had an English newspaper.

"We do indeed, sir," said the woman behind the counter.

"Would you like today's paper or yesterday's?"

"Today's, please."

"In that case, you'll have to come back tomorrow.

## Bullying

Once the preferred teaching method in traditional medical schools.

When I was a clinical student at St Thomas' Hospital in 1950, two years before the publication of Richard Gordon's *Doctor in the House*, there was always tension when the neurologist Jack Elkington took his students round the ward. Students who hadn't done their homework, and occasionally students who had, were icily humiliated before their colleagues. And God help the patient or nurse who made a noise while the great man was talking. One day when his entourage entered the ward, the Elk (inevitable nickname) paused and looked around. Sister had done her work well. Every patient was in bed, neatly lined up with nose the regulation number of inches above the sheet. No bed cover was wrinkled. The nurses stood silently at their posts. No sight nor sound intruded on serenity. The Elk gazed tetchily towards the window then said, "The birds are a little noisy this morning, Sister."

Since then students have learned how to fight back. Phil Hammond, a student at the same place thirty-five years later, described how his contemporaries responded. "One was so offended by the abuse he got from a surgeon, he nicked his shoes from the operating theatre changing rooms and wore them on every ward round for his eight-week attachment."

## Business plan

List of aspirational platitudes demanded, after the dawn of the internal market (qv), from all hospital departments, even the least likely.

In those halcyon days, Ted Cockayne, a GP in Bury St Edmunds, sent me the business prospectus he'd received from the West Suffolk Hospitals' Chaplaincy & Pastoral Care Department. It opened:

*The department provides a comprehensive service which seeks to meet the spiritual/religious/pastoral needs of patients, relatives and staff within a framework of client choice appropriate to their cultural or religious expression (or none), and/or spiritual and pastoral need in accord with the first standard outlined in the Patients Charter.*

And it closed:

*The department is committed to a developing quality strategy, departmental and clinical audit.*

Dr Cockayne asked, "How do you audit the chaplain?"

I suggested a ceremony in which the chaplains lined up on a suitable piece of West Suffolk greensward, the hospital chief executive prayed for divine intervention, and then stood back to see if any of his pastoral care providers were struck by a thunderbolt.

## Caesar

He unto whom doctors should render that which should be rendered.

One morning when Oliver Wendell Holmes Sr., American author and physician, arrived at a patient's home, he met a priest leaving the house. In grave sententious tones the priest announced, "Your patient is very ill and is about to die."

"Yes," said Holmes, "and he is going straight to hell."

"You must not say such things," said the priest. "I have just given him extreme unction."

Holmes shrugged. "You expressed a medical opinion and I have just as much right to a theological one."

## Cancerphobic seizures

Electrical storms of unreason on the surface of the brain triggered by overdosing on tabloids. Less common but more debilitating than the antonymous condition Miraculous Cure Euphoria.

Medical help is at hand. Dr Ben Goldacre offers preventive care on his *badscience* website where he tries to keep his readers up to date with the *Daily Mail*'s ambitious project to divide the world's inanimate objects into those that cause cancer and those that cure it.

For those already infected I've found the most effective treatment is constant repetition of a remark by Sir Richard Doll, one of the epidemiologists who established the link between cigarette smoking and lung cancer. When, in a televised interview, I asked him about the causes of cancer, he sighed, then paused, then said: "So many things in this world can cause cancer, it's a wonder any of us get out of it alive."

## Candidiasis

Variety of Candida infection discovered by Richard Wagner in the blood of the dragon Fafner. Makes people speak the truth without knowing they are doing so.

A family looked after by Tottenham GP John Nixon was suing the council because of its failure to re-house them. In search of a 'doctor's note' to support their claim, they invited Dr Nixon to inspect the children's bedroom. As they entered it, the mother said: "Just look at all that compensation on the walls."

## Care

(Obsolete)

To show concern. To look after. What doctors and nurses used to do for the sick and infirm.

My father was a GP in a Yorkshire colliery village and, during the 1930s Depression, my sister and I would help him load his car with cauldrons of soup that our mother had brewed on the kitchen range. "Soup not medicine. That's what most of them need," he would say as we staggered out with yet another tureen. To him, what is now called "social care" and medical care were indivisible.

(Now)

To allocate resources.

Rarely used without qualifying adjective. As in:

### Nursing care

Helping the sick and the debilitated with the daily tasks of living they can no longer manage for themselves.

### Social care

Same as nursing care except that, if the patient is old and doesn't live in Scotland, the NHS won't pay for it.

### Emergency care

A great nuisance to hospital administrators. According to the National Association of Health Authorities and Trusts: "Emergency admissions to hospitals have been rising. Such increases are disrupting the contractual system, distorting priorities by causing a shift in resources to pay for the increase, and making it difficult to plan for the future with confidence."

## Career counselling

Pastoral advice that medicine's educational establishment gave to 21st century junior doctors on how to career... i.e. accelerate rapidly downhill out of control.

In 2005 a bunch of Great Medical Thinkers proposed a radical reform of postgraduate medical training with a 'does what it says on the tin' style title: *Modernising Medical Careers* (MMC). The response of doctors who practised rather than preached was that the reforms hadn't been thought through and could damage medical training.

The preachers paid no attention. In 2007 they implemented MMC and provoked allergic reactions characteristic of medical schemes with "modernise" in their title: junior doctors marched in mass protest in London and Glasgow, senior doctors decided to boycott the programme; the website at its centre couldn't cope, leaked confidential information, and had to be taken down; the Secretary of State apologised to Parliament; and the *Lancet* published an article headlined: *Medical training in the UK: sleepwalking to disaster*.

There was also the usual trouble with modernised mathematics: the sums didn't add up. Critics, using unmodernised maths, claimed there weren't enough training posts to implement the scheme and doctors would be forced to emigrate or leave the profession because they would be unable to find jobs in the UK.

By mid or late 2007 every senior member of MMC Programme Board had been replaced. In 2008 the reconstructed Board cancelled some of the contentious proposals and agreed to make no further attempts to introduce new selection methods without first piloting and evaluating them.

Five years on the anger lingers. The fiasco damaged not just the careers of young doctors but the reputations of senior academic doctors who got involved in MMC's creation.

## Caring community

Expanding agglomerate of institutions, quangos, task forces, think tanks, study groups and working parties where conspicuously caring persons meet to discuss the philosophy of care and its delivery, explore opportunities, devise initiatives and strategic frameworks, draw up roadmaps, highlight the need for greater awareness and improved communications, organise workshops and social media campaigns, sponsor walks... indeed everything except going out, rolling up their sleeves, and physically helping those in need.

The impressive growth in the caring community over the past two decades has been matched only by the decline in the quality of actual care offered to the old and the poor. In 2012 many old people were terrified of going into hospital or a private 'home' not just because of what they learned from the media but because of what they saw for themselves when they visited their incarcerated contemporaries.

## Caring language
1.  Words that bring more comfort to those who utter them than to those who hear them.

2.  The professional lingo of those who refer to themselves as 'caring professionals' implying that, though engaged in a simple human activity, they are members of a professional elite. The users of Professional Caring Language favour it not just in discussions, documents, and declarations, but in informal conversation between themselves. A few key words offer the flavour:

### Catalyst
Title awarded to a senior professional caring person skilled at browbeating disparate groups on caring committees into accepting the catalyst's own opinions.

### Creative workshop
A meeting of professional caring people where ideas are acknowledged to emerge only from group activity, the notion that an individual might have a 'good wheeze' being dangerously elitist. Presumably called 'creative' to distinguish it from a destructive workshop such as a knacker's yard.

### Ethnic
Used not because of its meaning but as a 'caring' decoration. The most memorable feature I spotted at a Creative Workshop was a kiosk labelled *Ethnic Sandwich Bar*.

## Caring occasions
Meetings of the faithful where the proceedings are conducted in Professional Caring Language and everyone behaves in the approved caring professional manner.

When, as a journalistic adventure, I attended one, I was put in a 'working group' charged with defining desirable characteristics in a medical or nursing teacher. Our suggestions were sought in creative kindergarten style. We were each given a bundle of fluorescent Magic Markers, had to write the two characteristics we thought most important on ragged pieces of recycled paper, then walk to the front of the class and pin them to a piece of recycled cardboard set on an easel.

I thought hard about the teachers from whom I had learned most, and wrote 'Enthusiasm' in fluorescent pink and 'Imagination' in fluorescent green. In what I hoped would be seen as a creative gesture, I pinned 'Enthusiasm' to the board upside down to draw attention to it.

Only when I got back to my seat and looked at the gaudy display at the front of the class did I discover that my two suggestions stood out like a couple of jaundiced patients in a pale-faced ward. It wasn't a matter of colour but of vocabulary. My single words were surrounded by phrases like 'situation awareness', 'pedagogic restraint' and 'feedback sensitivity.'

Our self-appointed leader, a fat middle-aged man with beard, pebble glasses, and a liking for denim, walked to the board, pointedly turned 'Enthusiasm' the right way up and demanded a word with the perpetrator of the solecism.

In an inspired moment I turned to the woman in the seat behind me, told her to own up and, in the confusion that followed, made my escape.

## Chairmanship

A skill doctors find difficult to master. At too many medical meetings, the most intransigent waffler is the one in the chair.

Even at international symposia the presiding men or women forget that their duty of care is not just to the subject and the speaker but to the audience. Few are prepared to stop speakers who bore on beyond their allotted time and I doubt I will ever see a doctor emulate the physicist I heard chairing a scientific symposium. When a tedious speaker murmured the traditional, "I fear I may be running out of time," the chairman intervened: "You are already trespassing upon eternity." The remark won spontaneous applause.

Lesser cases respond to prophylaxis. I learned the best technique for curbing garrulity from Baroness Williams of Crosby when she was mere Shirley Williams. The trick is to nominate speakers in batches, putting those who need restraint first in the list. "First you, Dr Gush, then Mr Waffle, then Dr Garrulous, after that Mrs Sane, and finally Dr Sensible." The shame of holding up the queue seems to curb the most insensitive of wafflers... even at medical meetings notorious for the dominance of speakers who are generous only with words.

One of the finest proponents of the ploy was the late Professor Sir George Pickering who devised another technique I've never dared try. He was chairing an international symposium somewhere the US. The audience had endured a tough morning and were eager to break for lunch; the self-important speaker showed no signs of winding up and failed to respond to two polite reminders of the time. While he continued in full bore Sir George leant close to the microphone and growled Mercutio's line from *Romeo and Juliet*: "The bawdy hand of the dial is now upon the prick of noon."

Under cover of startled audience reaction, Sir George sped from the podium and left the speaker at the lectern, silent and blinking, while the grateful audience poured through the exits. Later the official *Proceedings* solemnly recorded the quotation, without attribution, and drew complaints, I'm told, from members of the religious right.

## Changing face of general practice
Sometimes best expressed in verse

### 20th Century.
W H Auden, doctor's son:

*Give me a doctor, partridge-plump,*
*Short in leg and broad in rump.*
*An endomorph with gentle hands*
*Who'll never make absurd demands*
*That I abandon all my vices*
*Nor pull a long face in a crisis.*
*But with a twinkle in his eye*
*Will tell me that I have to die.*

**21ˢᵗ Century.**
Marie Campkin, retired London GP:

*Give me a doctor underweight,*
*Computerised and up-to-date,*
*A businessman who understands*
*Accountancy and target bands.*
*Who demonstrates sincere devotion*
*To audit and to health promotion.*
*But when my outlook's for the worse*
*Refers me to the practice nurse.*

## Character assessment

Psychometric technique used by large corporations and the armed services to categorise their recruits.

During the Vietnam war my friend George, a New York journalist, was summoned to a draft board interview conducted by a sergeant.

"Did you go to high school?" asked the sergeant.

"Yes," said George. "Then to Columbia. After my degree at Columbia I did postgraduate research at Cornell before getting a second degree from the University of Southern California."

The sergeant nodded, picked up a rubber stamp and after flourishing it slowly in mid-air, slammed it down on his dossier.

George, like every good journalist, was adept at reading print upside down and saw his record had been stamped with just one word: 'Literate.'

## Character dislocation

A post-traumatic disorder that affects communication.

The disorder originated in the days when all print was set in metal type. Workers carrying trays of type across the shop floor sometimes dropped them and put the bits back where they thought they should be. The *Guardian*, 'twas said, employed people to do this for them and people trained on the *Guardian* later moved on to work on other newspapers and magazines.

As with IT viruses (qv), true Character Dislocation should be diagnosed only if it actually enhances the message, as does the missing 'm' in this item from the *In Memoriam* column in the *Birmingham Post*.

> *If roses grow in heaven, Lord*
> *And you have one to spare*
> *Please place it in my uncle's ars*
> *To show that I still care.*

## Charming
The doctor's way to deal with warts. A fine example of the power psyche can wield over soma.

The first blow to the mechanistic attitudes my medical school instilled was a clinical trial that suggested the most effective way of getting rid of warts was not to cut them off or freeze them but to 'charm' them. Later, when I was a GP, I achieved a high cure rate in children by calling on the services of a retired surgeon who would stare intently at the wart while muttering Jabberwocky phrases in a broad Devonian accent.

Many traditional wart cures carry a whiff of witchcraft. A GP attending a postgraduate refresher course was foolish enough to ask Sam Shuster, then professor of dermatology at Newcastle, what was the best treatment for warts. Sam, lowering his voice to a sombre register, recommended burying the patient's GP at the crossroads at midnight.

In 1998, in a letter to *The Oldie*, Valerie Roseblade of Tetchbury suggested that wart-plagued readers might like to try a traditional Gloucestershire remedy: "Wish them up a piebald horse's backside." She first tried it many years before through a bus window. The horse looked startled and the wart went. She tried again when a black and white cowboy film was shown on television. This time the horse didn't react. Nor did the wart.

## Chekhov
Author of medicine's most valuable textbooks. Of all the doctor-writers, Anton Chekhov is the one who most clearly reveals how close the art of a writer is to that of a clinician.

When I speak at postgraduate meetings someone occasionally asks me to name a book I think essential reading for "GPs in training" (which I interpret as GPs at any stage of their career). I invariably nominate Anton Chekhov's short stories in the biggest collection the questioner can find.

Chekhov practised medicine intermittently throughout his life, indeed claimed that he felt guilty if he neglected it for too long, and Nabokov could have been describing a wise GP when he wrote of him:

*Things for him were funny and sad at the same time, but you would not see their sadness if you would not see their fun.*

The current quest for evidence-based certainty worries a lot of GPs, or at least those I meet at postgraduate courses. One reason is that evidence-based medicine classifies data in terms of disease while GPs have to deal with illness. The two are not synonymous. Diseases can be defined, their causes sought, organisms or mechanical defects identified; an illness is an individual event, the possession of one person whose physical condition and emotional state determine the way the disease affects that individual life.

Even with diseases where we have compelling data, and they are still sadly few, the clinician has to weigh the generality of the evidence against the particular needs of the individual and seek to understand the feelings of regret, betrayal, fear, loneliness – indeed all the perplexing emotions – that can turn the same disease into a different illness in different people.

Novelists and playwrights face the same challenge, succinctly defined by Philip Roth: "Keeping the particular alive in a simplifying, generalising, world." And that's precisely what Chekov does in his short stories, and in his plays, where the wise and observant doctor and the gifted writer become one.

Re-reading them now I remember how much I learned from them when I was a young insecure GP who feared I was the only confused inhabitant of a world that everyone else understood.

I also remember how much they taught me when I was a not so young GP who still found life more complicated than orthodox medical texts would suggest.

## Chemist's shop
Once found on every high street. Now found only down Memory Lane.

At some time while I was growing up, our friendly neighbourhood chemists emerged from behind their flasks of coloured water and transmuted into 'community pharmacists.' Boots the Chemist became just Boots and local shops became mere links in national and international chains.

I recently met a retired chemist – I beg his pardon, pharmacist – who owned his own shop – I beg his pardon, premises – in those distant days when chemists mixed ingredients rather than put labels on pre-packed pills and liquids, when customers asked for things like liniments and rubbing oils, and when condoms had to be kept under the counter and dispensed in brown paper wrappers.

Kind man though he was, he'd been trained to exploit prudery in a cruel yet profitable way. If, when his young woman assistant was behind the counter, they spotted a man hanging around outside the shop looking embarrassed and waiting for her boss to take over – defining signs of a condom seeker – he would send her into the dispensary behind the coloured flasks. Then, as their victim entered the shop he would quickly move behind the flasks and the young woman would emerge to greet the embarrassed customer.

That, he said, was how they sold most of their combs.

## Chocolate coating
Technique of covering inaction with a sweet glazing of Management Speak in the hope of making it more palatable. Rarely works.

From Hampshire County Council Social Services to James Willis, when he was a GP in Alton : *Please accept our assurance that having accepted this referral, we will ensure that it is allocated to the appropriate Care Manager, who will arrange to make an assessment at the earliest convenience. Whilst we would not want to delay this, I must point out that we are currently working to a pending list.*

From a body calling itself Community Health in Sheffield to local GP Trefor Roscoe: *Unfortunately owing to a crisis staffing situation the implementation time scale of this project has been dramatically reduced.*

Occasionally the chocolate glaze is decorated with the pomp and circumstance of minor office. A self-justifying message from a 'Locality Commissioner' (who he?) to Dr Charles Perrott of Brackley ended: *I have copied this letter to some key people, largely as a mechanism of communication and ensuring consistency.*

## Choosing a GP

A decision that demands cunning, an awareness of the games doctors play, and great good fortune. (See Consumer choice.)

Katherine Whitehorn has explained why GP medicine is so much harder to rate than hospital medicine.

*The best GP is not necessarily the one who gives the most inoculations or even does the most house visits but the one with the subtlety to see further into a brick wall than the next man.*

## Circumcision

Genital mutilation. Condemned if performed on females yet still inflicted on innocent young males to satisfy the demands of religion or bourgeois fashion.

The commonest surgically unnecessary operation performed in Britain and the only medically unnecessary mutilation condoned by the GMC.

A Chicago surgeon contributes to the debate with this conversation between two six-year-old boys having a pee.

"Your thing doesn't have any skin on it."

"I've been circumcised."

"What's that mean?"

"It means they cut the skin off the end."

"How old were you when it was cut off?"

"My Mom said I was five days old."

"Did it hurt?"

"You bet it hurt. I couldn't walk for a year."

## Cliché

The lingua franca of medico-political debate.

In the days when I sat at the Press table during BMA annual meetings, one of my antidotes to tedium was to imagine a BMA cliché committee catechising prospective speakers in the style of

Myles na Gopoleen to ensure they were properly equipped for
the rostrum.

Q: What is immutable about principles?
A: They are always basic.
Q: Or alternatively?
A: Fundamental.
Q: Where does this moment invariably reside?
A: In time.
Q: In what manner must our messages be promulgated?
A: They must go out.
Q: Whence?
Q: From this place.
Q: In what manner?
A: Loud.
Q: And?
A: Clear.
Q: What is the only form of analysis we favour?
A: The final.
Q: And in that analysis what will happen to the truth?
A: It will dawn.
Q: At what inappropriate hour will that dawn take place?
A: At the end of the day.
Q: And what rustic omen will presage the event?
A: The chickens will come home to roost.

I used to fight off the boredom with a trick I learned from
Horace Fleming, an Enniskillen surgeon. As each cliché was
uttered, I tried to express the sentiment in other words. Thus 'at
the end of the day' became 'at the beginning of the night'.

If you translate each phrase after it is uttered, just loud enough
for others to hear, you can occasionally stop the flow. But don't
count on it.

## Clinical confabulation
Rewriting a patient's story to fit the doctor's view of it.

There's sometimes a dangerous rift between the way patients
perceive events and the way doctors describe the same events
when discussing them with their peers.

In November 2009 the *BMJ* published the story of a sixty-two-year-old woman "bed bound with severe arthritis and in constant pain despite strong opioid treatment". She had signed "an advance directive stating that she did not want life sustaining medical treatment" and, after writing a detailed suicide note that "clearly expressed [her] distress at her longstanding pain and severe restriction of function and independence", she swallowed a potent concoction of sedatives and sank into what she assumed would be oblivion.

I can only guess at her assumption, because, as is traditional in our journals, her story is written by the doctors. We read in detail the ethical arguments they considered and the agonies they endured reaching their decisions. We hear nothing directly from the woman or her family. Their actions and attitudes are described not by them but as they were perceived by the doctors.

The first medical decision was to deny the woman the oblivion she sought. She received "lifesaving treatment" and awoke in hospital with the whole of her left side paralysed. Her doctors were, however, able to give her a drug to provide "excellent symptomatic relief from her arthritis" before she was "diagnosed with depression" and given an anti-depressant drug. Three months later she went home.

Six months after that the doctors who saw her described her as "cheerful." She "acknowledged" that her quality of life had improved but "considered" that it was still poor. She "maintained" that she would have preferred to have had her wishes respected, to have retained her independence and dignity, and not to have survived. "This position," we are told, "was confirmed in a subsequent letter." We don't see the letter, or even a quotation from it, so we can't read what she thought, only what her doctors thought she thought. Indeed we hear nothing about what happened to her and her family during those six months.

The story ends with a chilling sentence: "She lived almost pain-free for another eighteen months with some reservations but no resentment over her management and *unfortunately* (my italics) subsequently died in hospital in a manner which she had tried to avoid."

"Served her right," the Devil whispered in my ear, "for placing her trust in irrelevant fripperies like advance directives that fly in the face of one of medicine's traditional precepts: daddy and mummy know best."

Even worse than the euphemism (that use of "unfortunately" still challenges my vomiting centre) is the casuistry that infects much medical discussion of death and dying.

## Clinical experience
Making the same mistakes with increasing confidence over an impressive number of years.

## Clinical foresight
Commendable skill sometimes carried to extreme.

One of the attractions of general practice is that, if you keep your eyes and ears open, nearly everything is new under the sun. Or, as postgraduate tutors prefer to put it, primary care is a process of continuing education.

When, as a GP, you fear you're succumbing to routine, an unexpected new experience will shake you out of it. As when Martin Harris, a London GP, who'd been a practising for twenty years, received a letter from a genus of specialist he'd never before encountered.

*The above person who is registered with you has approached me, as a Foresight Clinician, with a view to preparing herself for a planned pregnancy.*

*Evidence is accumulating that the fitness or otherwise of the mother and the father at the time of conception can bear directly on the outcome of the pregnancy, both for the mother and her baby.*

*It is our view that prospective parents should have the opportunity of reviewing their health and fitness before conception. The Foresight Clinics offer to couples (sic), following a review of their past and present living habits, together with analysis of certain body tissues and fluids.*

*A 'family consultation' then takes place during which living habits, e.g. eating, drinking and smoking habits, are assessed together with the findings of physical and laboratory examinations. At this time any deficiencies or toxicities are made known to the couple whose responsibility it will remain to take action in rectifying them.*

*A summary of the findings will be forwarded to you in due course so that when the couple approach you with their early pregnancy, you will already have some idea of the conditions under which they conceived.*

At which point Dr Harris felt a profound sense of inadequacy. Nothing in his training or experience had taught him how to use this vital information.

## Clinical intuition
Knowing the answer without bothering to look.

Aristotle, the Greek philosopher, maintained that women had fewer teeth than men. Though he'd been married twice, it never occurred to him to check his claim by looking in his wives' mouths.

## Cloning humans
Attempting to repeat in a laboratory what letter writers to the *Guardian* and *Daily Telegraph*, and members of the Socialist Worker's Party appear to have achieved without scientific intervention.

## Coalface
Fantasy workplace evoked by medical politicians who want to stress that, unlike other pontificators, they still treat patients.

Typical usage is that of a *BMJ* correspondent, "Many of us working at the coal face of the NHS experience these problems."

Medical institutions are not averse to the phrase. The GMC, as you would expect, embeds it in portentous prose: "This work is underpinned by relationship building and awareness raising amongst the volunteers who deliver the service at the 'coal face'."

One *BMJ* columnist went an image too far when he wrote, "As a BMA politician I believe one must keep in touch with the grass roots at the coal face."

Such usage demeans the memory of an inhuman and degrading place where miners sacrificed their lungs, their limbs and occasionally their lives in the service of Mammon.

## Cocksure
Anatomical certainty that sustains the arrogance of the powerful.

Mohammed Al-Fayed, in a tape recorded conversation with Tiny Rowland: *You have six girlfriends. I have 24 girlfriends, right? This makes my (sic) difference that my cock is bigger than yours.*

Lord Melbourne: *I wish I was as cocksure of anything as Tom Macaulay is cocksure of everything.*

## Coitus interruptus

Contraceptive technique that, when Englishmen talk to their doctors, becomes a rich source of regional euphemism and a confirmation of their abiding love of trains.

| | |
|---|---|
| Cheshire and Merseyside: | *I get off the train at Edge Hill, doctor.* |
| Cambridgeshire: | *I get out at Saffron Waldon.* |
| Hampshire: | *I stop at Fratton.* |
| South east counties served by Victoria and Waterloo : | *I always change at Clapham Junction.* |

## Colon

Lower bowel where lurk noxious substances that threaten the vitality of celebrities.

By the turn of the century colonic irrigation had regained the social cachet it had in the 1930s. A 1995 *Sunday Times article*, after hinting that Diana and Fergie were regular indulgers, offered one of those contradictory sentences characteristic of a gossip column: "Discretion is a key word among colonic therapists, who insist that client confidentiality precludes them from naming their patients but celebrity converts are said to include the author and yachtswoman Clare Francis, the actress Joan Collins, and Vidal Sassoon and his second wife, Ronnie." It's odd how useful names can breach the confidentiality barrier.

The fashion can occasionally leaven the mundanity of more orthodox medicine. As in this letter from a consultant to a GP:

*You asked me to see this woman. I gathered from your letter that she had been using coffee for self administered colonic enemas. She tells me she now feels better. The reason apparently is that her husband has bought her a new coffee percolator.*

Could they, I wonder, have saved themselves the cost of a percolator if she'd just added an extra spoonful of sugar?

## Coloured water

A quack remedy but an alarming symptom.

Dr C. M. B Reid, a Lytham GP, had a patient who, while in London on business, thought he had cystitis. He went to a chemist who gave him some De Witts pills, warning him that they might discolour his urine. On his way home the man stopped at a service station and went to the Gents. A small boy in the next stall stared wide-eyed and unbelieving at the stream of bright blue urine.

"Hey, mister," he asked, "why is your wee blue?"

With calm authority, the man replied: "I am not of this planet."

Whereupon the boy rushed to the door shouting: "Dad, there's an alien in here."

## Combative

Traditional sporting relationship between Man and disease.

Journalists reporting from hospitals regularly evoke the imagery of war: doctors fight for patients' lives, victims battle bravely against illness.

Journalists writing about football use similar metaphors: Titans clash, strikers put goalmouths under siege, defenders take no prisoners.

So why was I startled by the image conjured up by the *Guardian* journalist who wrote, "Paul Ince will undergo surgery on Monday after losing his battle with a hernia"?

## Commitment

A professional obligation that all doctors bear though the weight of the burden can be affected by circumstance.

At a convivial meeting of the Kit-Kat Club, Sir Samuel Garth (1661-1719), physician and poet, announced he would have to leave early to attend to his practice. Yet, under the influence of the conversation and the wine, he stayed on and on.

When Richard Steele reminded him of his waiting patients, Garth pulled out a list of fifteen names and, after perusing it, said:

*It is no great matter whether I see them tonight or not. Nine of them have such bad constitutions that all the physicians in the world can't save them, and the other six have such good constitutions that all the physicians in the world can't kill them.*

## Common touch
What doctors think they're showing when at their most patronising.

A month or two ago, waiting my turn as a patient at a local hospital, I chatted with a man whom I reckoned to be in his mid-sixties. As an eager young houseman escorted him away he turned to me and whispered: "If this young whippersnapper calls me 'Dad' just one more time, I think I'll strangle him."

Time was when I was as guilty as anyone but I was lucky to get my cumuppence early in my career. On my very first morning as a school doctor, I assumed the traditional avuncular pose and asked my first patient: "And now, young man, what are you going to do when you leave school?"

To which he replied: "I thought I'd go straight home."

I fared slightly better than my contemporary Chris Cones when he was a house physician at the Doncaster Royal Infirmary. Loaded syringe in hand, he approached a young woman. "Just a little prick," he said.

To which she responded: "Are you bragging or complaining?"

## Communication aid
Any device that gets in the way of understanding.

The young GP was starting up in single-handed practice in a new town. On his first morning, before his receptionist arrived, he heard his very first patient enter the waiting room. After a pause, there was a tentative knock on the door and it started to open. He immediately grabbed the telephone and spoke into it: "I'm sorry. Life is pretty hectic at the moment but I might just be able to fit you in next week. I'll have to get back to you later this morning." He replaced the receiver and turned to the man who was standing in the door. "Sorry about that. Do come in and sit down."

"No need," came the reply. "I've just come to connect your phone."

Excerpt from a telephonic transaction recorded in Birmingham:

*GP: Yes I have arranged the admission and can confirm that the patient needs an ambulance. He is confused and semi-comatose and has bronchopneumonia. He suffers from malnutrition, has cellulitis of the left buttock from a pressure sore, is incontinent, and has congestive cardiac failure.*

Hospital box-ticker: *I see, doctor. And with which of those conditions are you admitting him.*

Excerpt from a letter from British Dental Association nabob.
*I apologise for not addressing you by name but I do not have the computer capability to personalise the greeting.*

## Community

A concept easier to admire than to define.

For thirty years I lived in suburban Surrey in the same house among the same people. Yet in each decade I inhabited a different community.

For the first seven years, as a local GP, I had privileged access to the lives of many of the people, far greater than that granted to lawyers or even relatives who think they have access to family confidences. I was allowed to see how individuals behaved behind their social facades, to know the anxieties and insecurities that plagued the lives of persons of seemingly brazen confidence, to be aware of secret unacknowledged acts of courage.

I was also aware of the diurnal patterns. As I drove around visiting patients, I might, at different times, see the same woman drive her husband to the station, drive her children to school, load her car outside the grocers, meet the evening train. I knew who played bridge with whom and often on which days; who would visit the sick and do their shopping; who was a helpful neighbour and who would make a great show of helping while being a hindrance; whose car was parked for a suspiciously long time outside a house where a husband or wife had commuted to London for the day.

Then one morning I hung up my stethoscope and, for eighteen years, worked in offices in London. The community became a base from which I commuted. I knew nothing of what happened there on weekdays; I was part of it only in the morning, in the evening, and at weekends which I tended to spend immured within my Englishman's castle. The people I met at the station, on the train, in the High Street on a Saturday morning, at an occasional party (once you cease being a GP, you lose an excuse for declining invitations), I had to accept on the terms on which they offered themselves. I was no longer privy to the fears, the anger, and the jealousies that lay beneath the surface. The community was more arid than that I had known but I was happy to be part of it largely because my children had made lots of friends and were happy at local schools.

Then I ceased to commute and started to work at home again; not as a GP but as a writer. Elements of both communities I'd known now came together. Once again I was aware of the diurnal pattern as I walked across the cricket green on my way to the post office to despatch an article or script, or when I rode my bike to the stationers in the High Street to buy paper-clips or rubber bands. I was no longer privy to people's secrets but I recognised individuals, knew what time they were likely to come out of the library, knew who would be playing bowls on a Tuesday afternoon, which rowdy kids would be on the swings when school was over, which cars were parked in suspicious places. I also became aware of things the community did as a community, the 'bring and buy's, the 'continuing education' classes, the enthusiasm for first aid, for archeology, for 'keep fit', indeed for a bewildering range of activities that brought people together.

People create communities for themselves. Wise politicians allow them to evolve and don't try to create them artificially.

## Community service
A phrase that charts changes in social attitudes.

> **1949.** Willing contribution that people, home from the war, made to the community of which they were members.

> **2012.** Punishment judges use as an alternative to prison.

## Compensation
Arrangement whereby lawyers get doctors to pay for lawyers' mistakes.

When Thomas Passmore of Norfolk, Virginia, thought his right hand was possessed by the devil, he cut it off with a circular saw. He had seen the malignant number 666 appear on it so he followed the biblical injunction: "If thine right hand offend thee, cut it off."

When he, and his hand, were taken to a local hospital, he refused permission for the surgeons to intervene because the Bible offered no authority for the surgical reattachment of offending parts. The hospital sought to override his instructions with a court injunction on the grounds that he was grossly deluded and incapable of making a rational decision. The judge refused to grant an injunction.

Mr Passmore later sued the hospital for $3.4 million for medical negligence.

## Competitive acronyming

A game that hospital consultants play with GPs in lieu of having a life.

When Dr W Denys Wells of Walsall was happy to confess ignorance and sought translation of a letter from a local consultant, his reward was a patronising letter.

I *understand that you found the initial BRD unsatisfactory because the abbreviation DKA was used. I believe this is a very commonly used abbreviation and should not result in a confusion.*

The reply included no translation of DKA nor, for that matter, BRD.

Cornel Fleming, a North London GP, encountered similar hauteur after a letter from the Whittington Hospital explained that one of his patients with back pain had been treated with rice. Sensing a new dietary approach, he sought more information. Back came a supercilious letter from the surgeon's secretary hinting that all well educated doctors knew that RICE meant rest, ice, compression and elevation, just as MICE meant movement, ice, compression and elevation. The message was couched in such condescending tones it tempted Dr Fleming to invite the surgeon to perform SIUYA, not a traditional Japanese gesture of contrition but a traditional British exhortation to place the ice in an uncomfortable repository.

Browsing through a copy of *Contraception News* hoping to raise his level of understanding to that of clever hospital doctors, Dr Ray Dawes, a GP in Gloucester, discovered that the cognoscenti described an act of unprotected sexual intercourse as an UPSI. He thought this a phonetic aberration. His patients who asked for the morning after pill attributed their need to a WHOOPSY.

## Complexity

The natural state of any human entity: the structure of a gene, the mechanical working of a human body, the inventive ideas created by a human mind.

Time was when science journalists described this complexity and tried to make it intelligible, interesting, exciting. In the age of rolling news, photo opportunity and sound-bite, all-purpose journalists seek to 'simplify' it and inevitably distort it.

Albert Einstein denounced attempts to 'simplify' his theory. When an American woman asked him to explain Relativity in a few words, he told her a story:

A blind man and a friend were walking down a hot and dusty road.

"Oh," said the friend, "what wouldn't I give for a cool drink of milk."

"Drink I know," said the blind man, "but what is this milk you speak of?"

"A white liquid."

"Liquid I know, but what is white?"

"White is the colour of a swan's feathers."

"Feathers I know, but what is a swan?"

"A swan is a bird with a bend in its neck."

"Neck I know, but what is a bend?"

The friend took the blind man's arm and extended it.

"That," he said, "is straight."

He then flexed the arm at the elbow.

"That," he said, " is a bend."

"Ah," said the blind man, "now I understand what milk is."

## Complications

What doctors fear but many patients treasure, particularly those who live well-upholstered lives.

Edith Wharton describes such a one in her novel *Ethan Frome*.

*She continued to gaze at him … with a mien of wan authority, as one consciously singled out for a great fate. "I've got complications," she said. Ethan knew the word for one of exceptional import. Almost everybody in the neighbourhood had 'troubles' frankly localised and specified, but only the chosen had 'complications.'*

## Concern

A rewarding emotional response to other people's distress. Less demanding than taking action but just as satisfying.

In the days when GPs fielded their own 'out of hours' calls they would often encounter Concern on a Sunday evening. Sons or daughters who had made a dutiful weekend visit to parents they hadn't seen for some time, and been alarmed by the old folks' decline, felt obliged to do something helpful. The least burdensome thing they could do was to ring the doctor before they left and, with anger tinged with guilt, demand that "Something be done."

It was an understandable human response and GPs tried not to let it irritate them, even if over previous weeks they'd expended much time and energy trying to organise what they knew was inadequate care for the unfortunate parents and had to rely heavily on the kindliness of their patients' neighbours.

Concern comes cheap: coping is more demanding. We all have plenty of things in our lives with which we already have to cope and we don't want any more drawn to our attention. We prefer to leave as much as we can to people like nurses, doctors, police, or others who have a duty to deal with unsavoury matters.

## Conditioned responses

Reflex verbal signals that fill the pauses in one-sided conversations when listeners feel the need to indicate they're still alive.

Like other self-defence mechanisms they're produced by the autonomic system without conscious intervention by their producer. The usual response is a grunt or a monosyllabic segue,

"Oh!", "Ah", or "Mmm" though, these days, persons overexposed to celebrity interviews respond with the multipurpose polysyllabic "Absolutely".

A few unfortunates, like me, are born with damaged verbal reflex centres. For all of my life, I've failed to respond automatically when I'm greeted with: "How are you?" My instinctive reaction as a doctor is to give a literal answer. "Blood pressure's under control. Spot of wax in the right ear. But mustn't grumble." I usually suppress the urge and mumble something inaudible, or launch into a boring explanation of how difficult I find it to respond.

Things were much easier in the day when the traditional greeting was a formal "How do you do?" Long before I was born the question had become meaningless and demanded no rational answer. Civilised people just had to repeat it, proffer a hand, and turn to the business of enjoying one another's company. But those days have gone and I don't want to end up like my friend Geoff Watts who, when lying in bed with a high fever, answered the telephone and responded to my genuine "How are you?" with an automatic "Fine, thanks."

What a pity our schools never conditioned my generation to respond to "How are you?" We had a fierce French master who merely had to bark *Comment allez-vous?* for us to respond in drilled chorus: *"Je vais bien, monsieur."* An equally fierce Greetings master could have trained us to react to "How are you?" with an automatic "Very well thank you, how are you" without that fatal pause that allows the brain to consider the meaning of the words.

I suppose I could say "Nicely thank you" or "Mustn't grumble" if they didn't tweak so irksomely at my class consciousness. I even flirted for a time with "As well as can be expected" but it sounded too like a hospital bulletin. The nearest I came to a useful answer was "Surviving." But these days it takes on political overtones and, instead of terminating what should be a ritual exchange, invites inquirers to argue or, even worse, give detailed accounts of their own struggles against adversity.

In 2011 I noticed that people who like to show they're ahead of the game, such as interviewers on Radio Four's *Today* programme, had imported the American response, "I'm good.

How are you?" Even seventy years on from a Catholic childhood, I couldn't say that. I'd need time to examine my conscience and possibly choose to die rather than claim to be good.

I've no problem in countries where the question differs. In the USA, for instance, when asked "How are you keeping?" I automatically respond "Out of trouble." Recently I encountered a new American technique. A US doctor was about to introduce me to his companion but before he could speak she drew a deep breath and said: "You're speaking to Melanie Orenstein, a psychotherapist with a special interest in the rehabilitation of those who've suffered a life-threatening incident of cardiac disease."

I heard my voice respond "How do you do?" The ancient reflex had clicked in and passed the buck. Painlessly.

## Conditioning

Psychological technique that can be turned to useful purpose.

As in a case history reported by Philippa Pigache.

Annoyed at the rowdy play of young boys outside his house, an old man called them over and explained that he loved the sound of children's voices but was growing deaf. If he gave them each 10p, would they shout even louder? The boys were delighted to oblige.

After a couple of days of noisy roistering, the old man told the children he was running short of funds and could now afford only 5p a day. The boys were not pleased but continued their noisy play, though with less enthusiasm.

The following day the old man told them he was broke and couldn't pay them. Angrily the boys said they weren't making a noise for nothing, not for no one, and departed to play elsewhere.

## Cone syndrome

Compulsive disorder that leads politicians to introduce legislation that seems to serve no real purpose.

Named after an outbreak that afflicted the British government in the early 1990s and featured a 'cones hotline' telephone number that motorists could ring to whinge about redundant traffic cones deployed for no apparent reason. Possibly the most ridiculed policy ever introduced by a British government, it survived for just three years in a state of lingering morbidity.

Other symptoms of that outbreak included a Citizens Charter and a Patient's Charter. A critic of the Citizen's Charter described it in the House of Commons as "a mixture of the belated, the ineffectual, the banal, the vague and the damaging." The Patient's Charter was a similar mixture though, if anything, more platitudinous. Politicians saw it as an alternative to spending money on public services; medical cynics saw it as a device for diverting money from the care of patients to the sustenance of government supporters in the public relations, advertising, and glossy paper industries.

Those beneficiaries exploited the opportunity with enthusiasm. When Dr Robert Addlestone dropped in at his local Lawnswood crematorium in Leeds he found a booklet entitled *The Dead Citizen's Charter*. Not only was it written in deadly earnest – if you'll pardon the expression – but was described by its authors as "a consultative document." In characteristic Charter style, its opening sentence revealed one of those great truths we would never have discovered for ourselves: "An individual's funeral will take place just once."

The 1990s outbreak of Cone syndrome faded away when politicians realised that Chartering didn't really work as as diversionary ploy. Twenty years later epidemiologists warned us of the danger of another outbreak with the proclamation of The Big Society.

## Conflict resolution
Difficult skill, easier to study than perform.

I know of only one medical researcher who hopes his finest achievement will never be recognised. In 1975 when working in Oxford he launched an ingenious experiment by ringing the police. In querulous tones he complained that some undergraduates, engaged on their detestable 'rag week', had dressed as labourers and were digging up part of the Cornmarket.

"They're being very aggressive to bystanders," he said, "so you'll need a number of officers to sort them out." The police thanked him for the tip-off and despatched a couple of van loads of Oxford's finest.

Their informant then nipped across the road and spoke to the

Wimpy labourers digging up the Cornmarket. Did they know, he asked, that rag week students was going around dressed as policemen and trying to make bogus arrests?

"Thanks for the tip," said the foreman. "But don't you worry, sir. We'll be ready for them."

Our hero then joined other students of conflict resolution at a window overlooking the potential learning opportunity.

Neither police nor labourers had noticed that the date was April 1st.

## Conjoint aetiology

A condition and it's cause equally dependent upon one another.

As in the *San Francisco Chronicle* report of a man who when questioned by police about his habit of walking backwards replied: "I like to see the surprised expression on the faces of the people who are following me."

## Conjunctionitis

A common symptom of addiction to DMG, Decorated Municipal Gothic (qv), the prose style which too many medical writers and lecturers believe adds dignity, scientific worth, or even grandeur to their utterance.

Enchanted by the sound of their own DMG, addicts discover that their words become even more resonant when linked in pairs, particularly if they are tautologous: hopes and aspirations, fears and apprehensions, help and assistance, higher and higher, lower and lower, so on and so on.

Conjunctionitis gives speech a remorseless, and for listeners a usefully soporific, rhythm, like waves rolling onto a beach.

Simple tautology without a conjunction produces the more abrupt rhythm that gives clichés staying power. I found four examples in just one medical article: "Future prospect", "Mutual consensus", "Forward planning" (as opposed presumably to backward planning), and "Final conclusion."

## Consolation

A soothing of the spirit sometimes available from unlikely sources.

When the sun shines on the Five Points district of Atlanta, Georgia, it brings out the Southern Bible thumpers who crowd the pavements, Good Book in hand, seeking to sell passers-by their version of God.

Some years ago, I discovered they're more pragmatic than they sound. One of them approached and explained that God, working through her, could solve any problem that weighed upon my mind.

Depressed and jet-lagged I growled: "My only problem is that I'm nearly 4,000 miles away from my wife and children whom I love dearly and have no prospect of seeing for another two weeks."

"You don't need God," she said. "You need transportation."

## Conspicuous abstemiousness

Behavioural disorder afflicting those with a mission to reform the rest of us.

When the television producer Royston Morley was invited to lunch at the Beaconsfield home of Sir John Reith, BBC director general and conspicuous abstainer, his host asked, when the fish was served, if he would like a glass of white wine and, with the steak, if he would like a glass of red. He accepted both though he noticed that other BBC underlings around the table drank only water.

After lunch, while he was browsing though the books in the library, he heard Reith's voice behind him: "I see, Mr Morley, that you are a drinking man."

## Constructive solution

Helpful suggestion that sounds logical in an administrator's office but less so in the front line.

A fine specimen appears in the minutes of the Accident and Emergency Committee at the Royal Free Hospital, London. *A request was made for more stethoscopes in A&E. It was not felt that this was possible but it was suggested that longer tubing be put onto the existing ones in the department.*

## Consumer choice

A dangerous way to pick a doctor. (See Choosing a GP.)

The most incompetent GP I ever met was also the one most loved by his patients and, most honoured by his community. I stood in for him while he was on holiday and soon found I needed to redefine my notion of ethical conduct. His patients' faith in his bizarre remedies was so powerfully therapeutic I decided not to change any treatment unless it was actually killing the patient.

That man would have topped any list of 'consumer favourites' if only because he spent a lot of time with each patient listening to everything they had to say. He had a large practice and all his patients loved him despite the fact he was incapable of coping with any pathology they might have about their persons, including the pathology he induced with the prescriptions he showered upon the healthy.

All his patients died happy. Earlier than they might have done, maybe, but happy.

## Contrariness

Commendable quality shown by doctors who brought about social change unpalatable to the medical establishment of their day.

A few have won posthumous acclaim, including John Snow, whose observations on the source of cholera were ignored for thirty years (see Romantic fiction), and Ignaz Semmelweis whose detection of the source of puerperal fever was dismissed by his Viennese betters as the sort of untutored thinking you'd expect from an uppity Hungarian.

Typical of the many who remain under-celebrated was William Price, born in 1800, who graduated at St Bartholomew's Hospital in London before returning to Glamorgan to live and practise in Llantrisant.

Price was non-conformist to an extravagant degree. He spurned all forms of transport and walked miles across the hills visiting patients, often at two or three in the morning claiming that at that hour a patient's resistance was at its lowest and disease more easily diagnosed. He was a dedicated chaser of women and fathered many children but condemned marriage because it led to the enslavement of women. He was a Chartist, a vegetarian, a vociferous opponent of vaccination and Methodism, appointed himself Archdruid of Wales, and liked to walk naked across the Welsh hills accompanied by groups of naked young women eager to share the health-giving exercise.

Yet none of these sins against decent society put him in the dock at Cardiff Assizes in 1884. He stood there charged with attempting to obstruct the course of an inquest by burning a body instead of burying it in hallowed ground. The body was that of his infant son who died at the age of five months and whom Price cremated on a hilltop in accordance with what he claimed were ancient Druidical rites.

At the start of the trial Price, wearing a white robe embroidered with cabalistic signs, announced he would be defending himself, and he did so with gusto. He challenged the prosecution to name the legislation that made burning a corpse illegal and when Llantrisant's minister said the Church required that bodies of baptised infants be committed to hallowed ground, he cried, "The Church is not the law."

Prosecution witnesses testified to his "madness." They claimed that his manservant and his housekeeper, mother of several of his children, drove away intruders with blunderbusses and that the doctor robbed graves and dissected corpses. Price treated the allegations with disdain and called as his witnesses the people of Llantrisant.

They spoke of his skill as a doctor, how he returned to Wales to practise among those who needed him most, his understanding not just of their ills but of the way in which they were forced to live their lives. Two phrases kept recurring: "He would always come willing" and "He only charged those he knew could pay." Women said he was "gentle as a bird" at their confinements and a miner who'd been trapped by a fall of coal waxed lyrical about the anaesthetising effect of the brandy Price gave him before amputating his leg.

The Cardiff jury failed to agree a verdict and Price was freed. The case did, however, establish the legality of cremation. The judge accepted Price's plea that though the law did not say that cremation was legal, nor did it say it was illegal.

The British establishment and medicine's nabobs were not pleased. The Home Office engaged in endless niggling over detail and a crematorium at Woking, "specially constructed with regenerative and reverberating furnaces according to the Italian models", remained un-reverberate for eighteen years.

By then Price was ten years dead. His will directed that his corpse be seated in an ancient Druidical chair and burnt on

Caerlan hill on top of two tons of Welsh coal. The Home Office, still quibbling with the Cremation Society, allowed the corpse to be burned but only if it were in a coffin. Twenty thousand spectators turned up and paid three pence each to watch the "hellish spectacle".

## Conversational deafness

A mild congenital disability that afflicts the English and causes them to end sentences with questions.

Just checking that their listeners have heard what they've said, what? Afflicts all social classes, know what I mean?

## Corporate snowbirds

Snowbird is a North American soubriquet for anyone who migrates south in search of warmth during the winter. Corporate snowbird is my soubriquet for retired executives from multinational companies, most of them men, who settle in sun-blessed resorts they previously enjoyed when on vacation.

A few years ago when making a documentary on ageing, I visited a handful of international 'retirement communities' where the entire population seemed to consist of former field officers in the corporate army who had earned their comfortable retirement by a lifetime of unquestioning support of the system. When I was young we called them 'yes men'.

They live, with or without partners, in cantonments located in warm climes – California, Arizona, Florida, Spain, Portugal – where their substantial villas are protected by high walls, electronic gates, and patrolling security guards to prevent intrusion by the less fortunate. They read a little, drink a lot, dabble in sexual adventure, and have loads of parties at which their conversation rarely strays from their performance that day on the golf course, recent advances in cardiovascular medicine and joint replacement, and the skill with which they manage their portfolios. (In truth, when it comes to finance they are often the suckers most easily ripped off by the experts.)

From outside the barricades, their's seems an arid existence and I was reminded of the price they pay for it when, the morning after visiting one of the gated communities in Southern California, I had breakfast in a local hotel. At a nearby table a corporate 'top executive', twenty stone of solid flesh configured like a hippopotamus, was conducting a 'breakfast meeting' with half a dozen subordinates gathered round his table. The 'meeting' was a boastful monologue delivered, between mouthfuls, by the hippo, and punctuated by humiliating verbal assaults on each acolyte in turn.

What intrigued me was the way his audience of seemingly intelligent middle-aged men tolerated this psychopathic rant. I concluded, sadly, that their dutiful listening was part of the price they paid for the dream that lay just over the horizon: the luxury retirement villa, the power boat in the harbour, and the endless rounds of sun-kissed golf. I longed to tell them to take a trip round the corner, have a look at the yes men of yesteryear, and ask themselves whether it was worth it.

## Corporeal chauvinism

Vision of the human body as a fortress under attack from malevolent outsiders. Endemic in Scotland.

In *Medicine & Culture,* Lynn Payer describes how, unlike French women who say they have reserves of health they can draw upon, Scottish women think they are either sick or well, with nothing in between. They reject such things as natural degeneration as causes of disease and favour causes such as infection, climate, damp, poisons, and adverse working conditions. Disease to them is an evil lurking outside them waiting to attack.

## Cosmetic surgeons

Plastic surgeons who trained to do good, then learned to do well.

By the end of the 20th century they had taken over from psychiatrists as purveyors of the 'dream' some people claim they want to live. Today physical image has the same attraction – and to the same sort of people – as mental cleanliness had in the 1960s: the secret of life is no longer a matter of letting it all hang out but of having it all tucked in.

I witnessed the first signs of change in the 1970s when women in Southern California started to boast about their cosmetic operations. Dammit all, the surgery was so expensive you wanted folks to know you could afford it. A woman who had a face job, a nose job, a chin job, or a boob job would give a 'show-off' party for her friends. The surgeon, in those days always a male whose role hovered uneasily twixt that of doctor and gigolo, was always invited and rarely failed to attend because that was where he recruited most of his future customers.

At one of these surgical Tupperware 'do's, a Los Angeles surgeon showed me the business card he handed to likely customers. On the back was a cartoon of a woman sitting *en negligee* in front of her dressing table. The caption read: "Mirror, mirror on the wall... lie to me."

## Counselling
Ill-defined therapy offered to people suffering from a condition for which medicine can't offer a quick fix.

The human transaction that 'counselling' describes was once an honourable and useful activity. The GPs to whom I was apprenticed in the 1950s listened sympathetically while their patients unburdened their fears and their worries, and tried to help victims of stress or tragedy by talking over their troubles with them, giving them useful information or even, whisper it gently, just by listening to them. But they would never have called it counselling.

The word has now been commandeered by a multitude of pseudo-professionals whose skills have yet to be satisfactorily evaluated. A small randomised controlled trial, reported in the *British Journal of General Practice* compared the results of counselling (usually involving up to six fifty-minute sessions) with routine care from a GP. Four months after treatment there were no differences in physical or mental health between those who'd had counselling and those given routine care.

Patients themselves remain uncertain of the value of counselling. One such was the subject of a letter Dr Hasnain Dalal, a GP in Truro, received from a local psychiatrist.

*There was no evidence of any psychiatric illness. When it was suggested that perhaps he should see a counsellor at the surgery to discuss his circumstantial worries, he said that all counsellors were do-gooders with third-rate qualifications. He thought that he was the best counsellor he knew. He felt that he would not harm anybody, but said that he might enjoy going bonkers.*

Needless to say the psychiatrist diagnosed the patient as being in the pink of sanity and in no need of help.

Instead of calling for counsellors, we need to re-learn the art of listening to one another and of befriending others. In his presidential address to the Johnson Society, Robert Robinson recalled the days…

*…when men actually turned to each other as Johnson first turned to Boswell, and in an exchange of words that celebrated and embraced the possibility of their joint existences, cried, "Give me your hand. I have taken a liking to you".*

## Creative dysarthria
Using an impediment to advantage.

A celebrated exponent was the humorist Patrick Campbell who transmuted from writer to national treasure as a team captain on the television game *Call My Bluff* opposite his old friend Frank Muir.

Campbell was an unlikely television performer because he had a serious stammer. Yet on *Call My Bluff* and *That Was the Week that Was* he used the impediment to great effect by making no attempt to disguise it. As an Irishman who loved to talk he saw the stammer as an enemy and he spent most of his life at war with it. When the enemy tried to interrupt him, he would encourage himself to fight back. As Frank Muir explained, "Locked silent by a troublesome initial letter, he would show his frustration by banging his knee and muttering *Come along! Come along!*" And the audience loved it.

He was not the only Irishman to make good use of a stammer. Back in the early years of the 'Troubles' I had dinner with a Dublin judge whose home was regularly picketed by political demonstrators. Most times the picketing was reasonably good-humoured but one day a more aggressive mob marched up the drive. As they approached the house the judge, watching from a window, saw them confront his bodyguard, a gun-toting but stammering police sergeant.

"S-s-s-stand right where you are," said the sergeant. "If one of you f-f-f-f-effers comes a s-s-s-step nearer, I'll blow his f-f-f-f-ing head off."

"Don't swear at these representatives of the people," said the self-righteous leader of the mob.

"With this s-s-s-s-stammer," said the sergeant, "I can't f-f-f-f-fing swear."

## Creative dysgraphia

Form of Malaproposis (qv) that affects letters that hospital consultants write to GPs. The diagnostic feature is that the surrogate word enhances the meaning.

As in a letter from a psychiatrist to Dr Stephen John Forsdick of St Austell: "I gather that she does have a habit of lying on the grass, which may predispose her to incest bites."

And most GPs could name patients who match the description a surgeon used in a letter to Dr A M McEwen of Buckhurst Hill. "Your patient is a keen player in her local bowels team."

## Cruciate position

Alignment that occurs when the patient is horizontal and the doctor vertical.

Neil Kessel, who coined the phrase when Professor of Psychiatry at Manchester University, pointed out that no useful communication could occur in this position.

### Modified Cruciate position

Gynaecologist's version of the traditional cruciate. The patient remains horizontal but the doctor sits with attention focused on places other than the patient's face.

An English actress who was once my patient had her first baby in a teaching hospital that prides itself on its teaching of communication skills. She'd had an episiotomy so her legs were raised into the stirrups when the houseman arrived to repair her perineum. He acknowledged her presence with a gruff "Good morning", then settled himself on a stool placed between her outstretched legs and stitched away, his attention, in her words, "wholly fixed on the site of his activity."

After several minutes of silent stitching, and no doubt feeling the need to exercise his communication skills, he asked without raising his head: "Haven't I seen you on television?"

## Cured

Any patient who has ceased to bother the doctor.

## Customised disease

Collections of symptoms masquerading as diseases.

Examples include claustrophobia, multiple personality disorder, social anxiety disorder, night eating syndrome, and frotteurism (better known to tabloid readers as dirty raincoat rub-a-dub disease).

An American psychiatrist recently pointed out that over 650 different types of phobia had now been described and documented. The strangest was Cherophobia, the fear of having a good time. Even as I write, I suspect a psychiatrist somewhere is inventing a name for the fear of getting a phobia.

The neurologist John Pierce has described how, when he was a consultant at Hull Royal Infirmary, many conditions he saw – including fibromyalgia, Chronic Whiplash Syndrome, concussion and post-concussional states – were not diseases but diagnoses. He called them Diseases by Committee Consensus. (This semantic distinction, significant for clinicians, does not deny that the conditions cause real pain or disability.)

The invention of disease is nothing new: sixty years ago doctors confidently diagnosed "masturbatory insanity" and sought cures for "sexual inversion" i.e. homosexuality. Today it is still easy – and often profitable – to convert any behaviour that conventional souls think 'odd' or 'unusual' into a customised disease. All you need is a committee and a consensus.

In 1952 the US encyclopaedia of mental disease, the *Diagnostic and Statistical Manual of Mental Disorders* (DSM), produced by a panel of psychiatrists, was a small, spiral-bound handbook. The latest edition is a 943 page tome. Most of the new diseases that give it bulk comply literally with John Pierce's definition of Diseases by Committee Consensus. Sceptical observers point out that most members of the editorial panel have financial links with the pharmaceutical industry and new diseases seem to appear, as if by magic, at the same time as drugs alleged to be useful in their treatment. (See Manufactured Diseases.)

Judging from the reverence the DSM receives from US doctors, courts, prisons, schools, insurance companies, and such like institutions, you would think it was based on analysis of a large body of scientific evidence. Yet a psychiatrist who worked on a recent edition told an interviewer:

*There was very little systematic research, and much of the research that existed was really a hodgepodge—scattered, inconsistent, and ambiguous. I think the majority of us recognised that the amount of good, solid science upon which we were making our decisions was pretty modest.*

During my professional lifetime, clinical research has disentangled the aetiology of many diseases, yet the list of what we used to call Diseases of Unknown Origin grows no shorter. For every disease doctors strike from the list, their patients seem to create a replacement. It's as if the human organism has an innate need for a specific number of demons to torment it. A sort of truth underlies the apocryphal medical tale of a patient complaining: "I'm still looking for a pill to cure my hypochondria. Everything I try seems to make it worse."

## Customised evidence

Essential knowledge for GPs seeking to practice evidence based medicine: evidence about individuals rather than populations. James Cave, a GP in Newbury, defined it in a letter to the *BMJ*.

*I have several hours' knowledge under my belt for almost all my patients and now know that Mr Jones gets backache when his teenage son comes home, that Mrs Franks does not want me to get her headaches better but just to acknowledge what an awful life she has, and that when Mrs Bloggs says she's a little worried about one of the twins you drop everything and go.*

When I read that, a warm glow suffused my cardiac cockles. Here was confirmation that the ingredient of general practice I found most rewarding back in the Dark Ages still retained its value. When I retired and left what I hoped would be a helpful note for my successor, it contained not one mention of population studies, mega drug trials, or meta-analyses but lots of information like that listed by Dr Cave, plus other mini-items such as how to chat up the person in charge of admissions to our local hospital, which health visitor to avoid, how to twist the arm of the local geriatrician, the name of the surgeon from whom sensitive patients needed protection... your own GP will know the sort of thing I mean. If she or he doesn't, maybe you should find another.

## C words

Words doctors use to describe commendable obedience in patients.

Occasionally, medicine's vocabulary acquires a word I find more irksome every time I hear it. High on my irking list is 'compliance' a word doctors use to describe the behaviour of patients who follow the treatment their doctors recommend. To my ears it carries echoes of a hierarchical world in which doctors issue orders which patients are expected to obey.

Another irking word, this time for patients, is one that most doctors take in their unthinking stride, the word 'consent.' When doctors use it, it sounds as if patients have been given a choice when maybe all they've been offered is the chance to acquiesce to the doctor's choice.

Another irker is 'co-operation,' which involves patients making changes in their lives just to please their doctors.

This treacherous trio is linked by definition: a co-operative patient is one who first consents and then complies.

A case of blatant non-compliance was described in a letter a hospital sent to Dr J Orr, a GP in Camberley, about one of his patients:

*Once her condition had stabilised we were discussing placement possibly in a Nursing Home. Mrs X was clearly not happy to pursue this option and in the early hours of 12 November she became unresponsive and passed away.*

Said Dr Orr, "She was always a determined soul."

Any doctor fool enough to think that seemingly co-operative patients are passively obedient should recall the clinical trial in which one of the subjects complained to the investigator that her double-blinded tablets had been changed. When asked how she knew, she explained that, unlike the previous batch, they floated when she threw them down the lavatory.

# D

## Data

Information published in medical journals in lieu of thought.

*The British Journal of General Practice* allocated five pages to a paper that concluded:

*In this pilot study, the null hypothesis that both treatments will show equal results cannot be confirmed or rejected because of the small number of participants.*

## Deafness

An even greater disability than blindness. The blind evoke immediate sympathy but, because we have problems communicating with the deaf, they are often a source or irritation and sometimes, sadly, figures of fun.

Despite the prejudice, deafness can be a source of salutary anecdote when the deaf person is not the butt but the hero of the tale. As in the story of a Worcester GP told to me by his son Robin Steel (one of the few medical politicians I met whom I'd have been happy to consult as a patient).

One day Dr Steel senior, visiting a patient at home, had to pass a deaf old woman sitting in a chair. As he went by, she stared at him with a puzzled frown.

"Who's this?" she asked.

"It's the doctor," said her daughter.

"Who?" repeated the mother a cupping her hand to her ear.

"The doctor, Mother."

"Who, dear?"

"The doctor," said the daughter, now shouting.

"The what?"

"You know, Mother. The man who killed Father."

## Death

1. Word that doctors have difficulty in pronouncing

Peter Archer, 47, was arrested for running naked down a street in Melbourne but released when the police discovered he was fleeing from a mortuary where a doctor had officially pronounced him dead.

Asuncion Gutirrez, aged 100, who'd also been 'pronounced dead' startled her mourning family and friends in Managua, Nicaragua, when she sat up in her coffin at her wake and asked for food. "This is the third time she has done this to us," said her grandson.

2. Concept that even clever doctors have difficulty comprehending.

First sentence of an editorial in the *British Medical Journal*: "People who walk faster are less likely to die than slow walkers."

3. Spectre in whose presence it is sometimes difficult to assume solemnity.

A GP friend of mine, Bev Daily, used to look after an odd couple – a middle-aged man and his elderly father who lived together in an isolated house and who were as dependent on one another, and as argumentative, as Steptoe and son. One day the son called the doctor to see his father who'd been asleep all day.

When Bev went into the bedroom he found that the old man was dead. He spent a minute or two trying to assemble the right words to break the news to a son whom he knew loved his father more than any creature on this earth. Yet when he went downstairs he found, as so often happens, that he lapsed into platitudes.

"I'm sorry to say," he muttered, "that your father has passed away."

"Bloody hell," said the son. "I've just made him a big plate of stew."

## Decisive

Traditional attribute of surgeons: sometimes mistaken but never in doubt. (See One of the Old School.)

Writing in the *Guardian,* Dr Luisa Dillner warned readers: "When considering the attitude of male obstetricians and gynaecologists, you have to remember they are predominantly surgeons. This makes them automatically autocratic. Many genuinely have difficulty with the concept that what's yours isn't necessarily theirs to remove."

In the early 1950s, when Richard Gordon created Sir Lancelot Spratt, Dublin could match London in autocratic surgeons. One of the most notorious would stride down his ward the day before his list, point at each patient in turn, and announce his intention in a single word. "Cholecystectomy… amputation… laparotomy."

The patients, better known as 'teaching material', were expected to respond with a quick tug at the forelock and a humble, "Thank you, sir."

In those days elderly men with prostatic cancer were offered treatment by physical rather than hormonal castration and one morning the surgeon went on his rounds, declaiming his intentions in his usual way.

"Laparotomy… castration… appendicectomy… "

"Hang on a second, sir," said patient number two with unforgivable impertinence. "This castration business? What exactly would that involve?"

The surgeon, perplexed by the interruption, barked a reply:

"A simple matter, my man. We'll just remove your testicles. At your age, they're no use to you."

"Oh I know that, sir," said the man. "But they are kind of… dressy."

## Decorated Municipal Gothic (DMG)

Prose style that evolves when writers eschew simple words that might express their ideas in a neat and palatable form, and use instead language they believe adds dignity, scientific worth, or even grandeur to their utterance.

Doctors evolved this style long before late 20th century managers imported Arcanian (qv) into NHS administration. Here, for instance, is an example of DMG from the 1960s.

*The pragmatic verity of the physiological concept of disease is established by its usefulness: with functional integrity our goal the no-thoroughfare of unattainable structural integrity leaves us no longer at a therapeutic non-plus.*

Clinicians draw on a well established DMG vocabulary to give their work what they think is a 'scientific' flavour. They write 'alimentation was maintained' when their patients would say they were fed. 'Speech' becomes 'verbal communication', 'many' becomes 'numerous', 'most' becomes 'the majority of'; people 'utilise' instead of 'use', 'facilitate' instead of 'ease', 'transmit' rather than 'send', 'locate' rather than 'find.'

Let just one of those words into a paper, or lecture, and the infection spreads with the abandon of bacteria alighting on a nutritious surface. The style is so addictive that syntax and meaning soon get lost in the scramble for prestigious words.

*Our implicit standards were confounded by retrospective analysis resulting in our outcome measures being invalid thereby blocking our impetus for change.*

Repeated exposure to the style so conditions us that we no longer pause mid-sentence to reflect on the barbarities being inflected on the English language. So authors continue to seek aggrandisement by camouflaging platitudes with portentous nouns and adjectives, as in this definition of educational objectives published by the Royal College of General Practitioners:

*If the collective and hierarchical qualities of an ordered list of objectives are not appreciated, the teacher may waste time reiterating material which could have been learned by the trainee by reading and fitting his new knowledge into the principles implicit in a higher order objective already achieved. This can also result in boredom for the learner.*

To which the only possible response is 'Hear, hear.'

DMG is not just a matter of jargon. When I edited *World Medicine* I saw authors, in search of readability, purge their articles of medical argot yet leave behind the contorted syntax and bizarre stylistic devices they'd been conditioned to accept as part of medical language but which readers find, at best, deterring and, at worst, impenetrable.

Oh how I wish we could rewind life's video recorder and take today's self-styled 'communicators' back to the time when people who wanted to be understood used simple words with well-defined meanings, those halcyon days when patients talked to one another instead of conducting a dialogue, when medical researchers wrote of the poor and not of socioeconomically disadvantaged subgroups, and when role-playing was something you did on a pianola.

## Decorations

Symbols of distinction that doctors in High Places once insisted be worn on ceremonial occasions. Maybe they still do; for some years now I have lived contentedly on lower ground.

The first time I was invited to a medical dressing up party, I felt disadvantaged. I'd never got round to claiming the Defence Medal – or was it the Victory Medal? – I won playing Private Pike in the Home Guard, trained to defend the Lancashire fells from Nazi paratroops disguised as nuns. Without a medal I feared I might be thrown out for turning up improperly dressed but, with characteristic kindness, John Rowan Wilson lent me a spelling medal he had won at school. It came on a royal blue ribbon that I hung around my neck and, though nobody showed any interest in it, it did save me from ignominious dismissal to the servants' hall.

I later developed enough self-confidence to turn up naked at Grand Occasions and did so for years, until along came an evening that really did demand a display of plumage: the celebration of the *BMJ's* 150th anniversary, to be held in the Whitehall Banqueting Hall from which King Charles stepped through the window to place his neck on the chopping block.

By then I had been inducted into the *Confrerie des Chevaliers du Tastevin*; an honour bestowed in my case for quantity of consumption rather than quality of perception. One evening after a magnificent banquet in the Chateau du Clos de Vougeot, I stood, head bowed, before the *Le Grand-Maitre de l'Ordre* who, cheered on by the wine-filled congregation, tapped me on the shoulder with a pre-phylloxera vine root, then hung round my neck a silken ribbon, striped with bands of old gold and russet red, from which dangled a silver sommelier's cup.

It lay in its box at the back of a drawer for many a year until the *BMJ* anniversary provided an occasion worthy of its display. When I tried it on, before setting off to Whitehall, the ribbon enhanced my starched white shirt with a hint, dare I say it, of regality; and the sommelier's cup lay hidden behind the meeting point of the lapels of my dinner jacket, save for a glimpse of the tip of its silver handle.

During the Reception before the banquet, the ribbon proved its worth. One of the Highest of the High, who usually ignored me, engaged me in a full five minutes of conversation while his eyes stayed focussed on the V of my lapels trying to divine what that tantalising glimpse of silver actually betokened.

Once he released me, I sought out every friend I could find and bragged about my social triumph. Eventually I spotted Larry Altman, the urbane medical correspondent of *The New York Times*. As I started on my tale, I saw that he too was wearing an impressive ribbon.

"Good God, Larry," I said. "don't tell me you go in for that sort of thing."

He undid his jacket to reveal... a medal won in a spelling bee at Harvard.

## Defiant resilience

Commendable quality which like wine – but, sadly, unlike memory – can improve with age.

A few years ago I spent a week in northern Florida investigating what happens to those who retire to the Sunshine State after busy working lives in the chillier north. My most memorable finding was a newspaper story I read over breakfast on my first day.

A seventy-year-old woman emerging with her shopping from a local Mall spotted four men preparing to drive off with her car. She dropped her shopping bags, drew a handgun, and screamed at the top of her voice: "I have a gun and I know how to use it. Get out of the car, you scumbags."

The men raised their hands, shouted "Don't shoot lady," and scuttled off like frightened rabbits.

The woman managed to load her shopping into the car and climb into the driver's seat but, still severely shaken, couldn't get her key into the ignition. After three failed attempts she realised why. She opened the glove compartment and found it full of unfamiliar objects. She was in the wrong car.

Her own car was parked a few spaces away so she transferred her shopping bags and drove to the police station.

As she told her story, the desk sergeant interrupted her and pointed to the far end of the counter. There, four ashen faced men were describing the person who'd hijacked their car: "Tough old boot, less than five feet tall, curly white hair, wearing glasses, definite psychopath."

No charges were filed.

## Degrees

Letters that eccentric (i.e. non-American) universities and colleges encourage doctors to put after their names to confuse information technologists.

A heavily 'personalised' letter from the British Medical Association and addressed to Mr J C M Strachan FRCS Ed, began "Dear Mr Ed."

A paper in the *Lancet* by E Farquhar Buzzard, MB Oxon, is referenced in the Cumulative Index Medicus as a joint publication by Buzzard EF and Oxon MB. The index also includes MB's elder brother, Oxon DM, and his cousins, Lond MB and Cantab ChB. Even more oddly, the South African authors of another paper are indexed as DuPlessis DJ and W'srand CM.

## Dermatologist

Medical adventurers in the skin trade. Ideal speciality for those who seek comfort and a regular income. The patients don't call the doctor at night and they never get better.

Dermatologists are masters of the art of description – a traditional form of diagnosis that is also therapeutic. The London physician Richard Asher captured the solemnity with which this art is practised.

*What is this strange skin condition with red rings which expand from the centre in widening circles? "That," says the dermatologist, "is erythema annulare centrifugum." He has spoken the words of power and the dignity of the profession has been upheld.*

## Detachment, Air of

Artificial attitude adopted by doctors when they write a scientific paper (qv) in the hope it will make their work seem more 'scientific'.

The world portrayed in scientific papers is entirely passive. The patient is admitted. She is examined. Tests are done. The appendix is removed. She is resuscitated. Nobody actively does anything, certainly not the 'scientifically' detached writer of the story.

When carried to extremes passivity can add an air of delicious uncertainty, as in this footnote to a multi-authored paper in the *Lancet*:

*Since this paper was written, one of us has died.*

## Detoxification

Gentler alternative to colonic lavage for ridding the body of those noxious substances that threaten the vitality of celebrities. (See Colon.)

GP columnist, 'Samantha Pepys', had quite a few patients who went to private nutritionalist clinics. "One woman was having a 'detoxification week'. She doesn't drink alcohol nor smoke (never has) and she doesn't have much stress in her life or a poor diet. What did she need to remove from her system? The only thing she had to lose was money."

## Diagnosis

The art of understanding.

A Californian physician Faith Fitzgerald was in a ward writing notes when two nurses asked if she would see a patient they were worried about – a seventy-five-year-old woman who'd been brought back to the ward after an operation. Within hours she'd started 'babbling incoherently' when on her own yet seemed fully oriented when they spoke to her. They wondered whether they should give her a sedative.

As Dr Fitzgerald approached the patient's room she could hear "unintelligible rhythmic speech which modulated in intensity from prayerful quietude to vigorous exhortations".

"There," said the nurse. "See what I mean?"

Through the window in the door they saw the woman lying on her back on the bed and declaiming at the ceiling. Then, as they watched, Dr Fitzgerald began to recognise words: Hrothgar, Herot, Beo, Grendel.

She walked into the room.

"Hello," said the patient brightly.

"Hello back," said Dr Fitzgerald. "You're doing Beowulf?"

The patient smiled. She'd been an English professor at a small university. Her specialty was Old English literature and, before her operation, she'd decided to recite Beowolf in Old English when she recovered just to check if "I had all my brain left after anaesthesia".

A different sort of understanding was shown by Dr Kumar Kotegaonkar of Manchester. One evening he had a phone call from a man asking for a visit to his elderly mother because she'd been 'squeaking' for two days.

An intrigued Dr Kotegaonkar made the visit and could find nothing abnormal until, as he removed his stethoscope from her chest, he heard a definite squeak. A repeat of the squeak drove him to even more diligent examination and eventually to triumphant diagnosis. Not only did he find the cause but was able to prescribe a cure.

Just a matter of fitting new batteries in the smoke alarm.

## Diagnostic smear

Diagnosis used as a political weapon.

When Robert Robinson was doing his National Service in West Africa, he discovered that the local newspaper's deeply ingrained anti-colonial attitude would sometimes surface at unexpected moments. He quoted the obituary of an Anglican bishop which "after many a lapidary flourish, ended on the grave and respectful note, *It is not generally known that for the last thirteen years of his life the bishop was a martyr to gonorrhoea.*"

## Dicing with death

Occupational hazard for medical students.

The night I discovered I was dying, I was a student in my second clinical year and had already learned enough to share my generation's fear of tuberculosis.

After smoking my fifty-second cigarette of the day I had a nasty cough and produced a gobbet of blood stained sputum. I knew at once I'd been invaded by tubercle bacilli because I'd seen the film *A Song to Remember* in which Cornel Wilde, as Chopin, coughed splatters of Technicoloured blood over the ivory keys.

I decided to face up bravely to the inevitable. How long had I left? Months rather than years I suspected, and perhaps only weeks. In those days, streptomycin was not even a twinkle in a chest physician's eye. In my dingy Victorian room across the road from the hospital, I sat beneath a purring gas mantle and reviewed the achievements of a promising young life about to be cut short. It didn't take long.

I decided that, before handing myself over to the doctors, I'd best put my affairs in order. I composed a rather touching letter to my parents thanking them for their love and for their moral and financial support, and apologising for the pain I knew I sometimes caused them. I suspect the apology was a touch over-poignant but I was still under Cornel's influence.

Next I drafted a list of bequests to ensure my closest friends would receive my most treasured possessions: my record of James Joyce reading from Finnegan's Wake, my new squash racquet, my virgin *Gray's Anatomy* (untouched by hand), and my framed exhortation, purloined from a golf club: *Will members please refrain from washing their balls in the basin.*

I realised that, at my age, Proust might have gathered more significant symbols of times past but the hour was too late for literary garnish. And it didn't matter because, once I'd disposed of these trappings of a brief life, I found peace of mind.

I picked up the frugal parcel I needed for my last journey – sponge bag and slippers wrapped in pyjamas – and, as I walked to the pillar box to post my letter and then through the hospital portico for the last time, my spirit rode the crest of a soaring Puccinian melody.

My re-ordering of my affairs had taken some time so when I walked into Casualty it was one o'clock in the morning. The only doctor allowed to examine students was a consultant-in-waiting, the Resident Assistant Physician. It never crossed my mind he might be irked at having to get out of bed to minister to a dying man. He wore a white coat over his pyjamas and seemed unimpressed as I unfolded my sorry tale. Indeed, he rudely interrupted it, ordered me to open my mouth, and brusquely flattened my tongue with a metal spatula. He then announced I'd abraded a small blood vessel at the back of my throat and shooed me off to the room I thought I'd never see again.

I remember no feeling of relief. All that sympathy I'd counted on receiving as one so young fighting so bravely and uncomplainingly had been dismissed with a short snarl. And my father never let me forget the more abject paragraphs of my letter.

## Dignitary
Captionese for "Worthies about whom there is little else to say".

At this moment I'm gazing on a newspaper photograph that's captioned *Mayor with medical dignitaries*. It's not a pretty sight. Anyone who has seen a clutch of our self-important colleagues tripping over their gold chains, or sweating it out under their ermine in the noonday sun, knows that the medical dignitary can be even more ludicrous than the civic variety.

Some quirk of medical anatomy makes academic finery sit uneasily upon our person. Lawyers can just get away with it because they wear wigs. Maybe doctors should follow their example because, whenever I see that collection of best suits and multicoloured robes that assembles for Grand Medical Occasions, I'm reminded of the chorus of an amateur Operatic Society standing by to give us an earful of Rudolf Friml.

In 1975, when the Royal Australian College of GPs held its annual meeting in the Sheraton Hotel in Perth, I witnessed what the programme called *The Procession Of Dignitaries*. After processing, they stood before us on the stage wearing clothes fashionable in nightclubs in the 1920s, overlaid with colourful robes and floppy velvet hats fashionable in Padua five hundred years before. Yet they stood at the heart of one of the world's most beautiful of modern cities. What on earth, I wondered, had this pseudoccasion got to do with the challenges facing a lively young specialty in a lively young continent.

Then the Musak crackled into life. And instead of the national anthem, we got the *Sugar Plum Fairy*. Suddenly everyone burst out laughing. The Key Speaker was so overcome with glee he snatched off his velvet hat and flung it on the floor. No longer were we dignitaries and plebs but a bunch of people laughing at the absurdity we'd all recognised but refused to acknowledge.

The concept of dignitary shares naught with that of dignity, save five consonants and two vowels, yet does seem subject to a natural law that the lesser the honour the greater the pride in its possession. Dean Acheson, the American statesman, was intercepted in the lobby of a Washington hotel by a flustered woman seeking assistance because she had jammed the zip in her ball gown. Acheson managed to unstick it and, after thanking him, she said: "I think I should tell you I am a regional assistant state vice president of the Daughters of the American Revolution."

Said Acheson: "My dear lady what a moment ago was a rare privilege now appears to have been a great honour."

## Disorientated
Even more confused than the doctor.

## Divine intervention
Convenient explanation for anything beyond our comprehension.

The patient sat in an armchair, a widower in his early eighties: Irish, grey-haired, affable, slightly confused but radiating a charm that bordered on charisma. It was the first time in his life he'd asked for a home visit and his GP reassured him that the fall down the stairs had broken no bones. "Indeed, you're in great shape for your age."

The patient nodded contentedly. "God has been good to me, doctor. I've been spared the afflictions visited on too many of my friends. 'Tis only in the last year, for instance, I've had to get up in the night to pass water. And even then God is good to me. In some strange way he offers light to guide me when the need is on me. And when the need is gone the light fades. But 'tis not for us to question His mysterious ways."

The GP bade him goodbye and, on the way out, had a word with his patient's daughter who'd called round from her home nearby.

"Your dad's a real charmer," said the GP. "And man of great faith." He told her about the divine illumination.

"Dear God," said the daughter, "don't tell me he's been peeing in the fridge again."

## Divine retribution

Phrase used happily by non-believers who accept only the second definition of divine, i.e. delightful. Often wreaked in unlikely places.

Today only a dwindling band of doctors born before 1940 can remember the days of National Service when the RAMC training centre at Cookham allowed itself six weeks to turn recently qualified doctors into officers and gentlemen. Many of the memories are of bizarre confrontations on the barrack square where a bellowing sergeant tried to drill often disinterested doctors.

Because we were non-combatant we didn't carry rifles but were expected to acquire the skills of stepping out with pride – chins up, arms straight at the elbows – turning left, turning right, and saluting by numbers.

Every squad had at least one member who appeared to lack the cerebellar control these tasks demanded. In one, the odd man out was taller than the rest and his slovenly gait a constant irritation to the sergeant.

"You are a shambles, sir," he would shout and shout again… but to little effect.

After one session even more dispiriting than usual, he dismissed everyone except the tall man. The time had come for a short sharp shock. He gave the 'shambles' a stern lecture on the virtues of obeying orders and of trying harder then, as a punishment, ordered him to do twenty circuits of the drill square "at the double".

"I want to see you run until you drop. And maybe you'll learn to use those legs like a proper human being."

The tall ungainly man set off like a gazelle and sped round the square with a long relaxed stride and determined smile. As he whizzed by on his second circuit, a member of the squad, from whom I heard this tale, let the sergeant in on a secret. The 'shambles' was Dr Roger Bannister who but a year before had run the first sub four-minute mile.

Sir William Stewart, the biologist who was the first head of the UK Office of Science and Technology, was born on Islay and liked to holiday at his croft on Barra. One year, clad in old overalls and wellies, he gave a lift to a pompous English medical student whose conversation revealed his low opinion of the local peasants.

"What are you doing here?" asked Stewart.

"I'm studying the island's seaweed. It may look all the same to you but it is extraordinarily variegated."

"Oh, I know," said Stewart. "Before you go, you must take a look at the *Ascophyllum nodusum* and the *Himanthalia lorea* on the south coast. On the west you'll find *Enteromorpha intestinalis* and, on the north, *Plumaria elegans* and *Chondrus crispus*."

"Whoever told you that?" said the student.

"Och," said Stewart, "everyone round here knows that."

## Doctor/patient relationship

Clunking phrase – in common use in journals, textbooks and lectures – that demeans a subtle, infinitely variable, melange of trust and understanding between disparate individuals.

As often happens in matters to do with the emotions, novelists are better than doctors at recognising its nature... and its irrationality.

Maurice, a character in Chris Paling's novel *The Silent Sentry* visited his GP only five times in eight years yet... "always enjoyed the old man's surrogate paternalism, his crumpled-suited kindliness. Maurice had long ago decided that doctors held the secret of eternal life but never prescribed it for fear of the side effects."

## Doctors at arms

The Geneva convention prohibits medical officers from bearing arms but the Royal Army Medical Corps has its own conventions. During World War Two it encouraged doctors, when in mufti, to carry a traditional weapon. A new recruit described his weapon training in the *Lancet*:

*As I had never possessed such an article, I decided to buy one when next in London. And this I did. It was an immaculate, thin, black pencil. The very epitome of the craftsman's art. I inquired how I should open and rewrap it.*

*The assistant looked at me in horror.*

*"One does not unfurl it, Sir," he said. "Never!"*

*"What will I do when it rains?"*

*"Quite simple, Sir. Hold it out at right angles to the body and shout 'Taxi!'"*

## Doctor's note

The ultimate verification.

From a letter to Dr J M Griffin, a Northampton GP, from a patient's executors:

*We completed the insurance claim form and forwarded this to the insurance company together with the original Death Certificate. The insurance company have, however, advised that the Death Certificate is insufficient for their purposes and have requested that the Medical Certificate on the reverse side of the insurance claim form be completed by Mr X's usual doctor.*

A family in Grassendale Park, Liverpool, made a claim for Disability Living Allowance on behalf of a healthy nine month old baby on the grounds of "inability to walk". Local GP John Winter told me the DSS paid his practice £16.40 for a professional opinion that the child's disability would likely improve with the passage of time.

Revd Donald Soper, in a letter to Hampstead and Highgate Express:

*I remember one Sunday afternoon at Speakers' Corner in Hyde Park being challenged by a heckler to prove that I was not mad. I found the situation somewhat tricky so, hoping to play for time, I challenged the heckler to prove that he was not mad which, to my discomfiture he did by producing his discharge certificate from a mental institution.*

## Doing Freddie proud

Phrase that once defined the purpose of an obituary in the *British Medical Journal*.

John Rowan Wilson, surgeon, journalist, and novelist, learned it when he was in charge of the *BMJ* obituary pages, in those days a useful post for writers in need of a regular cheque until they established themselves as authors.

A previous incumbent was Richard Gordon who distinguished himself by publishing the obituary of a prominent doctor who was still alive. When a doctor of music of the same name perished, Gordon rang a few friends of the putative corpse and persuaded them to supply a few kindly words. The subject of the obituary was not at all put out, indeed was amused. Anger was confined to the those who'd said flattering things they never would have uttered if they'd known the man was alive.

When Wilson took the job, the *BMJ's* editor Hugh Clegg assured him that, though he might find the work a little boring, he performed a vital function. Every doctor over fifty, said Clegg, turned to the obituary column in eager expectation. If he saw that one of his friends or rivals had finally hung up his stethoscope, he would rub his hands in triumph and his step that morning would have an extra spring. "Did you read about old Freddie ?" he would ask his friends, wagging a copy of the journal. "They did him proud. His wife will be so pleased."

Doing Freddie proud, said Wilson, was largely a matter of length. The content was of less concern than the column inches. Whenever he was rapped over the knuckles about an obituary it was always for giving someone more or less space than he or she was considered to deserve. Judgement on delicate matters of that kind, he claimed, was what separated the men from the boys in medical journalism.

In 1963 Wilson compiled a glossary of words and phrases plucked from obituaries submitted to the journal, adding a note of the truth that lay behind each cliché. For forty years or more his glossary survived, augmented down the years with phrases noted by others.

| | |
|---|---|
| A character: | A tiresome old man. |
| A perfectionist: | An obsessional neurotic. |
| Assertive: | A bully |
| Plainspoken: | Offensive. |
| Did not suffer fools gladly: | Damnably offensive. |
| A man of strong opinions: | A bigot. |
| Respected: | Feared. |
| One of the old school: | Hopelessly out of date. |
| Widely travelled: | Left juniors to do his work. |
| Many interests outside medicine: | His juniors did all his work. |
| Fond of the good things of life: | A drunk. |
| Lived life to the full: | A drunk. |
| Popular patron of the student rugby club: | A drunk. |
| Had all the irresistible charm of the Celt: | A talkative drunk. |

Wilson occasionally amused himself by rewriting a published obituary substituting the truth for the clichés. It remained a rewarding game to play until the first decade of this century. Then the *BMJ* decided it was a solemn international journal and Freddie no longer needed to be done so proud. Today the obituaries are shorter and more arid. Aficionados like me still try to play the Wilson game but much of the gusto has gone out of it.

## Domiciliary consultation

A traditional ceremony that fell from fashion in the last quarter of the 20th century.

I learned the ritual as a young GP acting as *locum tenens* for a Legacy Doctor (qv) while he spent a week in Deauville. My role, for which I was carefully coached, was that of acolyte. The central figure was one of my master's rich old ladies (ROLs) who enjoyed ill health and whose ego demanded regular attention. The occasion was her ritual monthly visit from a Great Man (GM) chauffeur-driven in a Rolls Royce from Harley Street to her country home.

On the appointed day, I stood in the hall alongside a deferential butler – a stranger would have difficulty telling which of us was which – to greet the visitor. The butler helped the GM unshed his overcoat then handed it, with hat and scarf, to an underling while I led the way upstairs to the bedroom, introduced the GM to a patient he knew better than I did, and moved discreetly to the background.

The GM sat on a chair alongside the ROL's four poster and generated a sonorous murmur of questions to which she responded with deep despairing sighs. As the questions drew peacefully to their close, the GM nodded at a uniformed nurse who stood at the far side of the bed. The nurse leaned forward and, while the GM turned to a washstand to warm his hands in a basin of hot water, she carefully rolled bedclothes up and down to reveal an impressive acreage of ROL, concealing only the forbidden territory that lay between the navel and the knees. A gentle clearing of the nurse's throat was the cue the GM awaited. He wiped his hands on a linen towel and moved to the bed to use them in gentle exploration of the ROL's available areas. Any hint of trespass on forbidden territory was signalled by a hiss from the patient.

There followed the ceremonial application of the stethoscope. The GM placed the business end on strategic points fore and aft on his patient's chest, listening with a stone-faced puzzlement that suggested he was in the presence of unique sounds, before demanding the ritual incantation of "Ninety-nine." He then prepared himself for a display of the percussive art. He placed his left hand flat against the ROL's upper back and rapped its middle finger with middle finger of his right to produce impressive resonance. As the last echo died away he nodded once more at the nurse who handed him another towel and rearranged the bedclothes while we retired to the bathroom to consult, the GM wiping his hands with the towel in the manner of Pontius Pilate.

In the bathroom the GM rewashed his hands while considering out loud what might be seemly for him to tell our patient. I listened attentively while he sought words that would express the rarity, indeed uniqueness, of her condition without reaching any definite conclusion. Other words hinted at her good fortune in having a doctor who really understood the depth of her suffering… referring, of course, not to the acolyte but to himself. No mention was made of a diagnosis. Further tests would, of course, be needed.

He finished by glancing half-questioningly in my direction. I obeyed my instructions and nodded silent approval before he embarked on another monologue about recent happenings within our trade, who had done what to whom at which Royal College. I listened politely though I knew none of the people he praised or castigated and nothing of the intrigues in which they might or might not have been engaged. Only when he judged enough time had passed to impress the ROL with the length of our consultation did we emerge. I stood respectfully in the background while he seated himself once more beside the four poster and muttered wisely to the ROL.

I'd been briefed on the signal she would give when she'd had enough so when, after one of her attenuated sighs, she gave three short dry coughs, I completed my duties by stepping forward and ushering the GM downstairs and into his Rolls.

I re-established contact with reality only when the chauffeur, having tucked a rug across his master's knees and closed the car door, gave me a broad un-enigmatic wink. The message was clear. "What sort of caper have we got ourselves caught up in?"

## Donner und Blitzen
Unusual late night injury seen in New Towns.

First reported in a Milton Keynes newspaper: "Police want to speak to anyone who recognises the youth pictured here beating up another man with a kebab."

## Doornail
Long established measure used to verify modern criteria for confirming death.

Two American researchers, Mike Dubik and Brian Wood, kept a large seven year-old doornail under close observation for twenty-four hours. They reported that, during that time, the nail showed no signs of vocalisation or volitional activity, exhibited no respiratory movements or spontaneous eye movements, offered no evidence of postural activity (decerebrate or decorticate), and made no spontaneous or induced movements. The doornail therefore met the established 'physical examination' criteria for the diagnosis of death.

They then moved on to the designated neurological investigations. They wired up the doornail to a standard machine designed to measure electrical activity in the brain and were able to record thirty minutes of electro-cerebral silence.

At the end of this exhaustive study, they concluded that "the criteria for death as described in modern medical literature are valid and may be used with confidence by clinicians."

## Dorian Gray syndrome

Wilde's fantasy achieved not with a picture in the attic but with an entry in Halliwell's film guide.

Though I've now passed most of life's recognised milestones there is one that will always lie ahead. I will never achieve the age of the actors I saw on the screen at my local Gaumont when I was a boy. Errol Flynn, Cary Grant, Betty Grable, Fred Astaire, Rita Hayworth et al. will always be older than me.

I'm now more than twice the age they were when they made those films yet when I see televised repeats of images of them captured when they were in their thirties and forties I still feel I'm in the presence of older persons.

The actors themselves are victims of this distorted perception. Fred Astaire said that, when he reached pensionable age people would approach him in shops and ask: "Weren't you Fred Astaire?" And James Mason looking in a shop window saw the reflection of two people staring at him from behind at from a number of different angles before one said to the other: "I'm sure it is. James Mason in later life."

## Doubt

Apart from death, the only certainty in medicine.

A lifetime of watching the world through medical spectacles leads me to suspect it would be a healthier place if fewer people had the courage of their convictions and more had the courage of their doubts.

Doctors, like members of all professions, are easily seduced by the comfort, pomp, and circumstance that reward conformity. Our profession has built so many institutions with marble pillars at the entrance and laurel-wreathed busts in the hall that we sometimes forget that the science that nourishes our craft is a subversive activity that expands our knowledge by questioning our 'certainties'.

The physiologist Joseph Barcroft was elected a Member of a Cambridge college when he developed a theory of respiratory control. I took a shine to him when he described the pride he felt when the college elected him a Fellow for disproving the same theory.

Though not given to swearing oaths, I'd happily pledge allegiance to the declaration of independence Thomas Jefferson wrote for himself after drafting a better-known one for his nation.

*I never submitted the whole system of my opinions to the creed of any party of men whatever, in religion, in philosophy, in politics or in anything else, where I was capable of thinking for myself. Such an addiction is the last degradation of a free and moral agent. If I could not go to Heaven but with a party, I would not go there at all.*

## Dramatic irony

Like comedy and tragedy, an inescapable ingredient of general practice.

Dr Gerard Flood was asked to visit a woman in a home for the elderly in Upholland, Lancashire. For years she'd had severe lung disease that caused her great difficulty in breathing. The staff asked him to see her urgently because her condition had deteriorated. Her lips were blue and her extremities cold but the symptom that most worried them was that she had lost the strength to use her cigarette lighter.

## Dressing to kill

Acquiring power over life and death by wearing the right clothes.

An uppity 'fashion guru' claimed recently that "using clothes to make a professional statement is an exciting new concept." What piffle. Doctors have been at it for centuries. Back in the 1880s our American colleagues, never shy of saying in public what Brits think in private, revealed that our motives were fiscal rather than aesthetic.

"If you dress well, people will employ you more readily, accord you more confidence – expect a larger bill and pay it more willingly."
D.W. Cathell. *The Physician Himself and What He Should Add to His Scientific Acquirements, Baltimore, 1882.*

"Never ride about town on your bicycle with short pants, coloured stockings, white shoes and a small cap stuck on the back of your head. Some doctors have actually ruined their practice by these childish actions. It looks more like second childhood than the doings of a dignified member of the profession."
C.R. Mabee. *The Physician's Business and Financial Adviser, Cleveland, 1889*

In the 20th century fashions changed but doctors still used clothes to signal their superior rank. Thirty years ago Sheila Kitzinger described the hierarchy of sterility that existed in a labour ward. The greater the hierarchical ranking, the fewer the sterile garments that needed to be worn. The least important people in the room, like the husband, had to wear boots or overshoes, sterile gown, mask, and cap. Yet a male consultant could walk in wearing outdoor shoes and might occasionally cover his clothes with a gown that he didn't bother to do up.

As for today, I'm not sure that things have changed as much as some believe. These tired old eyes detect a strange uniformity in the suits worn by consultants in private practice – rich but not gaudy – and even in the clothes favoured at the scruffier end of the profession by physiologists, biochemists and persons of that ilk whose meetings these days look like conventions of denim fetishists.

I also detect a uniformity of dress in GPs who wish to demonstrate their unconcern about appearance by wearing carefully considered 'casual' clothes. But then we live in an age when people were refused entry to a London nightclub because their casual dress was deemed too casual.

## Dual personality

Condition with which doctors often have a closer acquaintance than they would wish.

Ronald D Laing, the late and – to say the least – unorthodox psychiatrist, witnessed his first psychiatric interview as a member of an audience of medical students in a Glasgow hospital. In his autobiography *Wisdom, Madness and Folly*, he describes how he arrived late and found the psychiatrist and his patient sitting in comfortable chairs on a raised dais. The psychiatrist, impeccably dressed and with a cheerful flower in his buttonhole, was fluent and assured. The patient stammered, fidgeted, pulled faces, and wriggled in his chair. Only when the interview ended, did Laing discover that the man he'd identified as the psychiatrist was in fact the patient.

That ambivalence about who is treating whom stayed with him throughout his career. And I've a feeling it's a fairly common form of medical insecurity. Most doctors are aware of the vagaries and defects of their own minds. Small wonder we have doubts about using such uncertain instruments not just to define madness but to 'treat' it.

## Eagerness to help

Commendable human quality that does not always get its just reward.

An intern at New York City Hospital in the 1960s was rattling his way home on the subway, his eyes locked to the pages of a book. A young woman, strap-hanging alongside him, leaned down and asked: "Could you possibly give me your seat? I'm pregnant and I don't feel so good." The intern, a gentleman from the tips of his button-down collar to the toes of his two-tone shoes, leaped to his feet and ushered her into his place. Two stops later the coach began to empty and he sat beside her.

"Forgive me not offering my seat before you asked," he said, "but, let's face it, your condition doesn't really show. How pregnant are you?"

"Just an hour," she said. "But I'm so tired."

## Editorial changes

Decisions publishers make with exuberant abandon.

Thirty years ago new publishers took over *World Medicine,* a magazine I'd edited for fifteen years, and gave me four hours to clear my desk. I don't whinge about being made redundant; the condition was endemic even then. My regret is that I didn't have the theatrical send-off traditionally accorded to editors.

When Lord Beaverbrook wanted to rid himself of one he would send him and his family on a world cruise at the newspaper's expense. When the traveller returned, he would find his successor installed at his desk. Only once did the round-the-world ship return before Beaverbrook had found a replacement. So he cabled the editor: GO ROUND AGAIN.

Thanks to the compressed vocabulary that evolved when messages were priced per word, cables helped journalists to display similar panache when they decided to leave their jobs. Vincent Mulchrone, a revered newspaperman of that era, told me about a newly appointed Foreign Editor who noticed that one correspondent in a distant part hadn't filed any stories for some time. So he whizzed off a cable: WHY UNNEWS.

After a leisurely few days, back came the reply: UNNEWS GOODNEWS.

The angry editor replied immediately: UNNEWS UNJOB.

After an even more leisurely pause, came the reply: UPSTICK JOB ARSEWARDS.

In those days newspapers came in black and white; proprietors and journalists came in full colour. Some would say the positions are now reversed.

## Editorial corrections

Admissions of error that newspapers bury in remote corners of their organs.

Editors of scientific journals sometimes follow their example, which is a pity. Penitence is an attractive human quality; a pretence to infallibility is not.

Richard Smith, who was a lively editor of the *BMJ* before embarking on his third (or is it fourth?) career, put the case well.

*Readers sometimes observe wearily to me that "The BMJ seems to be full of corrections these days." The implication is that I'm running a sloppy ship: a little more discipline, and order would return. I'm wholly unapologetic. Great publications, I observe loftily, are full of corrections. Look at* The New York Times *or the* Melbourne Age. *It's crummy publications that don't have them.*

Richard has a fine collection of apologies editors have been forced to make. Most of them justify the abject grovelling.

> *Instead of being arrested, as we stated, for kicking his wife downstairs and hurling a kerosene lamp after her, the Reverend James P Wellman died unmarried four years ago.*

> *Due to an error in the preparation of this week's Gazette two photographs were transposed. We apologise to Cllr Ray xxxxx. for suggesting he was a vegetable and to allotment owner Mr Bernard xxxxx whose prize winning carrot did not make a speech at Faraday School prize giving.*

Just occasionally a forced apology can be used to reinforce the original story.

> *A report in the Evening Mail wrongly referred to the former Mayor of Frazeley, John Bird, as having a conviction for arson in 1992. In fact, the conviction was for blackmail. We apologise for the error.*

Richard savours a correction devised by H.L. Mencken because, he claims, the *BMJ* under his command narrowly escaped having to print something similar.

> *In my article last week on milk production please read cow for horse throughout.*

## Educationalism

Talk therapy for insecure medical teachers. Not to be confused with education.

Once upon a time when I had to attend conferences allegedly concerned with medical education, the waste bin in my hotel room slowly disappeared beneath a hillock of ill-written documents. The language that deterred me was that deployed by the director of a World Health Organisation programme centre to define his speciality. (Health warning: Reading this straight through without pause may cause breathlessness.)

*Palliative care is based in a multidimensional model of needs to which we can offer a systematic model of care and intervention, practised by a competent interdisciplinary team, with a based in ethical decision-making, and with several levels of the organisation of services, and inserted in every place of the Health Care Network, with a population-based approach. This model of care and organisation are (sic) the appropriate response to the needs of patients with life limiting progressive diseases and their families, with frequent crisis of needs, and there are excellent results of effectiveness, efficiency, and satisfaction. There are clear tendencies, towards the extension to other non-cancer conditions, early shared intervention, and presence in every setting of the Health Care system.*

Those conferences prompted me to formulate two Laws of Educationalism.

1. The greater the difficulty a lecturer has in keeping an audience awake, the more likely the lecture is about educational theory.
2. The more opaque the prose, the more likely the article will include an exhortation to improve 'communication skills'.

Teaching is a performing art that demands the skill to hold the attention of an audience and create the excitement that makes people want to know more. Those who don't have the talent to perform convince themselves that anyone who knows the subject and has a nodding acquaintance with the theory and jargon of 'communication' is automatically endowed with the qualities of a teacher. They create an elaborate palisade of educational theory behind which they feel comfortable, confident that they have acquired all the necessary attributes because they know how to set objectives, measure outcomes, and make the right noises in meetings.

Yet many teachers who, from behind the palisade, claim to know exactly what students need to be taught manage, when they actually engage in teaching, to bore their students into oblivion. The historian A. J. P. Taylor suggested: "It would be no bad thing if academic promotion were open only to those who could hold listeners or win readers."

I remember a sleepy summer afternoon in 1951 when I sat amid a bunch of fellow students in an outpatients clinic at St Thomas' Hospital. Our teacher was the gynaecologist Joe Wrigley and we listened while a tense, rapidly-speaking woman gave him a detailed account of her history of infertility and her own assessment of the possible causes and the investigations she needed.

After she departed to the examination room, Joe turned to us and said in earthy Yorkshire tones: "I don't know. I don't know. These young women today seem to know more than I do about the working of their genital apparatus."

A serious-minded know-all in the front row, angered by this seemingly reactionary approach, piped up: "Surely what you're saying, sir, is that anxiety can be a major factor in infertility."

"Of course I am, lad," said Joe. "But I thought I was putting it more interestingly."

## Emergency
No mere matter of life and death.

Report in *Medical Monitor*: *The patient was prescribed Viagra at the morning surgery. In the evening his wife phoned the emergency centre to complain that it hadn't worked.*

Comforting sign on the M40: *Emergency Toilets 20 miles.*

## Entitlement
Attempting to give a research paper a 'scientific' favour by stretching its title to reader-deterring extremes.

A characteristic example is this title to a *BMJ* article:

*Multifactorial intervention after a fall in older people with cognitive impairment and dementia presenting to the accident and emergency department: randomised controlled trial.*

## Environmental treatment
Negating the symptoms of an illness by changing the environment which the invalid inhabits.

Often achieved by the invalid moving to a warmer clime or seeking clearer air. Sometimes a less dramatic change can lead to a happier life.

One evening, at a dinner, I sat next to a retired Scottish businessman who had achieved harmonious equilibrium twixt illness and environment. When the symptoms caused by his enlarged prostate forced him to give up tennis, a game he much enjoyed, he took up golf. It was, he explained, the ideal game for him because while playing he could, when Nature demanded, nip behind one of the trees that lined the course and empty his bladder.

Playing one day with an old friend he took his dog with him for the walk. Half way down the second nine he turned to his caddie to check the score.

"How are we doing?" he asked.

"Still one down in the match, sir," said the caddie. "But I reckon you're eight up against the dog."

## Epiphany
Magic moment in which people unwittingly reveal something about themselves they've successfully kept hidden.

Dr Bodkin Adams, an Eastbourne GP, gained notoriety in the 1957 when he was accused, but found not guilty, of poisoning elderly women whom he'd induced to include him in their wills. Adams, who was not short on sanctimony, discovered that one way to impress lonely old women was to put on a show of piety. Sometimes when he entered a house he would dramatically drop to his knees in the hall and pray for the recovery of the patient he was about to see.

The younger sister of one of his patients described at his trial what happened after she admitted him to the house. As she started to climb the stairs to the sick-room, she heard a loud crash behind her and turned to see Bodkin Adams lying on the floor of the hall. He had knelt to pray and the mat had slipped from under him on the polished floor. The transcription of the court proceedings takes up the story.

Counsel: Could you hear what Dr Adams called out as he fell?
Witness: Yes I could.
Counsel: What did he say?
Witness: He shouted, "Oh fuck."

## Equanimity
Dangerous mental state.

A woman had to make regular visits to a Manchester diabetic clinic because she had a 'twittery' form of fluctuating diabetes: her blood sugar level jumped up and down rapidly and unexpectedly in a way that matched her twittery personality. Then, quite unexpectedly, her diabetes 'steadied'. The physician looking after her asked if she'd made any changes to her way of life. She explained that she'd taken up transcendental meditation and felt that it had made her less jumpy.

A year or so later her diabetes started twittering again so her physician asked if she were still meditating.

"No," she said. "I've given it up. I couldn't stand the peace of mind."

## Erudition
What doctors acquire from learned journals.

Effect of ale, garlic, and soured cream on the appetite of leeches.
*Anders Baerheim, Honge Sandvik. British Medical Journal*

Masturbation Using Metal Washers for the Treatment of Impotence: Painful Consequences.
*Rana A, Sharma N. British Journal of Urology.*

Copulation as a possible mechanism to maintain monogamy in porcupines, *Hystrix indica.*
*Sever & Mendelssohn. Animal Behaviour*

## Euphoria

Joyful feeling of well being.

Doctors trained to diagnose illness regard this as an undesirable state of mind. Medical textbooks record euphoria as symptom of twenty-seven diseases.

## Euthanasia

Literally a 'good death.'

Doctors disagree about the meaning of "good" and the debate often degenerates into adversarial combat between groups defending strongly held beliefs. Many seek refuge in ambivalence.

On January 20th, 1936, King George V was seriously ill with a chest infection. His doctor, Lord Dawson of Penn, dined that evening at Sandringham with the Prince of Wales, the Archbishop of Canterbury, and the Prime Minister.

During dinner Dawson composed a medical bulletin. Some claim he scribbled it on the back of a menu; more likely he wrote down a sentence he'd been marinating in his mind for days. The bulletin, issued at 9.25 pm and broadcast by the BBC, read: "The King's life is moving peacefully towards its close."

Yet the King's condition was no better or no worse than it had been for forty-eight hours. A suspicious person might conclude that the good doctor, having composed a series of solemn bulletins ushering the King towards a graceful exit, had decided the time had come to ease him off stage.

After dinner, the Archbishop, Dawson and the Prince of Wales joined the Queen in the King's bedchamber. Dawson already had the Queen's and Prince's consent for what he planned to do. At about eleven o'clock, after steering the Archbishop out of the room, he injected a massive dose of morphine and cocaine into the King's jugular vein and the King died peacefully in the presence of his wife and children.

Dawson admitted in his diary that the timing of the lethal dose had been determined by the deadline of *The Times*. He thought it more dignified that the King's death be announced in this traditional forum rather than in lesser prints or over the new and as yet undignified air waves. Lady Dawson phoned the editor of *The Times* advising him to keep the page open. Dawson didn't consult the two other doctors in the case and had to give the lethal injection himself because the nurse who was present refused to do so.

Later that year the second reading of a Bill enabling euthanasia was defeated in the House of Lords. By then Dawson had been created a Viscount establishing, as Richard Gordon wrote, "the going rate for regicide." During the debate the new Viscount was one of the Bill's most vigorous opponents arguing that legislation was unnecessary because "good doctors" already helped their patients to die.

Today, Dawson's paternalistic attitude is unacceptable and strict observance of the law is enforced in hospitals and reinforced by the presence of potential whistle blowers.

My wife was one of many who had the mode of dying she most feared forced upon her. During the fifty years we shared our lives, she often made me promise to protect her from a painful lingering death. She hoped that some compassionate doctor would intervene "in the way they used to." Like me she found it difficult to see the moral distinction between starving and dehydrating people to death and ending life with one painless intervention.

I tried to reassure her with talk of palliative care but, at the moment of truth, all I could do was pass on her wishes to hospital doctors who had no legal way to implement them. Having witnessed her cruel undignified death, I will never lose the feeling that I betrayed her, though I remain grateful to the nurses who cared for her with skill and kindness during the three days she took to die an undignified death. They tried hard to keep her at peace but the moments that dominate my memory are her spells of lucidity when her physical and audible signals were those of someone being tortured rather than comforted.

Compassionate doctors still break the law to honour patients' wishes, if they can do so surreptitiously. The decision should not be theirs. People should be allowed to make their own decisions, and offered more choices, about the ending of their lives.

## Evidence-based medicine (EBM)
Without doubt, the rational and effective way to challenge disease and ease suffering… but only if the evidence is evidence-based.

Re-examination of the details of drug trials sponsored by industry, and particularly of trials that were not published when the results were unhelpful to their sponsors, suggest that some evidence on which doctors are urged to base treatment is of the same quality as the evidence that Saddam Hussein possessed weapons of mass destruction.

A respected medical editor, Dr Marcia Angell, has written:

*It is simply no longer possible to believe much of the clinical research that is published, or to rely on the judgment of trusted physicians or authoritative medical guidelines. I take no pleasure in this conclusion, which I reached slowly and reluctantly over my two decades as an editor of The New England Journal of Medicine.*

Another problem is that careless usage of the phrase 'evidence-based medicine', particularly the downplaying of the role of individual expertise, has demeaned it into one of those fashionable phrases that read well in journals, go down well at meetings, and earn Brownie points on CVs.

The fashion was exemplified by a 'population expert' I caught on television talking tautologically about "evidence-based demography" as if there could be any other sort. Maybe he wished to disassociate himself from the method used by the great Tommy Cooper:

*One in five people in the world is Chinese. And there are five people in my family, so it must be one of them. It's either my mum or my dad, or my older brother Colin, or my younger brother Ho-Cha-Chu. But I think it's Colin.*

In its corrupted form, EBM drops easily from the lips of the unthinking but rarely consoles GPs trying to cope with the complexities of individual lives. I'm glad I retired from general practice before it arrived. I'm all in favour of evidence-based treatment; my problem would have been that so few of my patients suffered from evidence-based illness.

I remember, years ago, attending a postgraduate course when the fashionable notion of the moment was 'correlated data.' A visiting guru explained that when a new patient visited his surgery he fed his computer with a battery of physical and social characteristics plus a diagnosis keyed to a coded nomenclature. I was impressed. When I was in practice, I rarely knew the diagnosis on a patient's last visit, never mind the first. And many of the conditions I diagnosed never found space in a nomenclature. I wondered what he computed for the 'Gran-is-getting-on-our-wick-and-it's-time-the-doctor-did-something' syndrome, or the 'My-boss-is-driving-me-bananas-and-I-need-a-two-day-anti-suicide-break' diathesis, or a 'United-are-being-televised-live-tonight-so-my-breathing-is-playing-up-a-bit' certificate.

The guru, I suspected, would record those under Miscellaneous. I left the meeting wondering if mine had been the only practice in which Miscellaneous was the chief endemic disease.

## Excuses

A game in which players offer explanations in the hope of acceptance rather than belief. There are only two rules.

1. All parties recognise that a game is being played.
2. Pleas of "extenuating circumstances" need have nothing to do with truth or reality.

That second rule was a useful – come to think of it, the only useful – lesson I learned while doing my national service in the RAMC. I soon discovered that regular army officers, like modern NHS executives, expected an answer for everything; anyone who failed to provide one was assumed to be guilty. As a result, answers were what officers got: some were close to the truth but many were celebrations of human inventiveness.

The army had been at the game for so long, I saw it played to a high standard. One tradition that delighted me was that the more imaginative the excuse offered to a bored officer, the more likely it was to be accepted, though not, of course, believed. The *Lancet* reported a classic match played in the final days of World War Two.

An RAMC brigadier, inspecting the wards in a military hospital, spotted a cobweb on the ceiling and ordered the medical officer to put the orderly sergeant on a charge.

"Permission to speak, sir," barked the sergeant, as if addressing a parade ground. "We always keep one cobweb, sir. First-aid treatment for arresting haemorrhage, sir." Then he snapped his face back to attention.

The brigadier recognised a good move when he heard one. He may even have remembered the days when cobwebs were used to encourage blood to coagulate. So he nodded his head in approval and ordered the medical officer to erase the charge.

When they entered the next ward, he ordered the medical officer to re-instate it.

"Why, sir?" asked the doctor.

The brigadier pointed at the ceiling. "No cobweb," he said.

## Executive stress

Proud affliction of Top People. Another status emblem that goes nicely with the leather-bound diary and the key to the executive washroom.

Real stress is more common on the shop than the top floor but executives can afford the expensive remedies on offer, and the fees and time to attend seminars on the subject.

During the lotus-eating years before the banking crash we had many well-publicised reports about the stress of modern living. Professor Cary Cooper reported that 97 per cent of high-ranking civil servants said they suffered from stress and claimed a major cause was having to queue to use the office copier. Other publicised reports warned us of the stress modern living inflicted on the users of company cars and on families celebrating Christmas.

Small wonder that people come to regard all stress as a bad thing. Yet, in their haste to protect themselves against the strain, they forget that stress gives us the drive to be creative and to succeed. Complete suppression of stress, were it possible, could surely lead only to boredom.

Stress is still an affliction more often invoked than suffered. Listening one evening to the radio in New York I heard a woman tell a phone-in programme: "I read this article. It said typical symptoms of executive stress were eating too much, smoking too much, impulse buying, and driving too fast. Are they kidding? This is my idea of a great day."

## Exit lines

Memorable observations uttered by those granted a last word.

The playwright Brendan Behan died in a Dublin nursing home that was run by nuns. His final act on this earth was to look up at the young nun who sat by his bedside, clasp her by the hand, and whisper: "Thank you for all your kindness. May you be the mother of a bishop."

## Expanded cultural horizons
Ephemeral benefit promoted in international conference brochures to encourage participants to bring their families and boost sales of hotel rooms and sight-seeing tours.

When Jean Bousquet, a French professor of medicine, was invited to speak at a meeting in San Francisco, he took his ten-year-old son with him to experience the cultural differences between France and the US. On their first evening, when father and son went on a walk from their hotel, the boy tugged excitedly at his father's sleeve.

"Look Papa," he said, "a French restaurant."

He was pointing at McDonald's.

## Expert
Title medical schools award to anyone who visits from another place and brings slides.

David Sackett, a persuasive advocate of evidence-based medicine, advised doctors who became expert in one area of medicine to move swiftly to another before they become an Authority (qv) and start to obstruct ideas that don't coincide with their own.

## Exploiting the sick
For centuries the core business of inventive hucksters, fairground proprietors, and governors of lunatic asylums. Recently deployed by television producers who claim their programmes are not exploitive but educational.

No one doubts the need for education. A Home Counties supermarket manager recently banished a woman from his store because she had a patch of eczema on her neck and he feared she would infect the food. A woman with psoriasis, who'd hidden most of her skin with a voluminous track suit, was asked to leave a London store because the rash on the backs of her hands "could upset other customers".

These humiliations, regularly inflicted by people who don't know better, are the reason why groups like the Psoriasis

Association grab every opportunity to disarm prejudice with unembarrassed explanation of the realities. So, when my daughter Lucy, who suffered from psoriatic arthropathy, was asked to appear on a television programme, she was delighted. She was an energetic supporter of the Association and the programme, she was told, would give her the chance to talk about her condition and answer questions phoned in by viewers.

Luckily she was street wise enough to ask a few questions and discovered that the subject of the programme was "people with embarrassing problems" and she would share the session with 'victims' of two other conditions – smelly feet and flatulence. To the surprise of the producer she declined the invitation. Her psoriasis was not an embarrassing problem but a life-threatening disability, a consequence of Lupus, the disease that eventually killed her.

She accepted that the programme makers wanted to boost their ratings but thought it an inadequate excuse for exploiting the sick. Unfortunately, 21st century television viewers don't agree, or at least enough of them to make exploitation a profitable business.

Technological advance does not always mean progress. Sometimes it's a way to regress without discomfort. Today's voyeurs can sit in their own homes on their own sofas in front of their own high definition screens; their forebears had to travel all the way to Bedlam to gawp at, and if they felt the need, to mock the afflicted.

# F

## Face reading
An underused way of understanding the world and the folk who inhabit it.

I once did a radio programme with a Chinese woman who was by way of being a face reader. She told me I had a sensuous chin. I'd have been better pleased if she'd hinted the quality were more widely spread but I didn't mind. I knew the limitations. I'd done my share of face reading when I was a GP.

The interesting stories in people's faces come from within; facial expressions imposed by surgeons, dentists, and cosmeticians are near to inscrutable. Women who have their faces hoisted expensively into place may acquire a camera friendly veneer but, like the late Nancy Reagan, are stuck with the same facial expression whether they be confronted with stark tragedy or outrageous comedy. For readers, a doctored face becomes a closed book.

Faces left to fend for themselves mature along readable lines. Most people settle for what they've got and leave well alone. Others seek faces that they think will offer them an advantage. No surprise then that the highlight of the face reader's year is the party political conference season when otherwise intelligent people try to remould their facial muscles into an expression they call gravitas (qv). In most cases the demeanour they seek eludes them and they end up, like the rest of us, with the faces they deserve. Their solemn features never quite conceal what lurks beneath so what is written in their faces is not gravitas but pride. Or do I mean presumption? Whichever it is, it is based on an image of self that has escaped self criticism.

In some who wield great power, the contortions needed to conceal underlying motives and personality so exhaust the facial muscles that they eventually sag into a truthful expression that cartoonists are the first to spot. Richard Nixon was a good example. As his presidency stumbled towards its nemesis, his face grew more and more like that in the newspaper cartoons until, in the end, it looked as if it were about to melt and run down the front of his navy blue suit. He became a walking illustration of the phrase 'losing face'.

Even those more skilled at facial deception than Tricky Dickie cannot sustain a permanently unreadable face. The moment face watchers cherish is that when the "photo opportunity" is over, the television lights dim, and the tutored smile relaxes, maybe for only a second, into an expression all too easy to read.

People tell you more when you ignore the words and read the message in their faces. Even party political broadcasts grow informative when you turn the sound down.

## Faith
1. A valuable ally in achieving a 'cure' and a dangerous enemy in assessing it. (See Placebo.)

2. An urge affecting people anxious to bestow omniscience on benevolent authority.
A gentle GP I know was involved in a delicate consultation with an unmarried pregnant teenager. He'd been her doctor since she was an infant, had retained her confidence through the turmoil of her adolescence and, because he had once looked after her during a long and tricky illness, she had total belief in his omnipotence.
After he'd examined her and confirmed she was pregnant, he asked, as he turned away from the couch: "Presumably you know who the father is?"
"No," she said eagerly. "Who?"

## Family
An entity more often invoked than understood.

Some would claim we know more about families now than we've ever known thanks to information that social surveyors, market researchers, and opinion pollsters feed into their databanks. But databanks are like soap operas: the longer they run, the more they stereotype. And, as every GP knows, the stereotypes crumble as soon as you meet the individuals. That's why I mutter a bit when I hear politicians and folk of similar ilk talk about 'ordinary families.' The words are incompatible. Ordinary can be applied only to the inanimate. Once you breathe life into something you breathe in complexity.

I mutter even louder when the same folk say they are 'pro-family' as if 'family' were a well defined entity and all families shared the same values and behaved in the same sort of way. One thing I learned as a GP and from ten years of interviewing families on Radio Four's *Relative Values*, is that most of us have no idea what really goes on in other peoples families. As Alan Bennett points out in *Writing Home*, every family has a secret and that secret is that they're not like other families.

I can't define the quality that, when poured over a group of individuals, turns them into a family, though it's clear that blood relationship isn't essential and that most of us can recognise a family when we see one. The nearest I can get to explaining that quality is a sentimental tale that came my way in general practice when I looked after a family which, because of the father's job, was forever on the move from a rented house in one country to a rented house in another.

One day I overheard his seven-year-old daughter in conversation with an old woman in my waiting room.

"It must be very sad for you," said the old woman, "not having a home of your own."

"Oh we have a home," said the girl. "We just don't have a house to put it in."

## Family medicine
1. Treating patients within the context of their family. An ideal worth pursuing.

2. Treating patients within the context of the doctor's family. An altogether trickier proposition.

> When I was a GP's child in the 1930s and the early 40s, the whole family was expected to play for the practice team. As soon we were capable of opening the front door my sister and I were deemed capable of taking messages (few patients then had telephones) or calling our mother for assistance. She, who had no medical or nursing training, became adept at staunching blood, binding wounds, and other temporising measures while she waited for her husband to return from his rounds.
> We became rather blasé about our duties, even on occasion offering advice. One enduring memory of childhood is of my sister, aged all of ten, standing on our doorstep admonishing a huge barrel-chested miner. "No wonder you've got earache. Get your mummy to show you how to blow your nose properly."

> When my old friend John Oldroyd first qualified as a doctor he chose to work in the West Riding town in which he'd grown up. One day at the local hospital he was

giving an anaesthetic to a woman and, as he was about to inject the anaesthetising Pentothal into a vein, she asked:
"Did I hear the nurse call you Dr Oldroyd?"
"Yes," said John.
"So, is Mr Oldroyd at the Mill your father?"
"Yes."
As John gently pushed the plunger on the syringe, the woman smiled wistfully and, before slipping into oblivion, muttered: "You know, if I'd played my cards right I could have been your mother."

A GP described in a medical journal how, when her childminder went missing, she had to take her daughter with her into her consulting room. There the child scribbled on anything she could find: scrap paper, patients' notes and carpet. Luckily, the surgery was pretty uneventful. "One man, however, had a penile rash and found it very embarrassing to show it to a female doctor – let alone her daughter – so I examined him behind the screens. This was fine until Joanna pulled the screens back and shouted: 'Mummy, *what* are you doing?'"

## Family pets
Sometimes regarded as surrogate children.

Can also serve as surrogate spouses. The novelist Marie Corelli indulged in multiple surrogacy. When asked why she never married, she replied that she had three pets to replace a man: a dog that growled all morning, a parrot that swore all evening, and a cat that stayed out all night.

As surrogates, family pets come within the compass of any GP who presumes to be known as a family doctor. Raymond Greene, like his brother Graham, was a fine writer but better known as a neurologist. Early in his career when working as a GP in Oxford he looked after an old lady whose most treasured possession was a tom-cat who followed her like a dog and seemed to return the affection she lavished on him. One morning she telephoned Greene in great distress. The cat had had gone mad and had attacked her while she slept, scratching her and biting her around her waist. Greene called to see her and, when he examined her, found she had shingles. He explained that she must have had a nightmare and her loved one was innocent. She reacted not with joy but with bitter tears. She'd already summoned the vet and had the cat destroyed.

## Family resemblance

Indications of identity eagerly sought in babies. A source of embarrassment in adolescence and confusion in middle-age.

Bob Nevin, dean of St Thomas's Medical School in the 1960s, once described how, when the sons of his contemporaries came for interviews, he could recognise them immediately. They looked like their fathers and had the same attitudes and mannerisms as their fathers. Only later when he met their parents did he discover that the fathers no longer looked like the fathers.

## Family values

Any beliefs held or moral standards valued by the person who uses the phrase. I treasure the memory of a notice in a West Country B&B.

*Please do not wait to be introduced to your fellow guests:*
*we are all one big family.*
*Do not leave your valuables in your bedroom*

## Fancy

Discrete group of cerebral cells that triggers an unexpected response to selective sensory tickling.

One of the great mysteries of existence is why an occasional remark, incident, or even joke provokes me not just to smile but to laugh. Or, as we doctors put it in our technical jargon, why does something I would normally take in my stride suddenly become an allergen that tickles my fancy?

I'm normally unamused by jokes that depend on the double meaning of words like organ or intercourse; so why did I giggle when I read that C Bernard Rutley was following up the success of his children's book *Peeko the Beaver* with a new character called Shag the Caribou?

And why did a postcard, illustrated by the bit of the Bayeux tapestry showing Harold's fatal wounding at the Battle of Hastings, make laugh out loud when I read the caption: *I spy with my little eye something beginning with A*?

This, I fear, is personal territory I do not have the courage to explore.

## Fashionable doctors

Doctors who try to give the impression that the rich and powerful turn to them for advice.

The status is not easily won. First you must establish a harmonious relationship with gossip columnists, best done by feeding them unattributable titbits about your patients. Once they start to raise your 'profile' you need to follow the rules of the *demi-monde célébrité*: accept every invitation, pretend to hear what people say to you at noisy chattering parties, prepare witty comments on the passing show to unleash across dinner tables, and take every chance to convey, by hint or wink, that your clientele is international, powerful, and rich.

You must also learn to sit solemnly through mind-numbing luncheons and dinners in the City, to listen gravely to self-centred politicians, always remembering that the most boring are often the most influential, and to keep a notebook by your telephone listing 'cool' replies for journalists who ring you for answers to the great questions of the day such as: Does Lynda la Luxe have anorexia? What tracks do you have on your iPod? Do bald men have bigger testicles?

Fashionable doctors come in all shapes, sizes, colours, and levels of ability and intelligence. Their common denominator was defined back in 1923 by the American surgeon J Chalmers da Costa, "A fashionable surgeon, like a pelican, can be recognised by the size of his bill."

## Fear

The commonest symptom to drive patients to a doctor... and punters to a huckster.

Magazine advertisements from the 1930s and 40s in The London Museum of Brands, Packaging, and Advertising show how great was the fear of any form of illness in the pre-antibiotic era, and how shamelessly it was exploited.

In one an over-worried man tells us:

*I've got to have an operation.*

Beneath him is an explanatory broken sentence:

*More serious than most men realise...*

*... the troubles caused by harsh toilet tissue.*

Indeed the social revolutionary who invented soft lavatory paper – the coarser stuff is now found only in deprived places such as NHS hospitals – triggered a new genre of advertisement. In one, an authoritative yet kindly doctor explains:

*In nearly every business organisation a surprisingly large percentage of the employees is suffering from rectal trouble... Be safe at home and work. Insist on Scott tissue or Waldorf.*

I'm told that sort of exploitation wouldn't be allowed today and, though fear is still used to sell preparations purporting to relieve the dreaded teenage scourges – acne, halitosis and dandruff – today's commercials seem less cruel than the old magazine ads.

One I found in the museum looked, at first glance, like an advertisement for a horror movie. At its centre was a man who was clearly a social outcast: haggard, shamefaced, and unable to look the artist in the eye. Only when I read the caption did I learn the depth of his depravity.

*He took his girl to the swimming bath and gave her ATHLETE'S FOOT.*

*He was... A CARRIER.*

Madison Avenue has always been a fount of entertaining images of illness. One of them intruded for a moment on the life of Robert Robertson who recorded it with his usual felicity:

*I dearly love a non sequitur if it's operatic enough, and, marooned overnight in the city of Washington, I turned on the television and caught the opening lines of one of the commercials. The scene was a bus-stop and it was raining, and the man standing there with his umbrella turned to the camera and said, "In weather like this, diarrhoea's no fun." For sheer quality, no programme was going to match that, so I turned it off and went to bed.*

## Feemanship

The art of extracting payment from patients. A traditional ingredient of the bedside manner.

Anthony Trollope defined the 19th century British ideal in *Doctor Thorne*:

*A physician should take his fee without letting his left hand know what his right hand is doing; it should be taken without a thought, without a look, without a move of the facial muscles; the true physician should hardly be aware that the last friendly grasp of the hand had been made more precious by the touch of gold.*

American physicians established a more rigorous tradition. Thirty years after the publication of *Dr Thorne*, Dr J J Taylor claimed in his Philadelphia textbook *How to Obtain the Best Financial Results in the Practice of Medicine*:

*Never allow sentiment to interfere with business. The 'thank-you' is best emphasised by the silvery accent of clinking coins.*

Dr Albert V Harmon of Chicago reiterated the advice 20 years later in *Large Fees and How to Get Them*:

*One of the most potent causes of professional poverty is the mania of the doctor for a pretence of well-doing. He exhibits this in many ways. One of the most pernicious is an affectation of contempt for money.*

### Festival of regeneration

Ritual celebration held every four or five years when a new prophet appears with a revolutionary plan to reorganise the NHS.

Each prophet claims that his or her plans will fulfil the dreams of the founders of the NHS; the only thing the plans have in common is their claim to be the final radical solution.

One of the more memorable festivals took place on 31 January 1989, though it is remembered less for what it achieved than for the extravagance of the celebration. Department of Health officials claimed proudly at the time that it was the most lavish launch accorded to a government initiative. Over a million pounds was spent on a telecast from Limehouse to studios and hotel ballrooms in six British cities where sat an audience of 2,500 Health Authority chairmen, NHS managers, and carefully selected doctors and nurses.

The star of the show, Kenneth Clarke, Secretary of State for Health, was ferried in ceremonial style by river boat from the House of Commons to the Limehouse studio where he proclaimed yet another dawn of yet another era – a sure sign to reorganisation aficionados that they were about to endure intensified administrative muddle that would eventually produce deterioration rather than enhancement.

Two years later the NHS, a child of postwar altruism, was irreparably damaged by the imposition of an internal market (qv), a child of Baby Boomer greed. This ensured that future festivals would not be celebrations of hope but desperate attempts to disguise degeneration.

### Final curtain syndrome
Common form of numerical dyslexia.

When the *Guardian* published the headline 'Messerschmitt crashes on final flight' a reader wrote to point out that a disproportionate number of aircraft seemed to crash on their final flight.

A few weeks later the *Daily Telegraph,* not wishing to be outdone, published the sad tale of Mrs Hayward who had laboured for weeks to complete an 8,000-piece jigsaw only to discover that the last piece was missing. What an amazing coincidence, wrote a reader, that it was the last and none of the previous 7,999. My own childhood memories accord more closely with those of Joyce Scorer who wrote to the paper to confess: 'I usually give up because the second piece is missing.'

### Flattery
Well-tried, effective yet underused form of therapy; possibly because of the degree of shamelessness demanded of the therapist.

It is a truth universally acknowledged that the more impressive a person's record of intellectual achievement, the more likely he or she will be susceptible to flattery. I once looked after a young boy who was the only child of high-powered parents – one a lawyer, the other a top grade civil servant. The boy who lived a lonely life discovered that the only way to gain his parents attention was to develop mysterious symptoms. His parents' reaction was to expect the doctor to 'do something' about them.

During one bout of illness I suggested we got a second opinion and called in a street wise – and expensive – paediatrician. After he had examined the boy we, as was the custom, retired from the bedroom to the bathroom for him to wash his hands and for us to 'consult'. He suggested we treated the parents rather than the boy and the best treatment for them would be a hefty dose of flattery.

After returning to the boy's bedside, making consoling noises, then bidding him farewell, we joined the parents in the drawing room for a more sombre consultation. I kept my attention fixed on the ceiling as the paediatrician addressed them solemnly: "Some parents have carthorses, a few have racehorses. You, I fear, are burdened with a racehorse."

The carefully chosen flattery presented the relationship in a form the parents understood. They began to give the boy more attention and, where once they would have chastised him, they tried to respond with understanding. The bouts of mysterious illness grew fewer.

## Flexibility
Essential ingredient of relationships between members of the caring professions.

In 1995, the UK health visitors' official publication alleged that they were being told to "bend over backwards to accommodate everything GPs want us to do". Local representative Hilary Toyne explained, "It's putting us in a very vulnerable position."

## Folk remedies
Secrets that pass from generation unto generation.

Once upon a time, according to the late Sir Alec Guinness, a character actor in a touring repertory company told a colleague he had painful piles. His friend responded by passing on details of a remedy used in his family for countless generations. Every morning and every evening, the patient had to make a strong pot of tea, drink three cupfuls, then remove the tea leaves from the pot and pack them tightly in and around his anus. The actor tried the remedy for five days but his symptoms if anything got worse. He decided to consult a doctor.

An avuncular GP listened with grave interest to a description of the treatment. He ushered this patient onto the couch, carefully examined the affected area, then told him to get dressed. When the old actor had resettled himself uneasily in his chair, the doctor spoke: "I have two bits of news. First, I can confirm you have piles. And, second, you're soon going to meet a tall dark stranger."

## Forgetfulness
Charming feature of ageing. Best left untreated by doctors.

> When a Chester psychiatrist, walked into his home after a hard day's work, his startled wife asked, "What are you doing here? Aren't you supposed to be in Manchester giving a lecture on amnesia?"

> Christopher Meehan who practises in Paisley received a letter from a local hospital describing one of the more predictable events of the year: "Mrs X did not keep her appointment at the memory clinic."

> When it came to firing people, the American publisher Henry Luce, a notoriously forgetful man, would remind himself of his unpleasant duty by jotting "Fire X" in his desk diary. One editor, named Huntington,
> forewarned of his imminent dismissal, sneaked into Luce's office and altered "Fire Huntington" to "Dine Huntington". As a result, the two men enjoyed a splendid dinner in one of New York's best restaurants and Huntington kept his job.

## Foundation stone laying
Ceremonial NHS activity that allows political and municipal dignitaries (qv) to flaunt their importance and their priestly aspirations.

A press release issued by the Barnsley Hospital Management Committee describes the rubric with the unerring eye for detail of Charles Pooter Esq.

> *At the Foundation Stone, Mr P. P. Lund Dip. Arch., RIBA,*
> *as representative of the Architects Charles B, Pearson, Son and Partners,*
> *will ask the Chairman of the Board to place a stainless steel cylinder★*
> *in position below the stone.*

*The architect will present the Minister with a ceremonial trowel and maul
and ask him to lay the foundation stone.
When the stone is laid, the Minister will say the traditional words:
"In equity, justice, temperance and fortitude,
I declare this stone well and truly laid."
As the words are said, the Minister will tap each corner of the stone three
times
starting at the far right hand corner
and moving in an anti-clockwise direction.*

*★The cylinder is exactly twelve inches long, one and a half inches in
diameter, and, for the benefit of posterity, contains coins of the realm
minted this year and a parchment inscribed with the names of the
Chairmen and members of the Sheffield Regional Hospital Board and the
Barnsley Hospital Management Committee.*

Posterity will I'm sure be grateful... for the coins, that is.

## Freedom of the bedchamber
A liberating lack of concern about bedtime

A freedom which those who write for a living share with ageing folk – which means I'm doubly qualified to escape what starts as a punishment imposed on children but becomes a punishment imposed on adults condemned to work regular hours.

I'm also free of concern about getting-up time. When I'm writing a book, as at the moment, I choose to get up early and start work at 5 a.m. Experience has taught me that, if I can produce a few hundred words before I wake up and discover what I'm daring to do, I can mitigate the terror induced by a blank page. Once I'm out of the starting blocks the terror fades and, for the rest of the day, my anxiety level hovers as near as it ever gets to equanimity.

This early morning business wasn't inherited. I come from a long line of late risers, indeed an Irish cousin claimed he needed extra hours because "I sleep very slowly."And there's certainly nothing heroic about it. I do it because it happens to suit me.

It also suits me, when I'm starting early, to go to bed early – round about 9 p.m. – and so miss the wave of sex and violence that I gather from the *Daily Mail* sweeps across your television screens while I'm safely tucked between the sheets.

The only problem provoked by my sleeping habits arose when people who didn't know me telephoned after nine in the evening and my children were at the age when they assumed every phone call was for them. They would grab the phone before their mother could get to it and brusquely tell the caller: "He can't come to the phone, he's asleep." This I discovered is one of the euphemisms used to protect sad souls who, late of an evening, are incapable of conversation. I twigged what was happening when a woman whom my wife met at a parent/teacher gathering expressed her sympathy because her husband too was "overfond of the bottle."

It was a small price to pay because freedom from the tyranny of regular hours is one of the great pleasures of life and one of the true rewards of ageing.

## Functionary

Itinerant speaker invited to perform at medical society or postgraduate meetings, with or without slides, before or after dinner and, not so long ago, with or without Ladies.

My train was an hour late and I was actually running when I burst into the foyer of a Tyneside hotel. The receptionist, I remember, was cleaning the dirt from under her fingernails with a plastic knitting needle.

"Which way to the Fitzwarren Suite?" I cried.

"You can't go in there," she said. "There's a function on."

'Twas then I heard my voice proclaim a line of stunning pomposity: "I am the function."

At that moment I discovered my medical identity and for years was content to play the role of functionary. True I had to eat more than my share of Aylesbury duckling, Bombe Surprise, and slices of tinned peach with a blob of synthetic cream on the top but I also met real doctors who did real jobs and contrasted favourably with the medical politicians I met as a journalist.

The late Henry Miller defined two kinds of lecture: those that contain slides and those that contain original thought. I used to manage without either until I discovered that slides introduce a useful sense of uncertainty. This serves to keep the speaker awake while the warm darkness encourages the audience to sleep, an arrangement some would claim ideal.

Over the years I endured the full repertoire of slide misfortune: upside down, sideways, back to front. I even strung together an impromptu narrative to match slides left in the projector of a Lancashire hotel after a meeting of a camera club. I managed the first three without giving the game away but when the fourth turned out to be a picture of a young woman making an unambiguous gesture with a model of the Blackpool Tower, I took fright and confessed. The medical audience noisily demanded to see the next one but when it proved to be a moody shot of the sun setting over Morecombe Bay, they slipped back gently into the arms of Morpheus.

I also near exhausted the repertoire of chairpeople. Those who get your name wrong are commonplace, as are those who introduce you as last week's speaker or even next's. The most daunting are those who pass you notes while you are in full flow, such as she who introduced me at a Ladies' Club in California in the 1970s. I was well into my stride and felt I had my kindly audience almost under my spell when she passed me a note: *Forgive my intruding, but your stable door is unbolted.* I was living every speaker's nightmare, facing an audience with my flies agape. I blew my nose, dropped my handkerchief and, while bending to retrieve it, zipped my fly.

The saddest chairpeople are those who are also the meeting organisers. They greet you at station or airport, drive you to the appointed place, and park you in a room with a large mug of coffee while they keep popping next door to see if anyone has turned up. Their conversation consists entirely of hints that the audience is likely to be slim but their optimism is indomitable. Beryl Bainbridge told me of an author who thirty minutes after the meeting was supposed to start found himself sitting in a hall populated by the chairman, himself, and a caretaker rattling his keys.

"Shall we pack it in?" asked the author.

"Not yet," said the chairman. "Best wait for stragglers."

## Funeral

Sombre occasion that can be tinged with joy when the human spirit breaks free from solemn ritual.

The only time I've envied those who believe in the supernatural was the morning of my wife's funeral. Her death had intruded suddenly and unexpectedly on one of the happiest spells in the fifty-eight years we spent together.

The funeral was a non-religious affair: panegyrics from our two daughters, live music from our son and his quartet, and recorded music from my wife. I too was to deliver a panegyric and act as a sort of compere.

I arrived early and, as I set off from the car park to the crematorium, good fortune turned up in the shape of my old friend Francis Matthews, who features elsewhere on these pages. The two of us walked up the path together and stood listlessly outside the entrance waiting for our slot in the crematorium's continuous performance. Fran didn't say much. Indeed he didn't need to say anything. I drew comfort just from his presence because he understood: he was still mourning, as he always will, the death of his own wife. For half a century there had been four of us; now we were down to two.

He nudged my elbow and pointed to a plaque on the wall. I took a look. It was the sort of plaque, polished bronze letters on blackened bronze base, that marks the spot where some historic incident took place. This one announced with ill-disguised pride that Guildford Crematorium was runner-up in the Cemetery of the Year competition.

Like many actors Fran is a talented mimic and I suddenly heard Eric Morecambe whisper in my ear, "I wonder who came in first?"

More surprisingly I heard myself respond in flat-vowelled West Riding tones: "As chairman of the cemetery committee I would like to say how proud we are of you lads. But next year if we dig just that little bit deeper and cut our edges just that little bit straighter we could be up there with the gold medal…"

Fran kept it going, no longer Eric Morecambe, now a West Riding alderman : "I'll tell you straight. There could be no 'olding us once young Jimmie gets his eye in with that shovel…" And on we went in improvised dialogue. We spoke only in a whisper and managed to keep our faces straight, our eyes doing the laughing for us.

We stood some distance from other members of the waiting congregation, most of them younger than the two of us. And as our whispers turned to mumbling, they kept that distance. I suspect they didn't want to intrude on two old men reminiscing sadly about times that had gone.

I suddenly realised I had lost my fear of the coming ritual. And I no longer needed the supernatural. My imagination, unaided by belief, could hear the laughter of our wives.

# G

## Garden path

Byway up which children sometimes lead parents, teachers, doctors... indeed anyone who threatens to prevent them from getting their own way.

One of my party tricks after a lecture is to say to the audience, "Hands up those of you who at some time in your childhood knew more about the world than your parents thought you knew." Only rarely does a hand remain un-raised.

In the 1970s, the daughter of one of my friends, lets call her Annie, decided she would no longer go to school. Her father was convinced her imagination was too lively for the plodders who were trying to teach her. That's the sort of diagnosis you'd expect from a father but he did have plenty of evidence of her powers of invention. She had once taken just a weekend to convince a visiting hard-nosed businesswoman that her parents were on the point of divorce and that she and her siblings would soon be pathetic victims of a broken marriage.

Her refusal to attend any form of school brought the family into contact with the social services and I have little doubt Annie was the star of many an interview and case conference. I can't be sure because her mother and father were never invited to attend. Indeed they were given the impression that no one was interested in what they had to say, though I suspect they might have given a slightly different version of the 'client's' previous history than she gave herself.

The only person who wanted to hear the parents' side of the story was a psychiatrist they sought out for themselves. He told them Annie was suffering from schoolphobia, which sounded more like a description than a diagnosis. He also, on the strength of one interview and a few psychological tests, offered an analytic explanation for her condition which later events showed was entirely spurious. But it did the trick. An impressive diagnosis pronounced by an eminent authority was enough to get social services off the family's back.

Annie was then taught at home by a retired teacher and, despite the gap in her education, built a successful career in a highly demanding profession thanks largely to the determination she had shown as a child. Thirty years later she was still, as she had always been, part of a close and happy family. The episode of childhood deceit was naught more than an oft-told family joke and the source of occasional teasing.

I suspect Annie gained from the experience – a battle honour won early in her life. But what if the incident were replayed now? Annie, never a slouch at keeping up with news and fashion, might garnish her tale with a touch of parental abuse, or even Satanism, and her parents could find themselves in the Kafka world inhabited by parents deprived of their children on the say-so of professionals. The experience of watching Annie's family on the receiving end made me wary of professional arrogance. I'd like to think that the tragic death of Sally Clarke, who never recovered after her wrongful conviction for 'killing' her two baby sons, may dampen the enthusiasm of those who pontificate on the strength of selective knowledge and restricted experience.

I'd like to think so, but…

## Gender ambiguity
Identity crisis provoked by ambiguous signs on lavatory doors.

Michael Rubinstein, a distinguished libel lawyer (so you know that every word of this is true), couldn't decide whether the elaborate graphic on a door in a French provincial restaurant indicated it was the Ladies or the Gents but his need was urgent and he went in. He was slightly discomfited by the absence of urinals but luckily the place was empty and he made use of the available facilities. On the way back to his table, he saw another door with an equally ambiguous graphic. When he peeped inside, he saw the gender-defining bank of urinals. His response, which I will ever regard as the defining act of an English gentleman, was to return immediately to the cubicle he had used and lower the seat.

## Gender jargon

Words and phrases male doctors use when referring to women.

When Faith Fitzgerald was associate dean for student affairs at Davis School of Medicine in the University of California, she compiled a helpful guide.

> **Female**: Biological term describing those members of species of plants and animals capable of generating young from ova, usually in conjunction with a male of a like species. Applied to female human beings without designation of species in the attempt to sound more scientific.
> **Girl**: A female human being of any age.
> **Young girl**: A female human being aged 16 to 50 years.
> **Old girl**: A female human being aged over 50 years.
> **Lady**: Term formerly implying nobility of birth or bearing, now indiscriminately applied to adult female human beings who don't like to be called girls.
> **Woman**:Scientifically accurate, dignified, and respectful term for an adult female human being. Seldom used.
> **Old woman**: A human being of either sex and any age who doesn't want to agree to the procedure or operation you propose.
> **Person**: A neuter term, conveying little data, applied generally to female human beings when one wants pointedly to avoid being caught in a reference to gender.

## Genetic engineering

Practised by the highborn long before the discovery of genes.

Well-bred practitioners also knew how to reduce it's side effects if we are to believe a tale Earl Mountbatten told across many a dinner table, though he resolutely refused to name the family.

In the 1930s, when the only son of the family proposed marriage to, and was accepted by, a 'suitable girl', his mother was delighted but his father forbade the match. The son, saddened but defiant, announced he would go ahead and marry the woman anyway. Whereupon his worried father took him on one side and explained she was his half sister, the product of what in those days was called an 'illicit liaison.'

The son, deeply upset, told his mother.

"Go ahead," she said. "And don't worry. He's not your father."

## General Medical Council (GMC)

Oligarchy created by the government to regulate the British medical profession.

On the first day of January 2009, the newly created body replaced the old self-regulating one without changing its name.

Few mourned the passing of the old GMC. It was far too large and though its *raison d'etre* was to protect patients, many doctors thought it was a professional institution, and a few GMC members behaved as if it were. The council's attempts to play both roles, and its grotesque obesity, sent it staggering to its downfall.

To those who know what is best for the rest of us the old GMC had other grievous faults. It had flirted with the dangerous concept of democracy and graciously allowed at first a handful and later even half its medical members to be elected. This unfortunate lapse led to the election of members who not only failed to toe the BMA or Royal College line but whose careers were not dependent on the patronage of their betters. The oligarchs on the council during the years I was the rebel in residence may not have been "beholden to an electorate" – a phrase the creators of the new GMC used as a criticism rather than a commendation – but many seemed beholden to those who appointed them. Several had serious symptoms of Knight Starvation (qv) and the only member I know to have turned down an invitation to appear in the Honours List was an elected member. Anyone who examines the GMC's history before it is completely rewritten will discover that the cause of its obesity was the intransigence of the unelected appointees who refused to restrict their representation.

The new GMC with its membership "By appointment only", includes possibly the finest collection of Quango-sitters ever assembled by the Appointments Commission. The council boasts that they are all independent but, as anyone familiar with the world of Quango knows, their 'independence' is a bit like that of the non-executive directors on remuneration committees of banks and other giant corporations. The background noise when oligarchs meet is the sound of mutual back-scratching.

## Generalists
Doctors who treat what they assume you have. As opposed to Specialists who assume you have what they treat.

Generalists are no longer as generalist as they used to be. The sign outside the house of a 19th century English surgeon-apothecary read:

*I. Popjay, Surgeon, Apothecary and Midwife, etc.; draws teeth and bleeds on lowest terms. Confectionery, Tobacco, Snuff, Tea, Coffee, Sugar and all sorts of perfumery sold here. N.B. New laid eggs every morning by Mrs. Popjay.*

## General physician
Endangered species.

A specialist who hadn't the heart to become a cardiologist, the nerve to be a neurologist, wasn't cut out to be a surgeon, never dreamed of being a psychiatrist, hadn't the guts to be a gastroenterologist nor the itch to be a dermatologist, didn't hang around the right joints to become a rheumatologist, and didn't have whatever it takes to become a testicular surgeon.

## Gesundheitfuhrers
Those with a mission to impose good health on others.

The US Department of Criminal Justice banned the last cigarette for prisoners about to be executed in Texas, because it was bad for their health. As compensation, those about to die were given a stick of celery.

## Gideon therapy
Countering loneliness or depression by reading a familiar text. Named after the Gideon Society which places bibles in hotel rooms.

One evening a British cardiologist attending a conference in San Francisco flicked idly through the pages of the Bible in his hotel room and found two twenty dollar bills tucked between the pages. Clipped to them was a note:

*If you opened this book because you're discouraged, read the
14th Chapter of John.
If you're broke and this would help, take it.
If you've had a fight with your wife, buy her a present.*
                                        *A Wayfaring Stranger.*

*P.S. On second thoughts, maybe you should take it down to the
Lotus Room and try their martinis. That's where I got this idea.*

## Gift horses
Presents from patients that are best left in their stables, their teeth
unexamined.

One evening an American businessman arrived in the surgery
of a Surrey GP, Dr Henry Wilkinson, bearing a "token of gratitude"
for the care the doctor had given to his family. The token was in an
elegant gift-wrapped package which the donor insisted be opened
in his presence. When the embarrassed Dr Wilkinson complied he
found a velvet-lined box containing a gold pen and propelling
pencil engraved with his initials. His flustered thanks, expressed in
somewhat extravagant terms, were accepted with a modesty that
the doctor had not previously encountered in the donor.

Only a month later when the velvet floor of the box broke
free from its moorings did Henry Wilkinson find the gilt-edged
card that lay beneath. On it someone had written in elegant
script: *To Harry Watts in grateful appreciation of the great job you have
done in setting up the European operation.*

## God
Role to which some doctors aspire, others have thrust upon them.

Dr Randas Batista, though starved of resources, contrived
to work as a cardiac surgeon in rural Brazil. He once told
me how a patient had asked, "Why do we peasants want to
be doctors and you doctors want to be God? Yet God
himself wanted to be a man."

A small boy, treated at Poole General Hospital, is convinced
that his tonsils were removed by the Almighty.
"I was taken into a big room where there were two lady

angels and two men angels all dressed in white. One of
the men angels looked down my throat and said, 'God,
look at this boy's tonsils.' And He did.'

## Going through the motions

Activity based on the traditional belief that faeces offer insight
into mysteries hidden in dark corporeal depths.

Well into the second half of the 20th century, the ritual of
hospital ward rounds included nurses standing by to perform a
ceremonial unveiling of the bed pan containing a patient's latest
offering which the consultant would then inspect carefully, and
sometimes investigate further with the aid of a wooden spatula. In
1950 Reginald Hilton, a consultant physician at St Thomas'
Hospital, London, still taught students, "The ideal stool is one that
wraps itself twice round the bedpan and is pointed at both ends."

Hospital consultants' interest in faeces matched Britons'
traditional pride in the performance of their bowels. Doctors
were quick to learn they could flatter fee-paying private patients
by congratulating them on the quality of their stools. (See Bowels,
pride in control over.)

## Good breeding

Traditionally the consequence of self control.

*Hold, furious Youth – Better thy Heat assuage,*
*And moderate a while thy eager Rage;*
*For if the Genial Sport you now complete,*
*Full of the Fumes of undigested Meat,*
*A thin diluted Substance shalt thou place,*
*Too weak a Basis for a Manly Grace*
*To rise in Figure just, and dignify thy Race.*
*Advis'd, defer the Work, till Time produce*
*A more mature, and well-concocted juice.*
*Hard is the Rule, and Lovers oft complain;*
*Tho hard, yet proper for a vig'rous Strain.*

Claude Quillet.
*Callipaedia, or the Art of Getting Beautiful Children, 1656*

## Good fortune

Fickle jade who down the years has occasionally smiled upon physicians.

George Fordyce, educated in Aberdeen and Edinburgh during the 'golden age' of Scottish medicine, was elected a physician at St Thomas' Hospital in London in 1770. He became an authority on fevers and his work was highly regarded during his lifetime. Yet he was no great hit with the capital's medical establishment because he showed little concern for the social graces. The 1827 biography of Fordyce in the archives of the Royal College of Physicians regards it as a failing that he engaged in little private practice and continues:

*His manners were less refined, and his dress in general less studied than is expected in this country in the physician... In the earlier years of his life to render the enjoyment of its pleasures compatible with his professional pursuits, he used to sleep but little. He was often known to lecture for three consecutive hours without having undressed himself the preceding night.*

Fordyce earned his place as a footnote in medical history in one strange yet memorable incident.

One evening when dining at Dolly's chophouse in Paternoster Row he had already consumed a tankard of strong ale, a bottle of port, and a quarter pint of brandy when he received an urgent summons to a lady taken ill with an unspecified complaint. He arrived at his patient's house aware that he was far from sober. He put on as good a show as he could but when he tried to examine his patient he had considerable difficulty finding her pulse. And, when he did, he was unable to count the beats. Muttering under his breath "Drunk, by God," he wrote out a prescription and hurriedly left the room.

The following morning a letter arrived from his patient.

Fordyce opened it expecting a severe rebuke but instead found an apology. His patient confessed that she well knew the unfortunate condition in which he had found her and begged him to keep the matter confidential "in consideration of the enclosed".

The enclosed was a bank note for a hundred pounds which in those days would have been described as 'a considerable fortune'.

## Good offices

Premises where those with friends in High Places transact their business.

A former GMC president Lord Walton of Detchant describes them in his autobiography when he writes of his son-in-law:

*There was only one important snag; he had not held a traineeship in general practice in the UK and despite his very broad experience and multiple qualifications it was uncertain as to whether he would be accepted by the joint Committee for Postgraduate Training in General Practice as being qualified to become a partner. Fortunately, through the good offices of my friend and colleague, Dr Donald Irvine, then Chairman of Council of the Royal College of General Practitioners, the committee was persuaded that the experience which Andrew had had [was sufficient] for him to be accepted as being vocationally trained.*

## Good old days

Golden era when doctors really knew what was best for their patients.

From a letter written by a gynaecologist at Cheltenham General, Eye And Children's Hospital in 1958.
*There is no doubt in my mind that this patient should have termination of pregnancy and sterilisation, not only in her own interests because she is depressed and is unable to cope, but also on eugenic grounds. Continual breeding from such stock is one way of committing racial suicide.*

Dr Chris Scott of Exmouth, searching through a patient's notes, found a letter written by a consultant in 1945.
*Poor little Miss L! I quite agree with you that although she is only thirty-nine she looks much more; she looks bereft of all attributes both physical and mental with which a stable person is endowed. Physically she is under weight, flat bosomed and tight lipped with a large cross on her chest. Mentally, she has always been a weakling ever since she can remember, and has never been quite as strong 'in her nerves' as other people. She represents very typically what is known as a constitutional inferior. At this age you will be able to do nothing for it whatever, except to give her encouragement and persuasion. I put her on to a simple routine treatment and gave her*

*as much encouragement as possible. Try, if you can, to keep her off all active treatment, as it is only trying to convert her into something she can never be.*

Dr Scott says that fifty years later Poor little Miss L was "hale and hearty", lived independently at home, and had seen her GP only three times in the previous five years.

Hospitals also knew what was best for their patients.

Notice sent to patients about to be admitted to Ancoats Hospital in Manchester in the 1930s.

*If admitted you will be required to observe the following rules.*

*CLEANLINESS – Patients on admission are required to have a bath. They must be clean in person and clothing, and bring with them a change of linen, pair of slippers, soap, towel, tooth brush, comb and brush.*

*FOOD – Eggs, Butter, Jam, and Fruit can be brought for the patients at the discretion of the Ward Sister, except in the case of the Children's Ward, when all food must be handed to either the Sister or the Nurse in charge of the Ward.*

*CONDUCT – Persons are liable to immediate dismissal for serious misconduct, and for wasting or destroying the property of the hospital.*

*VISITING – Patients are requested to inform relatives and friends that visiting is allowed on SATURDAY ONLY, and except in serious cases, this rule is strictly adhered to. Two special permits are issued to each patient for Wednesday.*

*WORK IN WARDS – Patients who are able to do so may be required to assist in the work of the Hospital, but are not allowed to make up the fires.*

## Good Samaritan

Biblical character who is an example to us all. Not necessarily a good role model for junior doctors… or commuting dermatologists.

I met 'Harry' at a West Riding medical society. Soon after qualifying in the 1950s he had worked as a casualty officer at St Luke's Hospital in Bradford. One night, in those early hours when all lights are dimmed and hospital buildings seem themselves to sleep, a nurse came down to Casualty from one of the wards. She was in a panic because a disturbed old lady had vanished from her bed and could be found nowhere in the hospital. Harry, being a kindly soul, offered to get out his car and look for the absconder.

He'd travelled barely half a mile when he spotted his quarry wandering along the pavement in her nightdress. Though she was highly confused, he managed to get her into the passenger seat and drove her back to the hospital where he left her locked in the car while he went to find her keepers. As he re-entered Casualty the nurse rushed up to him, thanked him for his kindness, and explained there was no need to panic because they'd found the missing woman on another ward.

Were this an apocryphal story that is where it would end. In real life, Harry and his fellow casualty officer were now in a fix. The woman was confused and carried no form of identity so they had no address to which they could return her. Yet they were frightened to admit her because the hospital had only a couple of beds free for emergencies and the surgeon who was their boss had promised a slow and painful death to anyone who 'blocked' those beds with non-urgent cases.

Eventually at 3 a.m., after protracted negotiations, they managed to get the night wanderer admitted to a Salvation Army hostel.

The following morning the leader of Bradford City Council rang St Luke's demanding the names of the doctors who had abducted his aunt when she wandered out for a breath of fresh air.

At a meeting in New York I met a local dermatologist who uses the subway to commute between his apartment near Battery Park and his midtown office. One evening, during the rush hour, he was in a crowded compartment strap-hanging next to a weary looking woman whose pallor, bloodless lips, and permanent breathlessness suggested she was, at the least, anaemic. She found it difficult to keep a secure grip on the strap above her head and, with each sway of the train, emitted an involuntary groan. In a seat alongside them sprawled an obese young boy aged fifteen or sixteen unmoved by the woman's plight.

The dermatologist watched the youth with mounting anger and, having failed to stare him into shame, eventually said: 'I'll give you a dollar for that seat."

The youth accepted the note cheerfully and when he got up, the dermatologist told the woman to take the seat.

"Oh no,"she said. "You must take it."

"Madam, I don't want to sit. I just want to teach this boy some manners."

The woman sat down tentatively, casting a troubled look at the youth and at her benefactor. Then she smiled, settled back contentedly, and said: "Johnnie, thank the gentleman for the dollar."

"I already did, Ma," said the youth.

## GP Truisms

Defined by John Burscough, a GP in Brigg, as: "Meaningless phrases doctors use to help assuage people's resentment at being less than perfectly well." Examples include:

- There's a lot of it about.
- Of course, this weather doesn't help.
- This is the wrong time of year for you.
- What you need is a little sea air.

I suspect these comforting mantra have always been a part of medicine. I like to think that Hippocrates, had he existed, would have assured the islanders of Cos, "It's just something that's going around." And that 18th century physicians told the great courtesans: "Just stay on your feet for a couple of days and we'll have you back in bed in no time."

GPs sometimes use clichés in an attempt to defuse tension.

The patient, semi-comatose, lay on the bed. Her worried husband stood alongside her. While we waited for the ambulance, I searched my mental file of reassuring phrases.

"At least her age is on her side," I said.

"But she *is* fifty-two," said the husband.

From the bed came a croaky whisper: "Fifty one."

## Graveside

As rich a source of medical wisdom as the bedside.

My father was a GP in a Yorkshire colliery village and our house overlooked the village cemetery. He claimed it gave him a "healthy outlook" because it provided a daily reminder of his ultimate success.

When I was a medical student, he would suddenly say, "Let's take a stroll amid my mistakes" and, while we walked between the graves, he would pass on ideas about medicine that proved more enduringly practical than much I learned in medical school.

He would punctuate his tutorial by pausing in front of gravestones, sometimes to explain how the bones beneath might have lingered a little longer above the earth if he had been a little wiser, sometimes to illustrate the social history of the village.

Mary T., aged seventeen, who died of septicaemia after an illegal abortion, lying alongside her father who suffocated underground in the big fire at Yorkshire Main colliery the day before his daughter planned to tell him she was pregnant.

The simple headstone that carried just the name of a man, the date he'd been killed down the pit, and the inscription, *The price of coal*.

Ernie C. the colliery clerk who worked in the office and wore a stiff collar from Monday to Friday but on Saturday nights donned a black cloak and hood to wrestle in local working mens' clubs as The Rotherham Phantom.

Sometimes we paused just to adduce further evidence for my father's Law of Headstones: "The more unctuous the inscription, the more unscrupulous the rogue who lies beneath."

He delivered his most memorable lesson at his own funeral. A huge crowd had gathered on the outskirts of the village and, as the hearse approached, a broad shouldered man stepped into the road and halted it with an imperious raise of his hand. A group of miners stepped forward, took the coffin from the hearse and carried it on their shoulders through the streets to the church.

I remember the thronged streets around the church noisy with gossip until the coffin arrived, and then the silence that lasted until Mrs Tierney struck up *Abide With Me* on the harmonium and everyone in the church and in the streets began to sing with the sort of vigour they summoned when a West Riding team got to Wembley.

That morning I tried to analyse what a man had to do to earn such love. Certainly not big things; those were celebrated with honours and decorations and commemorated by Abbey choirs. A bare-headed crowd on a February morning, a loyal hymn, and an honest declaration of love were earned by smaller things; a monotonous accumulation of small acts of sympathy, kindness and understanding that the bestower rarely remembered because they were rarely offered consciously. That was the last graveside lesson I learned from my dad.

## Gravitas
Public relations substitute for wisdom. Public demeanour adopted in middle-life by doctors with political or academic ambition.

A startling change can occur in clever doctors when the Young Turk transmutes into the Old Fart. Those over forty will recognise the symptoms. Men and women who once were lively, witty and intelligent companions suddenly assume a public persona quite at odds with the character that previously served them well. Where once they would have enlivened conversation, they make observations of paralysing ordinariness. And, on the slightest of excuses, they rise to their feet to make solemn speeches. Drawn into public discussion, they rasp on earnestly and nod wisely as if naught but weighty thoughts were granted admission to their minds. Most grievously of all, they refrain from using their private wit in public places for fear that amusing or penetrating remarks might be 'politically inept'.

The condition swiftly degenerates into pomposity, the unavoidable fate of those who believe that in order to be seen to be serious, they need to be seen to be solemn. The flaw is grievous because it leads to misjudging others. Sidney Smith told his brother, "You must not think me necessarily foolish because I am facetious... nor will I comprehend you necessarily wise because you are grave." And Somerset Maugham, who knew a thing or two about preferment in the medical profession, wrote, "Make him laugh and he will think you a trivial fellow, but bore him in the right way and your reputation is assured."

A writer in the *Listener* neatly summarised the danger. "Gravitas, the heavy tread of moral earnestness, becomes a bore if it is not accompanied by the light step of intelligence."

## Group therapy

Profitable form of psychiatry. One psychiatrist assembles a bunch of patients and sits and listens while they treat one another.

In more progressive hospitals a psychiatrist eager to respond to the government's demand for increased productivity will only pretend to listen while making notes about more urgent matters such as shortfall control, clinical throughput, and the department's business plan.

## Guidelines

Helpful hints that since the coming of the 'internal market' (qv) have proliferated with the fecundity of rhubarb growing on a sewage farm.

Based on the belief that all life can be reduced to an algorithm, they are ideal for those who find it tedious to think for themselves.

Writer and doctor Theodore Dalrymple defined the problem:

*The more flow diagrams I receive, the harder I find it to go with the flow. I have now been given guidelines as to what to do in the event of fire, an epidemic, a gun-wielding patient, a gas leak, and all the other common emergencies in the life of a hospital. So many of them have there been that I can no longer remember whether, when nuclear war breaks out, I am supposed to lie in the corner under sandbags, usher patients down the fire escape without panic, or call the switchboard.*

## Handmaiden

Job description for a nurse in the good old days (qv).

Advice published in 1938 by Dr Douglas Hay Scott, holder of the impressive post of Lecturer in First Aid, Hygiene, Home Nursing and Anatomy at Morley College, London.

*No matter who the doctor may be, it has to be acknowledged by the home nurse that he knows more than she does and she has to agree to be completely subservient to him.*

*One of the first principles of good nursing is that of obedience and unqualified loyalty to the doctor. As a general rule, of course, the doctor in charge of the case is so obviously competent that the home nurse has no other choice but to agree to all that is ordained.*

*The best way to regard the relationship of doctor and home nurse is to say that as the home nurse has very little knowledge it is sheer presumption on her part to query anything in the treatment ordered by the doctor.*

## Harley Street

Valuable postgraduate qualification that demands no attributes or skills other than renting a room in the right location.

Louis Appleby described it as "a street that has grown rich on snobbery and second opinions." And, let us not forget, on exploitation.

Before he became a novelist, A J Cronin worked there. Most of his patients were rich, bored, idle women and, in *Adventures in Two Worlds* he describes how he established a reputation for being a clever young doctor by inventing a new disease and a treatment to cure it.

He called the disease asthenia and the most powerful ingredient of the curative treatment was a series of injections.

*Again and yet again my sharp and shining needle sank into fashionable buttocks, bared upon the finest linen sheets. I became expert in the art of penetrating the worst end of the best society with a dexterity which rendered the operation almost painless.*

Cronin admits he was a rogue, though no more so than many of his colleagues, and his treatment was often surprisingly successful.

*Asthenia gave these bored and idle women an interest in life. My tonics braced their languid nerves. I dieted them, insisted on a regime of moderate exercise and early hours. I even persuaded two errant wives to return to their long-suffering husbands and, within nine months, they had matters other than asthenia to occupy them.*

Gone are the days, I hope, when doctors sought to return women to their 'proper' place but today's Harley Street practitioners still favour a style created when doctors could do little for their patients save impress them. In *Last Chorus: An Autobiographical Medley*, Humphrey Lyttleton described "the real Harley Street touch": a big desk, plushy carpet, exquisite furniture, and his doctor dressed as if he had come from a wedding.

'Humph' wondered why his bill included an odd number of pence. He didn't realise it was a post-decimal translation of a fee calculated in the traditional Harley Street unit of currency, the golden guinea.

## Headstone

Underused medium for sending meaningful messages to posterity.

I feel guilty that, after my father's death, we didn't fulfil a wish he expressed after dinner with a couple of friendly GPs. Exhilarated by wine, he described the headstone he would like over his grave: a simple slab of Connemara marble with an electric bell embedded in its centre and, beneath the bell-push, the inscription:

*You can ring like hell but you can't get me now.*
*Yours in peace.*
*James Michael O'Donnell.*

In the cantonment cemetery at Peshawar is a headstone engraved with the message:

*Here lies Captain Ernest Bloomfield,*
*accidentally shot by his orderly,*
*March 2nd 1897.*
*"Well done thou good and faithful servant."*

## Healing art

Mysterious process whereby, given a happy synergy of personality, a patient can feel better just for seeing a doctor, without the prescription of a magic potion.

This healing quality, memorably explored by Michael Balint, has been recognised for centuries under a variety of names and, when I was young, was often called the 'art' of clinical medicine. To deploy it, doctors need a broader education than medical schools provide. The Cambridge computer scientist and biographer of the internet, John Naughton, once wrote,

*The things that really matter to us – the secrets of the heart, of what it means to be an individual, the depths and heights of human experience – all are accessible, if at all, only through literature and the creative arts. Science has no purchase on them.*

Luckily help is at hand from the novelists, poets, and dramatists who sit on bookshelves, ever ready to illuminate areas of life beyond our experience, ever eager to sharpen our appreciation of the humanity we share with our patients. Doctors should consult them more often because, just as the knowledge they acquire from observing and investigating their patients can enhance their knowledge of disease, the understanding they may absorb from literature, or indeed any of the arts, can enhance their perception of the nature of an individual illness. (See Arts, The.)

## Healing waters

You don't have to drink water or immerse yourself in it to get a healthy benefit. Just travel across it.

A few years ago I discovered the ideal distractive therapy. While my wife was, in the jargon of the trade, 'undergoing surgery', I took a short boat trip along the Thames on one of the *bateaux mouches* plying from Westminster Pier.

It proved a great assuager of anxiety. I don't want to analyse the effect too closely lest it crumble beneath my scrutiny, but I know the qualities I enjoyed: the unhurried, stately progress, the distanced view of life beyond the river banks, the alien light and alien sounds.

The trip revived my superstition that travel across water can have mystical effects. When I was a child, we spent most of our family holidays in Ireland and the holiday began with an overnight boat trip. Years later, when I was deep into middle age, I found myself in Liverpool and wandered down to the place where those childhood holidays began – the Prince's landing stage, hardly one of the world's romantic shrines. Yet as I stood there, gazing across the Mersea, there came a moment when I didn't just think, didn't just dream, but *knew* that if I went aboard the Irish ferry and fell asleep, the following morning I would wake up in Dublin in 1938 and my uncle, long since dead, would be waiting to drive us to his home and a large breakfast of rashers and eggs and Haffner's pork sausages.

In much the same way, I now know that if I cross the Thames by walking across Westminster Bridge I'll remain in the same old London, yet were I to cross the same narrow stretch in a boat I would, when I stepped ashore, enter a new, fresh, and exciting city.

My superstition is probably the product of an overheated and romantic brain but there's no doubt that gazing across water at familiar sights endows them with enchantment. And if you can visit them only by boat the enchantment endures. I suspect that's why so many people like to visit islands. Once they've safely crossed the water and are ensconced on terra firma they enjoy a spurious feeling of adventure. I once sat next to a holiday-making woman on a bus travelling across the Isle of Wight from Bembridge and, as we crested the hill above Ryde, she pointed across Spithead towards Portsmouth and asked excitedly: "Is that England over there?"

## Health

A fantasy created by the World Health Organisation (WHO): "A state of complete physical, mental, and social well-being."

I'm not sure I know what health is but I am sure that WHO lost its collective marbles when it produced its definition. I've met lots of people I consider healthy but I've yet to meet anyone who's achieved WHO's eupeptic state. Most of us for most of the time have some niggle or ache, some twinge of anxiety or depression, which we accept as part of the business of being alive.

My notion of health is that it's akin to happiness. I favour the definition offered in 1765 by John Morgan, a principal founder of the first medical school in America: "That choice seasoning which gives relish to all our enjoyments."

When I was a GP, I saw many people with chronic disabling diseases who lead more rewarding – in my book, healthier – lives than others who knew they were healthy because they'd had "check-ups" to prove it yet lived in uneasy conflict with the world around them.

An addiction to idealistic concepts of health has been responsible for many delusions in Western society. It's not surprising people grow confused and start to think that to be healthy you've got to suffer, give up things you enjoy, become a food faddist or, even worse, the sort of exercise freak, often a hard-driving business executive, who equates health with physical fitness and ends up Mens Insana in Corporate Sauna. (See Sport.)

An idealised concept of health is also the source of a great deal of confused thinking about medicine. Doctors learn early in their careers that neither the human body nor the human mind are in any sense perfectible. Doctors are not here to create "complete physical, mental, and social well-being"; they're here to make do and mend, to patch up imperfect bodies and disturbed minds, to comfort and console, and to help patients accept, even overcome, incurable disability. It's also their job to leave well alone when there's nothing useful to be done. Their purpose was well stated by H L Mencken. "The aim of medicine is surely not to make men virtuous; it is to safeguard and rescue them from the consequences of their vices."

Some claim that over-concern with health is itself unhealthy. The late Henry Miller, one-time professor of neurology and Vice Chancellor of the University of Newcastle-upon Tyne, wrote:

*The normal state of most people is to feel faintly tired, harassed, and under the weather and my clinical observations lead me to believe that an abounding sensation of positive health usually presages either a cardiac infarction or incipient hypomania.*

## Health bulletins
Detailed reports on the health of celebrities prepared by skilled journalists with a mission to keep the nation well informed.

In May 1998 when Esther Rantzen's husband, the television producer Desmond Wilcox, was admitted to hospital, the *Guardian* reported:

*Desmond Wilcox (57), producer of the BBC documentary* The Human Body, *was taken by air ambulance to hospital for an operation in which veins from his leg were grafted onto his coronary artery.*

Three days later a reader wrote:

*You have since reported he was in fact aged sixty-seven, was not involved in* The Human Body, *was not moved by air ambulance, and had a catheterisation not a graft. Would it not have been simpler to say you were not talking about Desmond Wilcox?*

## Healthful hints

Newspaper titbits designed to expand readers' knowledge of medicine.

An anonymous doctor, offering advice to readers of *The Leader,* warned them: "The first signs of heart disease – sudden death or fatal heart attack – often come too late for many women."

Dr Miriam Stoppard, hoping to ease feelings of guilt, assured readers of her column in the *Mirror*: "Six out of ten women you meet are likely to be masturbating."

## Health Tsars

Overseers appointed by politicians who believe one way to 'modernise' the NHS is to resurrect defunct titles.

The philistines who organise Britain's health services have inflicted many grievous wounds upon the English language but when their publicists announced the creation of "Health Tsars" they came close to scraping the bottom of the cesspit. I've nothing against those they appointed but why lumber them with a title created for absolutist Russian rulers some of whom, let's face it, were more than a mite unsavoury?

There was no need to go foreign. When I was a boy, the King still bore the title Emperor of India so why couldn't the DHS have appointed good old fashioned Emperors? Or if they really wanted Eastern exotica they could have turned to their childhood story books and created Sultans or Grand Viziers. Though, once you start exploring the possibilities, you realise the most appropriate title would be Grand Panjandrum.

## Healthy exercise

Any form of exercise you enjoy.

Unhealthy exercise is exercise you don't enjoy but force yourself to do because you think it is making you healthy. (See Sport.)

As the American essayist Simeon Strunsky pointed out:

*The beneficial effects of the regular quarter-hour's exercise before breakfast is more than offset by the mental wear and tear in getting out of bed fifteen minutes earlier.*

## Healthy indulgence

The only truly healthy pursuit. A determination to get the most out of the joys and opportunities of life. Sometimes confused – but only by the unhealthy – with hedonism.

In his column in the *New Statesman*, Professor Laurie Taylor recorded his father's view of the value of indulgence:

*"Wait till you get to my age, Nicola. Then you'll realise getting old isn't a laughing matter. It's a confidence trick. They tell you not to smoke and drink so you'll live to a ripe old age, but they don't tell you that ripe old age is terrible. If I had my time over again, Nicola, I'd drink and smoke as much as I could so I'd never have to put up with any of this stuff."*

*As soon as Nicola had cleared away the sandwiches and filled up the regulation space in the Report Book – 'Mr Taylor enjoyed his hot tomato soup but left two chicken sandwiches. He was in good spirits but complained about his legs' – Dad pulled me into the firing line.*

*"I can't understand why young people like Nicola should have all the drugs. All I get from Dr Hughes are pills to stop my legs swelling and pills to make me sleep. None of those happy drugs they were talking about on the wireless last night."*

## Heartsink patients

A label GPs use for patients who, as they enter the consulting room, precipitate the defining symptom: the doctor's dominant hand clenches into a fist beneath the desk.

A veteran doctor-watcher, Ruth Holland, described them thus:

*Patients that doctors dread to see; at the sight of whom lurking in the waiting room strong men twitch like a hamster's whiskers and women with nine O levels, five A levels, degrees in medicine, husband, children, au pair, dogs, goldfish, Volvo, microwave, and secretary of uncertain temperament feel inadequate and unable to cope.*

*Heartsink patients are not the ones with the most unpleasant characters or indeed with the worst diseases, in fact most of them usually haven't got much wrong with them; it just happens that there is a particular type of person who causes your average general practitioner to break out in a rash of helplessness, hopelessness, and what-is-the-point-of-it-allness.*

Some cases of Heartsink arise from incompatibility of temperament and can be cured by a change of doctor. Most cases, however, cannot be resolved; they are the fault of neither patient nor doctor and their existence bears testimony to the imperfectability of human existence.

## Herbaceous fever

Also known as Alan Titchmarsh Disease. Obsessional state induced by overexposure to television gardening programmes.

Someone once gave me a 'gardening calendar' that listed rewarding things to do on each day of the year. In January, as I recall, I was expected to mulch my asparagus, sow my Shorthorn carrots on a hotbed, and force my rhubarb. Come the spring, when younger men's fancy might turn to thoughts that some of us never wholly abandon during the winter, mine would be directed towards pruning my forsythia, thinning my hardy annuals, and spraying my gooseberries. While others lay in summer shade, listening to the chock of leather upon willow, I would be busy stopping my carnations, pricking off my primulas, and syringing my runner beans. And come December while jovial men sat beside roaring fires supping mulled wine, guess who would be the lonely figure out there in the gloom protecting his celery and pruning his Clematis Jackmanii.

The calendar had one glaring omission. Search as I might, I could find no time off, no day allocated to just sitting in the garden and enjoying it. Yet one of the greatest rewards that gardening can offer comes to the man who settles comfortably in a deck chair, glass of wine in hand, and watches his wife, silhouetted against a fine sunset, hack her way through a thick bed of nettles.

## Heredity
Natural law that determines that all undesirable characteristics come from the other parent.

## Heretic
Tricky accolade in medicine. Can be valuable but needs careful handling.

If handled well, heresy gets your name known and is a useful launching pad for those aiming to reach the upper layers of our profession. Some of the most influential people in medicine are former heretics.

But you mustn't go over the top. The ideal identity is not that of a true subversive but of an altogether more reassuring soul, "a bit of a heretic." Medicine being what it is, yesterday's heresy all too often becomes today's received truth. Then the wise warriors, those who didn't go over the top, can sheath their swords and enjoy their rewards. As a profession we tend to treat yesterday's heretics with respect, even load them with an honour or two.

Hospital consultants with no political ambition but striving to escape the boredom of middle age sometimes project themselves as heretics because the role nourishes the ego and makes life more interesting. They recognise that a heretic needs a Them – a bunch of misguided, intransigent believers they can rail against – so they invent St Elsewhere's (qv). Once a Them has been identified, the fight is always fun and often profitable; one of the most rewarding reputations in private practice is that of someone who cures Their incurables.

## Heroic treatment
When used in medicine, implies courageous conduct on the part of the doctor though the heroism is, in truth, demanded of the patient.

One doctor who won applause from an audience for his 'heroic action' was the anonymous physician who responded to "Is there a doctor in the house?" and saved the show at Glyndebourne.

The 'show' was the opera *Macbeth* and the doctor was called because the singer playing Banco, David Franklin, was suffering from renal colic. In the story as David told it, the treatment that sustained him consisted of morphine to dull the pain, benzedrine to counter the depressive effect of the morphine, and champagne because Glyndebourne's owner John Christie thought it was good for everything.

David managed to keep going until the first interval but had to be carried to his dressing room where the doctor examined him. Mrs Franklin, watching anxiously, was worried by the doctor's demeanour.

"Should he really go back on?" she asked.

"What's he got to do in this next act?" asked the doctor.

"A death scene."

"That'll be all right then," said the doctor.

## High falution

The use of portentous words and phrases to create an impression of profundity. Recommended by Richard Asher in the 1960s as a way to rise quickly in the medical profession:

*Much sensible medicine is obvious, but the obvious does not impress. If only you will trouble to learn the art of putting obvious or trite things in a quasi-profound way then the world will be at your feet.*

In an article entitled *Medical Salesmanship,* he suggested the best way to convert the obvious into the profound was to use key words and expressions. His recommendations included: broadly based, dynamic, integrated, in perspective, socio-economic, environmental, psycho-social, psycho-biological, psychodynamic, indeed psycho-almost-anything.

The academically ambitious should never study diseases, but "observe the natural history of the disease." Nor should they study patients but "view the individual in perspective against his economic and psycho-social background", or, better still, "consider his dynamic status within the group."

Fifty years on the phrases remain much the same.

## Hiltonitis

Environmental disorientation that afflicts business travellers. (See Rolling Stone Syndrome.)

Every major city has hotels flung from the same giant concrete mixture and furnished from the same 'executive' catalogue. Every room has identical bedside lights, chairs, occasional table and trouser press. The same magazines are sold in each lobby, the same recorded music plays in each lift, and the same prawns or steak are flambéed in each restaurant. Each hotel lies at the centre of a cantonment of identical international airline offices, car hire firms, travel agents, and expensive shops selling identical goods by Gucci, Dior, or Dunhill so the globe trotting 'executives' who stay in these places have to walk several metres, versts, or rods, poles, or perches to discover whether they're whooping it up in Berlin or St Petersberg, or spending an aberrant weekend in Pittsburgh.

## Hippocrates

Ancient Greek physician venerated by doctors who believe their work invests them with religious mystique. Ideal role-model for that kind of doctor: part priest, part physician, never portrayed as young, paternalistic, jealous of his privileges, and addicted to pious utterance.

Thought to have lived in 5th century BC on the Greek island of Cos where hagiographers claim he lead a long and virtuous life. Yet, as the medical historian Roy Porter pointed out, everything we know about him is legend. This putative Father of Medicine is a man not of history but of fable. No one is sure of his dates to within twenty or thirty years and scholars claim that none of the texts of the Hippocratic corpus, many of which are contradictory, were written by the man after whom they are named.

## Hippocratic oath

A catalogue of restrictive practices dressed up as a solemn promise to Apollo. An oath that luckily for mankind is rarely sworn or even read.

Dr Robert Reid described it as a bigoted and dangerous document that embraced hard-line trade union practices such as the closed shop, and sought to invest those who practised the healing art with a religious mystique that separated them from other beings. Not only does it encourage nepotistic incompetent hierarchies but the ethical advice it hands out is wholly ambiguous.

The oath is a rich source of medical mythology. Despite what many people believe, it is not a fixed and definitive statement of medical ethics but has been modified relentlessly down the centuries. It has never been widely sworn by medical students or graduands, indeed most British doctors have never seen it. Nor has the swearing of it been imposed as a condition for obtaining a medical degree or entering practice.

The earliest certain evidence of the oath being sworn in a university comes from 1558, but not until 1804 is there evidence of it being sworn by newly fledged doctors. As Vivian Nutton, Professor of the History of Medicine at University College, London, explained in a lecture at the Royal College of Physicians:

*The demand for medical oaths and declarations is largely a feature of the second half of the 20th century, favoured by physicians but often viewed with suspicion by patients.*

## Hip replacement
NHS unit of currency favoured by politicians.

When government ministers defend increased health charges such as a hike in prescription fees, they claim: "This will allow us to do x thousand more hip replacements." The hip replacement unit has a lot going for it. It conjures up visions of elderly cripples throwing away their crutches and disguises the reality of the NHS 'internal market.' You can't expect politicians to say: "This extra income will allow us to employ x more management consultants or be ripped off by x more computer companies."

## Holier than who?
*Cri de couer* difficult to suppress during meetings of self-regarding specimens of the *Genus Medicopoliticus.*

One of many depressing experiences I suffered while a member of the General Medical Council was witnessing the relish with which some doctors, free from public gaze, discuss the shortcomings of their colleagues. A nasty sniff of sanctimony pervades the air when doctors indulge in dismissive scorn. Contempt for others should never come easily to professionals whose social usefulness depends on their being able to deal with people as they are, rather than as we would wish them to be.

Two things we learn from our patients, our colleagues, and indeed ourselves, are that most people have secrets they hope to hide and that most people find their own misdemeanours less heinous than those of others. We find reasons to condone our own offences but, when we judge others, we compare them not with our real selves but with the image of ourselves we like to present to the world.

My experience as a GP confirmed the verdict of our colleague Dr William Somerset Maugham:

*There is not much to choose between men. They are all a hotchpotch of greatness and littleness, of virtue and vice, of nobility and baseness. Some have more strength of character, or more opportunity, and so in one direction or another give their instincts freer play, but potentially they are all the same. For my part I do not think I am any better or any worse than most people, but I know that if I set down every action in my life and every thought that has crossed my mind, the world would consider me a monster of depravity.*

## Holistic

Oddly spelt word coined in the 1920s to define the long standing medical tradition that doctors should treat each patient as a 'whole person' and not as a collection of symptoms.

The concept has a strong appeal to those who are ill and therefore to those prepared to exploit them. Purveyors of treatments which have little scientific evidence to support claims for their success often say they use a 'whole person' approach. The idea of being 'More holistic than thou' transmutes the treatment into a 'cause', an article of faith to be promulgated with religious fervour and defended vigorously against all criticism regardless of its merit.

It has also helped create a popular myth that 'scientific medicine' is incompatible with the 'caring medicine' we want from our doctors. Yet, as a journalist who's had the good fortune to interview some of the brightest medical scientists of the past fifty years, my experience has been that the greater the scientific achievement the more I would have liked the scientist as my GP. Intellectual activity doesn't blunt understanding of the human condition; more often it enhances it.

I offer in evidence a passage from the closing pages of *Science and the Quiet Art: The Role of Medical Research in Health Care* written by Sir David Weatherall, whose scientific credentials are irreproachable: Fellow of the Royal Society, founder of Oxford's Institute of Molecular Medicine now renamed the Weatherall Institute of Molecular Medicine, Regius Professor of Medicine at Oxford.

*It is, then, the sheer complexity and unpredictability of the manifestations of illness that is responsible for the notion of medicine as an art. Apart from clinical and pastoral skills, good doctoring requires an ability to cut through many of the unexplained manifestations of disease, to appreciate what is important and what can be disregarded, and hence to get to the core of the problem, knowing when scientific explanation has failed and simple kindness must take over. This is the real art of clinical practice.*

## Homeopathy

Irrational treatment, originated in 1796, and dependent for its effectiveness on the placebo effect.

For the first 100 years of its existence, homeopathy was more effective than mainstream medicine which was based on equally irrational beliefs. In those years the harm done by orthodox treatments (bleeding, purging and blistering) outweighed the good done by the placebo effect. In the late 19th century, mainstream treatments started to be based on rational evidence and by the early 20th century were less harmful and more effective than placebo. So in its second 100 years homeopathy has been less effective than mainline medicine.

Its survival depends on the size of the congregation prepared to worship at the shrine of unreason. The history of religious belief suggests it may survive for another century or two.

## Home visits (USA: House calls)

Strange habit doctors once had of visiting the sick. In those days ingenuous doctors thought that seeing the conditions in which people lived might help them advise patients how best to help themselves. Home visits might even allow them to assess the support patients could expect from family and neighbours, and what other services they needed to ease their suffering.

Modern doctors, whose transit from school to university to hospital to retirement is monitored by the very best of educationalists, gain so broad an experience of real life they no longer need to waste time on such irrelevancies.

Even GPs – I beg their pardon, primary care providers – know, because spread-sheet experts have told them, that they're at their most effective when they're in their offices surrounded by the technical tools of their trade, their minds uncluttered with non-computable distractions.

If a patient's troubles can't be defined, digested, analysed and treated in a ten minute interview at a GP's surgery, the patient needs to go elsewhere. Next, please.

## Honour

(Once upon a time.) High respect, esteem, or reverence accorded to exalted worth or rank.

(Today.) Commodity supplied by a Royal medical institution in exchange for cash.

In 2012 the Royal Society of Medicine (RSM) reminded us that the plate glass screens surrounding its "stunning atrium" were, in truth, a Wall of Honour and we could nominate anyone, dead or alive, to have their names inscribed on it. We could even nominate ourselves.

In the spring of 2012 the price of honour was £2,500.

But, as the RSM helpfully explained, if you were a taxpayer, you needed to send only £2,150 because your fellow tax payers would make up the difference and, if you paid tax at a higher rate, your donation could be "tax efficient".

Those who felt they were of exalted worth but were also feeling the pinch could acquire honour by monthly direct debit, though this would increase "the overall cost".

Shoppers were warned they needed to hurry: there were only sixty-five spaces left.

## Hope

That which springs eternal.

*New Scientist* reported a discovery it claimed could provide hope for impotent men: a gel which, when rubbed on the penis, stimulated erection.

"The gel", said the report, "is being tested on seventy-five impotent men and results are expected by the end of the year."

A reader, Jacqueline Rowarth, wrote to the editor: "I have done a survey among female colleagues and we don't think it is worth the wait."

## Horticulture

Rewarding pastime for retired surgeons. Operations such as dead-heading, trimming, and pruning help them to turn skilled fingers and old instruments to less lethal purpose, and sometimes bring unexpected rewards.

When the urologist Terence Millin retired, he and his wife moved to a country village in Ireland where nobody knew who he was. A man of great energy, he immediately set about re-establishing the garden. A rather grand lady who lived nearby spotted what a diligent worker he was, if a bit scruffy. So one day, when she was passing, she called him over to his garden gate, asked how well the new owners of the place were treating him, and offered to pay him 50 per cent more if he came to work for her.

"Oh, I couldn't do that," said Millin. "I have a special deal here. They feed me well and I'm allowed to sleep with the lady of the house."

## Hospice

Archaic institution wholly out of place in a market-led service. Wastes valuable skills and resources when the only outcome is a patient's death.

The 20ᵗʰ century saw many great advances in medicine. One of the greatest – up there with the discovery of antibiotics and the extraordinary advancement of anaesthetic and surgical techniques – was the development of the hospice movement. An order of nuns, the Sisters of Charity, founded the first modern hospice for the dying, St Joseph's Hospice in London, and their ideas were energetically espoused by Dame Cicely Saunders who founded St Christopher's Hospice, also in London.

The nuns and Dame Cicely identified a group of patients who didn't have the right credentials for our modern metropolitan hospitals so they created hospitals of their own. In doing so, they started an international movement which has helped remind Western nations that we still need hospitals dedicated simply to caring for people, sustaining their spirit, and relieving their pain.

One of the glories of the hospice movement is that the care it offers is founded not just on kindness and good intentions but on scientific knowledge and on skill. Hospices quickly developed methods of care that revolutionised basic medical practices such as the relief of pain, demonstrating for instance that painkillers could be given in much higher doses than had been the custom.

They also allowed doctors to rediscover skills doctors acquired in the days before the Second World War when most of their time was spent on the prevention and alleviation of illness rather than on trying to 'cure' disease. In 1976 the British actress Sheilah Hancock revealed the way things had changed in a moving account of the way her first husband, who was dying of cancer, spent his last months in a hospice. He was free from pain and, on the evening before he died, they went out to dinner and the theatre.

Thirty-five years ago that news caused great surprise. Now we take it for granted. Today's tragedy, verging on scandal, is that that level of palliative care is still available to so few people. In too many general wards, the 'care' meted out to old people who are dying would have been unacceptable in those self same hospitals even before the coming of St Christopher's.

## Hospital
Once a place of sanctuary, now a site for photo opportunities.

One Christmas, the toy makers Hasbro donated a Cabbage Patch Doll to Mount Alvernia, a private hospital in Guildford. The occasion had all the makings of a five star promotional wheeze. A grand press show on Christmas day would provide not only pictures of little girls admitted over Christmas cuddling the toy but of doctors demonstrating the value of the gift by using it to show children where their incisions, bandages, and drips would go.

Come the day, the photo opportunists discovered that the Christmas intake were all boys. Never mind, the doll could be used for the demonstrations. Or could it? According to the *Surrey Advertiser*, the doll was undeniably female and the boys had all been admitted for circumcision.

## Hospital party

A contrived decompression of the pressure cooker in which junior doctors work immediately after they qualify.

The tradition may well have started with Dr Francois Rabelais. He certainly seems to have left his mark on it, or at least his name.

Another doctor, Peter Mark Roget, in his *Thesaurus of English Words and Phrases* offers, in the section on *Emotion, Religion and Morality*, a list of synonyms which define a traditional hospital residents' party: "Sensual, carnal, gross, beastly, hoggish, overindulgent, licentious, and debauched."

## Hospital trolley

New style NHS bed.

Eager to help, Dr John Townend wrote to *BMA News Review* urging the NHS to take advantage of this reality. A simple label, he suggested, could dramatically reduce waiting times for admission.

Both a trolley and a bed have wheels, both have sides to prevent you falling out, both can be bent in the middle and both give you back ache. If we had small labels reading *This is not a trolley, it is a bed,* we could stick them on trolleys when patients had been lying on them until the targeted time and thus admit them to a hospital bed.

## Hotline

Source of automated advice to the afflicted. Unencumbered with the intrusive human presence that hampers satisfactory discourse and, and in accord with the best marketing principles, delivering what callers want rather than what they need.

*Welcome to the psychiatric hotline. If you are obsessive-compulsive, please press one repeatedly. If you are co-dependent, please ask someone to press two. If you have multiple personalities, please press three, four, five and six. If you are paranoid-delusional, we know who you are and what you want. Just stay on the line so we can trace the call. If you are schizophrenic, listen carefully and a voice will tell you which number to press. If you are depressed, it doesn't matter which number you press – no-one will answer.*

## House names
Cabalistic phrases carved on pieces of wood that middle-class patients place in obscure corners of their properties to ward off GPs seeking them by torchlight on rainy nights.

When I was a GP, the easiest night calls – in terms of actually finding the patient – were to working class terraced houses that abutted the pavement and had numbers prominently displayed above the door knocker. The most elusive patients were those who considered it a social necessity to drop the numbers from their homes and give them names like The Maltings, The Cedars, or The Old Rectory. I often got a hint of the sort of people I was going to meet by the degree of pretension in the naming of their homes. One family called their house Halton Hall which, no doubt looked more impressive on their notepaper than on their pebble-dashed semi-detached bungalow.

The only place where people used imagination was the local caravan site. The Macbeths called their caravan Cawdor, the Salt family called theirs The Cruet, and quiet little Mr Twigg, who lived on his own, called his Strangeways Jail. When I asked him why, he said it provoked interesting conversation whenever he had to give his address.

## HSI
Hypersensitivity to Syntactical Infelicity. An immunological defect that afflicts many who earn their living by writing. Its most tiresome characteristic is that minor irritants can provoke a major allergic response.

With me, the allergen most likely to produce an outburst is the ambiguous adjective. Whenever a newspaper describes a journalist as a "Royal correspondent" and he or she turns out not to be a Royal – not even the ubiquitous Princess Michael of Kent whose versatility is confirmed by a plaque commemorating her opening of a Happy Eater on the A3 near Ripley – my T cells grow agitated. My unseemly reaction compares unfavourably with the stately demeanour of the hacks on whom the title is conferred who develop an hauteur so grand you'd swear they were born to it.

Radio and television are rich sources of ambiguous adjectives. Ne'er a month goes by without a BBC newsperson offering a variation on the theme, "We are getting reports of a man being shot in the Bexley Heath area"... as if Bexley Heath were an anatomical euphemism for the parts the BBC dare not reach.

I suspect this usage is an English rather than British phenomenon. I can't imagine a Glasgow newsreader solemnly announcing that a man had been shot in the Gorbals... unless, of course, he *had* been shot in the testicles.

One consolation for those who suffer from HSI is that an ambiguous adjective can occasionally provoke a pleasurable response. As when I read in the American magazine *People*: *For sale. Four-poster bed. 101 years old. Perfect for antique lover.*

## Hubbub
International signal of inattention.

The televising of Prime Minister's Questions has revealed how, when the last answer has been given and some hapless member gets up to speak, no one can hear him or her because of the hubbub that others create as they leave the chamber.

The same sound now afflicts large international scientific meetings where, unless one of the star speakers is at the podium, there's a continual undercurrent of noise as people join or leave the audience, chattering as they go.

When the American College of Cardiology met in a huge hall in Atlanta, I heard a lowly speaker rebel against this constant interruption.

"Mr Chairman," he said, "I've been on my feet for nearly ten minutes but there's so much noise I can hardly hear myself speak."

The chairman banged his gavel and induced a moment of silence into which floated a comment, in Southern drawl, from the back of the auditorium.

"Cheer up, my friend. You ain't missin' much."

## Humility
Debilitating affliction of doctors too sensitive to make a show of their healing skills. A sad condition that deprives doctors from displaying the bombastic self confidence that many patients find reassuring. (See Bedside Manner.)

Humble doctors can console themselves with the thought that not all patients respond to bombast. Samuel Johnson recognised the value of medical humility in his tribute to his friend Robert Levet, whom the snobbish Boswell dismissed as "an obscure practitiser in physik among the lower people".

*When fainting nature called for aid,*
*And hovering death prepared the blow,*
*His vigorous remedy displayed*
*The power of art without the show.*

## Hydrophilia

A bizarre addiction to bottled water that swept across the Western world in the last decade of the 20$^{th}$ century and the first decade of the 21$^{st}$.

Its victims were young people who grew afraid to wander far from home without a bottle of water clutched in one hand, lest they be struck down by an attack of dehydration. The fact that none of them had ever seen such an attack did not shake their belief in its existence. Indeed the longer the addiction lasted the greater their belief that pure bottled water, as opposed to the nasty raw stuff, alleviated those indeterminate symptoms we all suffer when we're feeling less than sprightly.

Hydrophiliacs' fear of bodily harm is akin to the panic seen in Koro epidemics in China, when men are seized with a conviction that their genitalia are retracting into their abdomens and will eventually disappear. Bottled water has yet to be prescribed as Koro preventive but China is a rapidly developing country and may soon come to see the light.

Hydrophilia's impact on British life has been considerable. Before its arrival Britons were rather proud of the water that came from British taps, often referring to it as Adam's Ale. Bottled water was something you consumed only when venturing south of Dover, particularly if you ended up in France, a country whose inhabitants were notorious for an un-British attitude to hygiene.

It's no surprise that hydrophilia is sustained by regular ex-cathedra statements from the purveyors of bottled waters. In 2011 Hydration for Health, an 'initiative' sponsored by the giant French food company Danone which produces Volvic, Evian, and Badoit, launched an advertising campaign in the medical press exhorting readers to encourage "healthy hydration" and claiming on its website: "Many people, including children are not drinking enough."

When the Glasgow GP and journalist Margaret McCartney asked Professor Stanley Goldfarb, a physician and nephrologist at the University of Pennsylvania who knows a thing or two about dehydration, where was the evidence that we needed to drink more water, he replied, "The current evidence is that there really is no evidence."

So, unless you're in the Tropics, the only way to justify wandering around with a bottle of water in your hand is to regard it as a fashion accessory.

## Hyperactivity
Antisocial activity in one's own children.

As opposed to *Parental Control, Lack of …* antisocial behaviour in other people's children.

# I

## Ibrahim's law
The most effective route to health is not always the most obvious.

I've named the law after the Egyptian poet and physician Ibrahim Nagi (1898-1953) who told the tale of a poor man who had saved enough money to visit him. When he examined the man, he realised the symptoms were of hunger rather than disease. Ibrahim explained to his patient that he didn't need medicine but a good meal; he refunded the fee, added a considerable sum from his own pocket, and told the man to spend it on meat which would provide the protein he needed.

Two months later patient and doctor met again by chance.

"How are you feeling now?" asked Ibrahim Nagi.

"Great and fighting fit thanks to you."

"How do you mean?"

"With your money and mine I could afford the fees so I went and saw a really good doctor."

## Identity

Ephemeral persona bestowed on you by others. Dangerous to bestow upon yourself.

One night after I'd dined with a bunch of ageing contemporaries at a medical reunion, I happened upon a cruel piece of architectural design. The wine had been good and there was lots of it, so for an hour or two we had the illusion that we were indulging in highly spiced and witty conversation, that our minds had recaptured the zestful irreverence of youth, and that, all in all, we were a pretty sharp and sophisticated bunch.

The organisers had sensibly hired a bus to return us to our hotel and, as I stepped from its platform, I confronted an architectural discomforter. The hotel wall in which the entrance doors were set was made of mirrored glass and suddenly this brittle, suave, and lively man-about-town came face to face with full frontal reality: a paunchy, balding, and bleary eyed old buffer in a rumpled dinner jacket. It was a literal 'sobering experience'.

Since that evening, whenever life grows excessively competitive and threatens my sense of security, I console myself with the thought that when Charlie Chaplin impishly entered a Charlie Chaplin look-alike contest in Monte Carlo he came in third.

## Illusionist

Professional entertainer who uses the placebo effect to bemuse an audience in the way others use it to exploit the sick.

That's why professional magicians, trained to deceive, are more effective detectors of charlatanism than professional scientists.

Any child with a 'Junior Conjuror's Set' learns two simple lessons about magic. The first is that audiences yearn to be deceived; the second is that audiences are disappointed when told how the trick is done.

The disappointment comes because the secret is usually simple and banal. Good magicians camouflage the banality with showmanship and convince their audience it has witnessed something that defies rational understanding.

Conjurers' instruction leaflets first describe the Effect, which is what the audience thinks it sees, then the Method which is what actually happens while the watchers' attention is diverted elsewhere, often by exploitation of their longing to be deceived. When scientists examine phenomena that are beyond our comprehension they tend to concentrate on the Effect, analysing it, dissecting it, hypothesising about it. A professional magician, out of habit, goes straight for possible Methods and is unimpressed by the anecdotal evidence of Effect.

That's why magicians are better than scientists at persuading audiences that deception has taken place. They reproduce the same Effects as fraudulent operators by using the simple devices of their trade, then announce not how the trick was done – which would merely disappoint – but that it was no more magical than the other illusions in their stage acts. Audiences find these demonstrations more convincing than intellectual argument. Harry Houdini used them to expose fraudulent "mediums"; the Amazing Randi still uses them to challenge fraudsters more likely to be found these days on television chat shows than at back room séances.

An effective way to deflate a charlatan's claim to possess mystic powers is to mock it with an anecdote. As in the tale Karl Sabbagh told me of the ventriloquist who was encouraged by his agent to cash in on the popular enthusiasm for the paranormal and set himself up as a medium. His first customer was a widow who wanted to contact her late husband.

"No problem," said the ventriloquist.

"And what will be your fee?"

"For £100 you will be able to talk to your husband. For £200 he will talk to you. And for £300 he will talk to you while I drink a glass of water."

"Ridicule," wrote Thomas Jefferson, "is the only weapon that can be used against unintelligible propositions. Ideas must be distinct before reason can act upon them."

## Image

Significant characteristic of individuals or institutions in an age more concerned with shadow than with substance.

A matter of great concern to 'Leaders of the Profession' who keep organising meetings to discuss ways of improving the profession's 'public image'. Whenever I'm invited to take part I suggest that a 'good public image' is akin to other abstractions like dignity, a sense of humour, or sex appeal: if you find yourself worrying whether you've got them, you've probably got something to worry about.

Doctors have never been short of advice from image-makers.

William Osler kept it simple: "Look wise, say nothing, and grunt."

Another American physician Dr D W Cathell was more expansive in his mighty work published in 1882, *The Physician Himself and What He Should Add to His Scientific Acquirements*.

*Prefer to spend your idle hours in your office, or at the drug stores, or with other doctors at the medical library, instead of lounging around club rooms, cigar stores, billiard parlours, barber shops, etc.... What shall I say of debauchery with harlots and association with concubines? Of drinking and gambling? My dear sir, if you have entered either of these roads, turn from it at once, for either will blast your career, will be fatal to every ambition.*

The traditional British approach has been less messianic. A Victorian handbook published in London suggested a doctor needed only three accoutrements to look the part:

*A top hat to give him authority; a paunch to give him dignity, and haemorrhoids to give him a concerned expression.*

## Immortality

More easily achieved by doctors than by their patients.

A doctor's easiest route to immortality is a well-chosen eponym. A Thurber cartoon shows a man rushing into a doctor's surgery shouting, "I've got Bright's disease and he's got mine."

GPs are ideally placed to achieve fame through eponymity because they see vast numbers of patients with indeterminate symptoms. All they need do is make a collection of a few, label them as a syndrome, and then attach the labeller's name. It's prudent, however, to show discretion in the choice of symptoms. No one wants to suffer the eponymous fate of Thomas Crapper.

Doctors who don't mind sharing immortality can share an eponym with a chum. The more names that are attached to an entity, the more impressive it becomes. A chum with a complicated name can make it even more impressive because syndromes that are difficult to pronounce are thought to carry conceptual weight. The very name Creutzfeld-Jakob Disease endows the condition with gravitas.

Once again, however, doctors need to show discretion and refrain from going over the top as in "The Finsterer-Lake-Lahey-modification-of-the-Miculicz-Kronlein-Hofmeister-Reichal-Polya-improvement-of-the-Billroth-II-gastrectomy."

A doctor is more likely to achieve immortality as an individual than as a multi-hyphenated group.

## Importance of not being earnest

A lesson that GPs, if they're lucky, learn early in their careers. At its worst, earnestness deadens empathy with patients; at its most trivial it makes a GP sound like a prat.

My late and much lamented friend, the cartoonist Mel Calman, based one of his drawings on a moment from my days in general practice. It shows a woman saying to her GP: "I'm very worried doctor. My husband hasn't spoken to me for three days."

And the earnest young GP, who once I was, replies: "Maybe he's trying to tell you something."

## Impotence

No laughing matter. Hence a fine exemplar of the medical tradition: 'The sadder the condition, the richer the source of *double entendre.*'

A letter from a community psychiatric nurse to Dr Douglas Howes, a GP in Chudleigh, Devon, explained: "This patient's impotence is causing relationship difficulties and therefore contributes to his feeling of disconnectedness."

A sixty-five-year-old man complained to Dr Charles Ward of Bristol about the side effects of his treatment: "They warned me about kidney and eye problems but they never told me impotency would raise its ugly head."

A urologist at Dudley Road Hospital, Birmingham, who'd seen a man with the condition, wrote to his GP Brian Dicker: "With regard to his erections, these seem to have settled down." Which, as Dr Dicker points out, was hardly reassuring.

A Braintree hospital eager to conserve its resources wrote to a local GP: "We should appreciate it if you would not refer further patients with impotence to the Urology Department to avoid the disappointment of raised expectations."

## Impression

As in 'making a good impression': an odd yet lingering tradition of patients putting on 'good', sometimes even 'best', clothes for a visit to the doctor, as if they were going to church.

A Glasgow woman attended her GP for a cervical smear. During the procedure the doctor (male) mentioned, in a kindly way, that she had obviously gone to some trouble to prepare herself. It seemed an unusual comment and, on her way home she wondered what he meant. She later mentioned the remark to her daughter explaining that all she'd done before going to the surgery was to have a wash and use her daughter's Fem Fresh spray. Only then did she discover that, by mistake, she had used her daughter's disco glitter.

## Improvisation

A skill doctors must master to be accepted as credible performers. One of the sterner tests of medical ingenuity is deciding what to do when chance elects you to be the first doctor on the scene of an accident without even a stethoscope in your pocket.

A sporting solution came from a surgeon at the Mayo Clinic who, on his drive home, encountered a small crowd gathered round a man lying unconscious in the road. He discovered to his relief that an ambulance was on its way but, having declared himself as a doctor, he felt he should be seen to do something. As a urologist he used the only expertise he possessed that was in any way appropriate, and the only piece of equipment in his bag that was in any way relevant. He inserted a urinary catheter.

When the paramedics arrived they took him quietly on one side and asked why he'd done it.

"Goddamit," he said. "I couldn't just stand there. I had to do something and it might just be useful when you get him to hospital. I'll tell you one thing, though. It's a hell of a crowd pleaser."

## Imputationism
The habit of attributing beliefs to adversaries in order to bolster our own.

A common feature of 'debates' about medical ethics.

When I was editor of *World Medicine* I collided with a Law of Human Perversity which decreed that, when I published opinionated pieces from opposite sides of a vigorously contested argument, each side assumed I shared the views of their opponents.

The deeply committed gave the impression that they rarely read articles with which they agreed – maybe they gave them a glance but found them too boring – but gave assiduous attention to those with which they didn't, as if in need of a regular fix of self-righteousness to nurture their beliefs.

Over the years I published articles in which writers expressed nearly every shade of moral and ethical opinion about abortion, family planning, euthanasia, genetic engineering, and so on and so on. Just as I published articles that expressed most shades of political opinion on private medicine, 'socialised medicine', the pharmaceutical industry and so on and so on.

Like most people I do have political and ethical opinions and, when I wanted to express them, I did so under my own name. But those were not the views attributed to me as an editor. In the eyes of some imputationists, I was pro-abortion; in the eyes of others, my religious beliefs – determined apparently by the O' in my name – blinded my attitude to abortion law reform. I still have a letter that accuses me of being "a killer of unwanted babies" which I keep stapled to another that arrived in the same post accusing me of being "responsible for the misery suffered by unwanted children".

In the eyes of other equally passionate people, I was a lackey of the wicked drug industry, an enemy of private enterprise, a fascist, a communist, an anarchist... think of a well-worn label and, at some time, an angry person wanted to hang it around my neck.

That experience led me to conclude that most of the ethical issues that generate insecurity in practising doctors – who have to make real decisions affecting real people rather than juggle with hypothesis in debate – will never be resolved by consensus agreement as long as doctors hold divergent political, moral, or religious beliefs. Points-scoring imputationist debate is nothing more than an entertaining sideshow.

## Incapacity

Disability which, unlike the genuine article, exists only in the eyes or ears, or even in the feet, of the beholder.

Margaret Weslake, a Staffordshire housewife, wrote to her local newspaper to complain that "in this International Year of Disabled People, insufficient media attention has been devoted to people incapacitated by flat feet."

Her complaint struck what for me was a tuneless chord because the media have been equally inattentive to the incapacity from which I suffer – tone deafness. I am, like Charles Lamb, "sentimentally disposed to harmony but organically incapable of a tune".

All through my life I have been victimised because of my incapacity. I was kicked out of the school choir and denied choir privileges like strawberry jam sandwiches for Sunday tea. (The choirmaster claimed, and at the time I believed him, that the school spent good money re-tuning the organ before they discovered the fault lay with me.)

When I left school I was denied entry to certain occupations like opera singer, chorus boy, or crooner with the Henry Hall orchestra. The discrimination was blatant because I know I produce the right notes but some strange force, possibly gamma radiation, distorts the sounds before they reach my listeners' ears.

Even my own family turned against me and wouldn't allow me to join in the hymns at weddings or funerals or the community singing at pantomimes.

Maybe Ms Weslake and I should get together. With her feet and my ears we could get an International Year all to ourselves. And, if we don't, at least we have the makings of an unusual song and dance act.

## Incognito
How a wise doctor always travels.

In a Richard Gordon novel a hotel manager calls a young doctor from his bed on the first night of his honeymoon to examine a sick guest. Later the doctor explains, "The marriage was consummated, but only just."

That incident stirred the medical journalist David Delvin to record some of his adventures travelling as an undisguised doctor. Holidays provided the worst. On one package tour the people at the next table engaged him for the whole two weeks in "a shouted dialogue about the state of British medicine or the state of their bowels – both, apparently, in much the same condition."

In an another hotel dining room the manager appeared at his elbow. "Excuse me, sir, but are you a doctor of medicine?"

"Er... yes?"

"I wonder if you happen to have anything with you for the chef's tummy. He keeps having diarrhoea and vomiting, and he's having difficulty doing the cooking."

Wise doctors take preventive measures. Jeannie Stirrat, a psychiatrist in Poole, commended a stratagem used by a friend when he was one of only twelve passengers on a cargo boat. When asked "What do you do for a living?" he replied, "I sell life insurance."

A Hampshire GP, Rachel MacSparron, used a ploy I regard near to perfection. The landlady at her holiday B&B in Scotland was inquisitive and chatty so when inevitably she asked, "What do you do for a living?", Dr MacSparron replied: "I work for the government and don't like to talk about my job." The subject lay buried for the rest of the holiday.

## Infantilism
Regressive behaviour in young children causing them to act like MPs during Prime Minister's Questions.

## Infirmary
Institution originally established to care for the infirm.

Technology has since transmogrified it into a place where treatment consists of mechanical things doctors can do to patients to improve their physical health. Hi-tech treatment of the 'treatable' leaves little space or time for non mechanical treatment of the infirm, such as restoring morale or confidence, or re-instilling a zest for life.

Infirm people who need too much non-mechanical care are unwelcome in modern infirmaries where they are known as Bedblockers (qv).

## Information
Digitised strings of Arcanian (qv) exchanged between medical 'information technologists'. As in this paragraph from *Information for information users* issued by NHS Executive South Thames:

*The project is envisaged to roll-out to a comprehensive range of pilot groups who will test the various functions of the new system before wider roll-out throughout the organisation. A key aim will be to monitor the comprehensive benefits realisation programme by the project subgroups during the implementation period.*

## Innocence of childhood
Myth perpetuated by sentimental adults who've forgotten how easily they manipulated 'grown-ups' when they themselves were children and led their parents up the garden path.

Dr Benjamin Spock pointed out that there are only two things a child will share willingly: communicable disease and the age of his mother.

I was once called to see a boy aged about eleven. I was worried that he might have acute appendicitis. True his mother had said that, despite her warning, he had eaten a bagful of green apples but every GP knows how dangerous it is to make a 'green apple' diagnosis in a child of that age. As I dithered at the bedside, trying to make a decision, I asked the boy what was so great about green apples.

"I didn't eat them because I liked them," he said haughtily. "I ate them to find out why my mother didn't want me to."

## In sickness or in health?
The most difficult decision a GP has to make.

When I went into general practice, my GP father told me there was one condition I'd need to grow skilled at detecting. It was pretty common, he said, but the diagnosis was tricky and I might need a year or two to sharpen my perception. In the meantime I'd have to rely on my GP friends. Hospital doctors couldn't help me because they didn't see enough of it, indeed they relied on GPs to diagnose it for them.

The condition was, of course, normality and I soon learned what he meant. Just as pathologists define whether biochemical measurements are normal or abnormal, GPs have to decide whether the odd symptoms and aberrations that people bring to their attention fall within normal limits. But, unlike pathologists, they can't look up the normal values in a book.

John Harman, a consultant physician at St Thomas' Hospital, London, claimed the most useful letter he could get from a GP was "one that says, 'I don't know what's the matter with this patient except that he's ill.' The GP has made the difficult diagnosis and left the easy one to me."

GPs learn this skill because their clinical experience differs, in one significant way, from that of hospital doctors. Steve McCabe, a GP in Portree defined the difference in the *BMJ*: "The great advantage we have as GPs – which our hospital colleagues don't have – is that we often know our patients inside out and can tell when something is 'not right'."

John Harman was not the only hospital consultant to recognise this difference in clinical experience. A paediatrician described in the *Lancet* how, when travelling on a train, he'd tried to diagnose what was the matter with an infant sitting on the lap of the woman opposite him. Only after twenty minutes' careful observation did he recognise a condition he rarely saw. The child was perfectly normal.

## Insight

Occasional glimpse that life affords us of not just who but what we are.

Whenever I feel a crisis of identity coming on I think back half a century to when, as a newly-hatched medical journalist, I made a brief appearance on the BBC's early evening television news.

If I remember aright, the sewer workers were on strike and I was there to reassure the punters that when the sewage seeped up into the streets the main threat would be not to their health but to their aesthetic sensitivity.

As I left Television Centre, I met my old friend and godfather to my son, the actor Francis Matthews who was on his way home after his day's stint as Paul Temple. He lived near us and offered me a lift. As we walked out of the main gates on our way to the car park in Wood Lane, two small boys approached and asked for our autographs. Impressed by the transient fame bestowed by a few authoritative words on sewage, I proudly signed my name. Then as we walked away, I heard one boy say to his chum: "I got Francis Matthews. Who did you get?" The boy whose book I'd signed replied: "A load of old rubbish."

It was a defining moment and I have since cruised through life comfortably aware of what I am. There's a lot to be said for being a load of old R. If you play the hand skilfully, you can draw advantages from the endeavours of the stars around you without having to suffer the anxieties that so often afflict them.

It is also, whisper it gently, a crafty role to play as a GP.

## Insignia

Trappings that can cause confusion when the professions mix.

Soon after World War Two, the BMA invited a bishop to conduct the Sunday service at their Annual Representatives Meeting and booked him into their VIP hotel for the previous evening.

He had planned to bring his wife but she had to cancel at the last moment so he had the double room to himself.

When he retired after dining with the doctors he discovered his pyjamas had been laid out one side of the double bed and his surplice neatly laid out on the other.

## Intelligent design
Helpful fantasy for those who don't like the implications of evolution.

One day in the Garden of Eden, Eve calls out to God, "Lord, I have a problem. I know you've created me and provided this beautiful garden, all these wonderful animals, and that hilarious snake, but I'm just not happy."

"Why's that, Eve?"

"I'm lonely. And I'm sick to death of apples."

"If loneliness really is a problem, I could create a man for you."

"What's a man, Lord?"

"He'll be bigger and faster than you and he'll like to hunt and kill things but he'll have flaws. He'll revel in childish things like fighting and kicking a ball about. He'll lie and cheat and be conceited. And, because he won't be too smart, he'll need your advice to think properly."

'Do I really need such a creature, Lord?"

"He'll have one redeeming feature. He'll be able to give you physical pleasure I think you'll enjoy, though he may look a bit silly when he's aroused. And you did say you were lonely."

'Well, it is pretty boring here on my own. Some excitement could cheer me up. Let's give it a go."

"You can have him on one condition."

"What's that, Lord?"

"'Because he'll be proud, arrogant, and self-admiring, you'll have to let him believe that I made him first. So remember, this is our secret… woman to woman."

## Internal market
Artificial market imposed on the NHS in 1991 during that strange interlude when John Major claimed to be Prime Minister and Margaret Thatcher's supporters claimed she was driving from the back seat. (See Themarket.)

As health systems go, the NHS was relatively cheap to run and, thanks to the ancient British tradition of 'muddling through', worked reasonably well. But in the Thatcherite revolutionary handbook it was guilty of a capital offence: it didn't conform to market principles. As a publicly funded monopoly it was by definition inefficient, so its administration was restructured to create an artificial market using theories that had been tried – and failed – in the United States which, unlike the UK, faced a real crisis over the cost of health care.

In opposition the Labour party claimed it would dismantle the internal market but, once in power, successive New Labour governments reinforced it. As a result, much of the increased spending on the NHS was used in monitoring and administering this artificial structure.

Twenty years after the market's launch many doctors remained unconvinced of its benefits. In June 2011 Michael Schachter, a senior lecturer at Imperial College London, lamented the way people no longer questioned the concept but claimed it was more efficient in ways that no-one seemed able to measure. He wrote in the *BMJ*:

*It has generated another layer of bureaucracy involved in commissioning, often consisting of people with little or no experience of patient care. It also introduces a potential conflict of interest, in that the purchasers may have an incentive to purchase less to safeguard their budgets and indeed their own incomes…*

*Several generations of healthcare professionals have been brainwashed into believing that this is an inevitable state of affairs but of course it is not, just the imposition of dogma by health economists who know little about health and apparently not much more about economics.*

The first effect of the ersartz market was to bring chaos to hospitals conditioned to cope only with confusion. The medical reaction was summed up in a jaunty graffito I found in a London teaching hospital at the time. At eye level above a urinal in the staff Gents I read: *At this moment you're the only man in this hospital who knows what he's doing.*

## Internal marketese

The enigmatic language of the sect that worships Themarket (qv).

When the internal market was imposed on the NHS, its supporters exploited the advantage of speaking a language that other people didn't understand. Only later did we discover that they didn't understand it themselves. But that didn't matter because they were motivated not by the meaning of words but by their sound.

The management at the East Surrey Hospital explained how the market would work:

*The planning process will consider the volume of each critical resource consumed by each episode and will produce load plans by specialty over an appropriate horizon. It will then aggregate these upwards into an overall resource plan so that capacity and production levels can be set to meet the level of demand.*

## International authority
Someone who has travelled overseas to give a lecture.

One of life's lesser known facts is that the late Auberon Waugh was an international authority on breast feeding. Alexander Chancellor has described how, when Waugh was editor of the *Literary Review* he received an invitation to address a distinguished gathering in the former French colony of Senegal. The subject of his hour-long lecture was to be breast-feeding and there was a generous fee attached.

According to Chancellor, Waugh found it difficult to resist any offer of free travel so with the help of his impressive collection of medical encyclopaedias he prepared his lecture and flew off to Senegal. There he spoke with grave authority before an audience of politicians and other worthies who seemed more bemused than bedazzled by his erudition. Only later did he learn from his hosts that he had misheard the original phone call and they had been expecting his views on 'Press freedom'.

## International medicine
A myth.

The incidence of heart disease is the same in Germany as in Britain yet Germans consume six times more heart drugs than Britons and their doctors diagnose Herzinsuffizienz on grounds that would not mean heart disease elsewhere. In Germany the acceptable national mood is pessimism so Germans are allowed to enjoy bad health and businessman take their 'heart medicine' publicly and with pride because it enhances their status. British businessmen take theirs in secret fearing that the knowledge they were 'flawed' could inhibit their advancement.

French doctors, influenced by Descartes, are often more concerned with the intellectual process than with its outcome. They take rectal temperatures because these are more accurate than oral ones. Others claim that such precision is unnecessary but French doctors revere the intellectual quality of accuracy for its own sake. It's not only doctors who are influenced by cultural tradition. French patients, as every Briton knows, are obsessed with their livers. An ingenuous American researcher comparing survival rates in intensive care units was alarmed by the high death rate attributed to liver disease in France. What he was measuring, of course, was the incidence not of the disease but of the attribution.

Elaine Duncan, a British doctor working in Galicia, has described the differences between the illnesses that Spanish and British women bring to her door. In Spain she never hears the common British complaints of pre-menstrual tension, "abdominal bloating" or being "tired all the time." Instead Spanish women consult her about "varicosities" – tiny veins in the thigh, "low blood pressure", which in Britain would be regarded as normal blood pressure, and "mareos" – a catch-all condition embracing vertigo, vomiting, fainting, anxiety crises, and generally not feeling well.

In Canada an inhaler for use with infants has to have bilingual instructions printed on its side. They read:

Keep mask in place for two breaths

*Tenir le masque en place pendant six respirations*

Does this mean the drug action differs if the infant's parents speak French rather than English?

## International scientific meetings

Periodic migrations of medical researchers from laboratories into darkened rooms where they read scientific papers (qv) at one another and compete to see who can be the most boring.

The undoubted highlight of an international congress of the Transplantation Society came at the end of a long, boring paper read in soporific tones by a speaker who never once raised his eyes from the script in front of him. When he finished the chairman turned to the stuporous audience and asked the traditional: "Any questions?" After a pause, a lethargic hand was raised at the back of the room. The chairman nodded and the questioner was handed a microphone. He rose slowly to his feet and asked: "What time is it?"

Sound advice offered in the 'Press Pack' at a meeting of the American College of Cardiology: *Do not photograph the speakers while they are addressing the audience. Shoot them as they approach the platform.*

## Intuitive response
Dangerous reaction in medicine.

A London gynaecologist was leaving the bedside of a young French woman after a post-operative visit. His patient with a shy smile beckoned to him to lower his head close to her mouth. She then whispered in his ear: "Can we have sex?" For a long and flustered moment he failed to realise the question concerned not him but her partner.

## Irritable vowel syndrome
Phonetic uncertainty that, in a more class conscious age, afflicted people who migrated from the North to the Home Counties.

The journalist Jill Tweedie described how when she came south and was faced with phrases like 'dance band' or 'Stafford Castle', she could never remember in which word to posh-up the vowel sound.

Although this syndrome is usually associated with the vowel 'a' – should it remain flat or be drawn out to an 'aaaah'? – it can also occur with lowlier vowels like 'u', especially in the North West. At about the time Jill Tweedie made her journey south, the chairman of a Lancashire exploration society had to introduce, as visiting lecturer, the Antarctic explorer Sir Vivian Fuchs. After he repeatedly referred to the guest as Sir Vivian Fucks, an agitated committee member leaned forward and whispered: "The man's name is Fooks."

"I know that," said the chairman, "but there are ladies present."

## Itinerant aspirate
Disorder of articulation in which aspirates migrate from one word to another.

This disorder is thought by some to afflict only Northerners but it occurs also in Bedfordshire. Jim Aylward, a GP in Ampthill, had a patient who always gave his first name as, "Orace with a Haitch." Another opened a surgery conversation with: "Sorry to trouble you doctor but I've got a problem with my harse."

Apparently this usage is built into some fine old Bedfordshire sayings: another patient ended her lively description of uncontrollable bowel turbulence with, "As my old mother used to say, doctor, it's a sad harse that never laughs."

## IT viruses
Organisms, similar to computer viruses, that target medical dictating machines, word processors, and typewriters. The diagnostic feature of a true virus infection is that it enhances the original message.

The **Type O** virus penetrates the DNA of a single word and enhances its meaning by altering its spelling.

Letter from a consultant to Dr Anthony Abrahams of Oxford.
*We had an expensive discussion of his symptoms.*

Letter from consultant to Dr Margaret Thomson of Luton.
*They should also consider using lubricants to re-juice the resistance when Mr X penetrates his wife.*

Report sent to Michael O'Ryan, a GP in Prescot.
*Dr X felt that the distended colon was related to his chronic consternation.*

Letter to Paul Sackin of Alconbury.
*This lady finds herself pregnant for the third time, the last being a normal delivery under Jim's car.*

The **Syntactical** virus penetrates the DNA of whole sentences and determines the order of words. As with Type O, the diagnostic feature is enhancement of the original message.

Guardian headline.
*Diet of premature babies affects IQ.*

British Society of Gastroenterology Newsletter.
*Barium enema symposium fills auditorium.*

Bulletin published by the Novartis Foundation.
*We have convened a distinguished panel of genetically modified food experts.*
(The group photograph revealed that a genetically modified expert is indistinguishable from the standard suit-wearing variety.)

The **New Style HIV** (Homophone Insinuating Virus) is a retrovirus that integrates with a word's chromosomal DNA to produce a homophone or near homophone that enhances the original message.

Letter found in patient's notes by Dr Kiaran O'Sullivan of Northwich.
*Contraceptive pills are not suiting her and other methods make her soar.*

Hospital letter to a Sheffield GP.
*He suffered this bazaar attack while at the Antiques Roadshow.*

Letter from a surgeon to Joe Speer, a GP in Bath.
*Vaginal examination was not performed as the patient was masturbating at the time.*
(Unusually discreet behaviour for a surgeon.)

# J

## Jargonism

Communication disorder that occurs in people who use the same phrases so often and unthinkingly that their brains grow insensate to the meaning of the words.

A typical example is sign I spotted inside the main entrance of Macey's department store in New York: *Elevator to the cellar*.

In clinical medicine the condition often occurs in those who grow used to emphasising the caring aspects of their work and fail to appreciate that stringing jargon phrases together does not necessarily instil them with meaning. A characteristic victim was a pain management consultant who wrote to the *BMJ*:

*I am so pleased that as a body of pain management we respond from all ends of the country with a universal response to this with some degree of incredulity yet understanding with a will to educate.*

More often the phrases are used to clothe a platitude in the ceremonial dress *de riguer* in NHS top management. As in *Focus on Health* issued by the Lothian Health Board.

*Health and "disease" are normative concepts. That is to say, they are polar terms in a continuum between optimum functioning and malfunctioning of an organism. When we consider the World Health Organisation definition of health… we are clearly dealing with health as a value-concept.*

The disorder has its compensations and occasionally produces life-enhancing messages such as one from a Romford Hospital:

*On Monday, 12th March, at 10.50 a.m. in the Conference Room at the Medical Centre there will be a meeting of the Bedpan Steering Committee.*

## Jarming

Activity promoted in the US in a commendable attempt to clear the streets of joggers.

The idea was proposed by Dr Joseph D Wasserug of Quincy, Massachusetts: "Everyone knows that violinists and orchestra conductors have unparalleled longevity, so why don't we stress the merits of exercising the arms instead of the legs? ... It is about time that the proponents of jogging were silenced. We should proclaim the therapeutic merits of jogging with your arms – jarming."

Like all innovators Dr Wasserug ran into reflex opposition. First to object was Hans Neuman, medical director of New Haven department of health, who, while admitting jarming could be helpful, said rather sniffily: "One cannot advise hiring an orchestra for physical training purposes."

Undaunted, Dr Wasserug replied that people could buy an orchestra on tape or disc and, like Walter Mitty, mount the podium, baton in hand. Indeed, jarming's big advantage over jogging, he said, was that it could be performed at any age, no matter how fit or unfit the performer. Not only that. "Like the tai-chi of the Chinese, jarming may be a sport of beauty and grace when properly performed. Indeed, the hand motions of leading symphony orchestra conductors rival those of prima ballerinas."

## Jaunty

Irritating manner assumed by doctors who think themselves 'good with patients'.

Joan Rivers, comedienne and doctor's daughter, has been on the receiving end. "My feet are in the stirrups, my knees are in my face, the door is open facing me and my gynaecologist does jokes: 'Doctor Schwartz at your cervix', or 'Dilated to meet you'. With that level of joke, there's no way you can get back at the son of a bitch unless you learn to throw your voice."

# K

## Keeping up appearances

Essential activity for doctors whose patients have more money than sense.

Bruce Sloane, the expatriate British psychiatrist who introduced me to the concept of Saniflush (qv), was a distinguished academic at the University of Southern California and lived in Beverly Hills near to an area popular with Hollywood psychiatrists: a canyon dotted with villas, all outrageously expensive but designed to give the casual laid-back appearance that the rich of Los Angeles expect of their psychiatrist.

Bruce loved to send up the fashionable image of the 1970s Beverly Hills psychiatrist: new age liberal, casual in dress and behaviour, rich but not gaudy. One evening, as he drove me though the canyon on our way to his home for dinner, he spotted a brand new Rolls Royce parked in one of the drives. "Oh my Gawd," he cried. "There goes the neighbourhood."

## Keep taking the tabloids
Essential step if you want to keep abreast of medical breakthroughs and scandals.

Tabloid readers of a nervous disposition need an antidote. I would prescribe a regular read of Ben Goldacre's *Bad Science* blog.

In June 2008 a front page story in the *Sunday Express* claimed that research by a government adviser Dr Roger Coghill showed that all those who had committed suicide in Bridgend lived closer to a mobile phone mast than average. When the indefatigable Goldacre contacted the researcher, he discovered Coghill wasn't a doctor, wasn't really a government adviser, couldn't explain what he meant by "average", and had, in what Goldacre describes as "a twist of almost incomprehensible ridiculousness", lost the data.

## Kennel psychiatry
Psychotherapy designed to foster meaningful relationships between dogs and their owners.

The world's first combined canine and human psychiatric service was established in Los Angeles, a city whose citizens would rather admit their true age than concede that any form of human behaviour was outlandish.

In 1955, Dr Dare Miller put up his plate on a modern Tudor-style residence on the outskirts of Beverly Hills and within a few years established a flourishing practice among Californian dogs in the higher income bracket. His panelled consulting room, with framed diplomas on the wall, was furnished with a thick piled rich gold carpet, which must have been a grave temptation to his patients. It also housed a more practical legless desk and a black plastic-covered psychoanalytical couch.

Sadly he didn't allow the dogs to stretch out on the couch. For him the "owner-pet situation" was a "parent-child relationship" and the couch was where the parents "familiarised" him with the child's problem. "The child's environment is the most important thing and the parent is the most important factor in that environment. Change the environment, and you have a happy blooming child."

When I first encountered Dr Miller in the late 1960s his most effective therapy was his Concentrated Course, made up of six forty-five minute sessions at $250 dollars a time. This Concentrated Course sometimes needed reinforcement with occasional 'touch-ups' at $50 a go. Touch-ups were needed, for instance, to cure "postman's syndrome" in a beagle, the child of a "major star."

Film stars and their dogs often trod Dr Miller's rich gold carpet. He treated Kirk Douglas's apricot-coloured poodle, Teddy, for "severe regression" and his cure of Katharine Hepburn's dog, Lobo, was one of his proudest moments. The athletic Miss Hepburn enjoyed running but Lobo could run even faster and regularly outdistanced her. "It is necessary for the child's happiness that the parent be the dominant personality in his life," said Dr Miller. So he set up a harmonious non-competitive relationship between Lobo and Miss Hepburn, though he wouldn't specify its nature for fear of breaching Lobo's right to confidentiality.

Dr Miller attributed his success to an ingenious device, developed at a cost of some $30,000 – a jeweller's chain that incorporated a tuning fork which, when struck or thrown, vibrated at 34,000 cycles per second, the upper range of a dog's hearing. He named the device Hi-Fido and used it, in Pavlovian style, to establish new behaviour patterns in dogs. The sound emitted by the chain, he claimed, dominated any idle thoughts wandering through a dog's mind. It was also a useful wake-up call when hurled at a dog.

He marketed the chain as part of a do-it-yourself Hi-Fido kit which also included his major work *The Secret of Canine*

*Communication*, widely regarded at the time as the "Dr Spock" of the dog owner's world.

When I met him, Dr Miller, though married, had no children. Nor did he have a dog.

## Key communication skills

Behavioural platitudes taught to budding doctors, and some who have already budded, in lieu of teaching them how to learn more about themselves, their motives, and their attitudes.

Doctors love communicating about 'communication'. In the first decade of this century the *BMJ* published 406 articles or letters with the word in the title or abstract.

Doctors also enjoy communicating about 'non-communication'. 'Breakdown in communication' is one of the commonest excuses for failure or ineptitude.

Yet much of the medical teaching of 'communication' never gets beyond the Janet and John stage, concentrating on superficial and often banal 'key communication skills'.

One of the most quoted is: "Establish eye contact at the beginning of the consultation and maintain it at reasonable intervals to show interest." (I love that "reasonable." I reckon I could diagnose unreasonable eye contact but reasonable is a trickier proposition.)

Still you can't argue with it – and I advise you not to get drawn into argument with the solemn proponents of this line of teaching. Of course, eye contact is important, as are other Key Skills such as regularly checking that patients understand what's being said, asking open questions, not interrupting, and so on. But grown ups regard all this as pretty obvious.

What worries me about the Key Skills is not just that they are platitudinous but that they are a beginner's guide to role-playing. And when you diminish the art of communicating to the mechanics of role-playing you ignore the limitations imposed by the individual quirks of doctors and their patients.

Even the most versatile of actors know there are limits to the range of parts they can play, imposed not just by their physical characteristics but by their personality. The same techniques don't work for everyone and doctors, like actors, need to nurture their individual gifts rather than try to ape the performances of others. As Samuel Johnson said, "Almost all absurdity of conduct arises from the imitation of those we cannot resemble."

Take the business of eye contact. Clearly it's a Good Thing to establish eye contact with a patient. Yet, as any intelligent grown up knows, the quality of eye contact – and how long it is held – varies with the age, sex, and cultural and social backgrounds of those engaged in conversation.

To accommodate this variance yet maintain the illusion of a mechanical skill, the academic assessment of medical communication skills is peppered with equivocating adjectives like 'appropriate', 'reasonable', and 'proper'. 'Appropriate' crops up seven times in the schedule for the MRCGP video exam. These adjectives would be more at home in a guide to Victorian etiquette than to a creative human activity.

People who empathise with others aren't plagued by equivocation. For them the need for and the nature of eye contact spring from a deeper level of sensibility and are not measured acts imposed by protocol.

This distinction has significant implications when doctor meets patient. The notion of communication as a mechanical skill implies that a doctor's personality makes a lesser contribution than a learned technique to the ability to understand and be understood. Yet a doctor's personality is sometimes the most powerful generator of empathy and understanding. (See Listening.)

## Killer bugs
Ravaging marauders that periodically attack British newspapers. No respecters of class, they infect broadsheets as readily as tabloids.

After the 1994 outbreak of flesh-eating killer bug disease, the former editor of *New Scientist*, Dr Bernard Dixon analysed the rampant non-epidemic for the *BMJ*. Dr Dixon, a microbiologist before he became a science journalist, catalogued the misinformation that fuelled the hysteria in tabloids and "serious" papers and concluded by asking four questions:

1. Why did journalists ignore the textbooks?
2. Why were medical microbiologists reluctant to help them?

3. Why did some editors ignore good advice which they received from their specialist writers?

4. Why did the Public Health Laboratory Service or the Department of Health not issue a succinct briefing paper at an early stage in the whole nonsensical nightmare?

I was tempted to supply the answers:

1. Because they contain long words like 'conscientious' and your modern newshound has no time to waste on consulting dictionaries.

2. Because they remembered what was published the last time they tried to enlighten the unenlightenable.

3. Because it would have spoiled a good story.

4. Because, in the time it would have taken for a briefing committee to be chosen and for its members to agree dates for a meeting, define an agenda, draft a statement, seek approval from the appropriate officials etcetera, etcetera… the Black Death could have swept across Europe and be coming round for the second time.

The effect of the outbreak on general practice was summed up by Niall Robertson, a GP in Bo'ness, West Lothian.

*I swear by Apollo et al. that during National Flesh-devouring Deathbug from Hell Terror Week, a man arrived in the morning surgery with a sore throat. After I'd thrown light on his tonsils and offered him an explanation of his symptoms, he turned anxious eyes on me and asked: "It couldn't be that necrophilia, could it, doctor?"*

## Knight starvation
Deficiency disease that afflicts senior doctors in their early to mid-fifties.

A progressive condition that deteriorates with the publication of each Honours List.

Treatment is awarded arbitrarily. One doctor may be offered therapy while others more erudite, more attentive to their patients, and altogether more agreeable, are denied. At least in the days of James I, Pitt the Younger, and Maundy Gregory, sufferers knew how to get treatment, indeed knew the exact price.

One of the sadder sights in medicine is to see senior doctors so troubled by the condition they're prepared do almost anything to get the antidote… forgetting in their eagerness that if someone wants to buy your support – be it with a free lunch or a knighthood – you must have something that's worth selling. Often it's your integrity.

Some years ago, in an article in the *BMJ*, I referred to an unnamed doctor who achieved the knighthood he coveted with "an act that denied the very qualities for which he'd won my respect". When the article appeared, the editor and I received pained complaints from three people who assumed I was writing about them. I was in fact writing about someone else but I still wonder what those three had been up to.

## Knowing your place

A skill less common now than it was in the days of Empire… as is the art of dealing with those who don't possess it.

A recent newspaper hou-ha over a local councillor who tried to jump the queue in A&E by pulling rank reminded me of a technique that ought to be known to receptionists in hospitals and health centres. I discovered it in a magazine provided in my dentist's waiting room.

The central figure was a B-minus celebrity, an 'actor' best known for his appearances in gossip columns and advertisements, who arrived at an airport and seeing a long queue at check-in strode boldly to the first-class desk.

The polite young man behind the counter looked at his ticket. "I'm sorry sir. This check-in is for first-class passengers only. You'll have to join the queue at the next desk."

The 'actor' raised what passed for his hackles and in a suitably outraged tone bellowed: "Do you know who I am?"

Whereupon the airline official picked up the public address microphone and announced: "There is a passenger at Desk 17 who doesn't know who he is. Could anybody who might identify him please proceed to the desk as soon as possible."

The only evidence I have for the event is anecdotal, but the dentist is, in all other matters, wholly reliable.

## KOL

Acronym coined by pharmaceutical salesmen for their most rewarding target: a Key Opinion Leader.

KOLs define themselves by their activities. They appear as authors on a spectacular number of scientific papers, including those written for them by junior colleagues or drug company 'ghost writers'; contribute chapters to textbooks; sit on government advisory committees and the boards of medical societies; advise politicians on protocols and guidelines; maintain a presence in the top echelons of medico-political and scientific institutions; give keynote lectures at international conferences and lownote lectures at meetings and dinners sponsored by companies that sell medical products or services.

In return they are rewarded not just with personal fees but with research grants to their institutions making them valuable – and powerful – academic assets. They also get a lot of Grade A pampering. Pharmaceutical companies fly them first class to conferences held in exotic places where a company 'minder' is at hand to ensure that they and their 'accompanying persons' get tables at the most fashionable restaurants, enjoy private tours of the 'sights', and don't have to dip their hands into their own pockets for the most trivial of purchases.

KOL-ing is an international activity but seen at its most brazen in the US. In 2008, Melody Petersen, a former reporter on *The New York Times,* described how KOLs had helped the sale of Neurontin, a drug approved by the Food and Drugs Administration for use in epilepsy but only when other drugs failed. Helped by a whistle-blowing scientist who worked for the manufacturers she revealed how the company paid KOLs to put their names on articles recommending the drug for other uses: insomnia, bipolar disease, tension headaches, sexual dysfunction, hot flushes, restless legs, and a long list of chronic ill-defined conditions. (See Manufactured Diseases.)

The KOLs also helped expand the market by speaking at meetings of doctors held in classy restaurants, hotels, and resorts where the audience enjoyed a gourmet meal or a weekend vacation and often received a $500 attendance fee. KOLs, some of them trained by the company's advertising agency, used these meetings to encourage colleagues to use the drug in conditions for which it wasn't approved, so called 'off-label' prescription. Meanwhile the company monitored doctors' prescriptions and lavished gifts on those who wrote the most for Neurontin.

In 2004 the company's new owners agreed to pay 430 million dollars to settle claims that the drug had been marketed illegally. But, by that time Neurontin sales had reached 10 billion dollars, mostly from 'off-label' prescriptions.

The whistleblower David Franklin was dismayed that so many doctors seemed eager to join in the deception. Ms Petersen commented: "We have a law in America that says radio disc jockeys can't take cash from music companies. But when it comes to something like medicines… doctors can take as much money as they want from the drug companies."

# L

## Laboratory
(Now) Fluorescent-lit office filled with computers, other electronic gadgetry, and a coffee machine.
(Once) Wizard's den crammed with bubbling retorts, high tension and… *romance!*

The fantasy world of science I inhabited in my youth – fostered by the comics I read and the films I saw – was perfectly captured by S J Perelman:

*I guess I'm an old mad scientist at bottom. Give me an underground laboratory, half a dozen atom-smashers, and a beautiful girl in a diaphanous veil waiting to be turned into a chimpanzee, and I care not who writes the nation's laws.*

## Labour saver's neurosis
Obsessional disorder induced by appliances that victims welcome into to their homes with the enthusiasm of Trojans greeting a gift horse.

If manufacturers construct a dishwasher, a lawnmower, a motor car, or a ratchet screwdriver, and issue instructions with it,

I assume they know what they are doing. If the manual says the car owner should check the tyre pressures and battery level every week, then that's what obsessional creatures like me will feel obliged to do.

In the early days, the obligatory routines can be refreshing, an opportunity to give outward sign of the inner pride of ownership. When I got my first car, never were wiper blades more solicitously examined, never was chrome more lovingly lathered, never were tyre treads more assiduously inspected. And I revelled in the challenge to keep our first family lawnmower in fighting trim. Adjusting the height of the cut, adjusting the spark-plug gap, cleaning the rollers, even draining the sump: those were tasks I tackled with the quiet enthusiasm of one who cared.

The obsessional burden grew as, deluded that we were making life easier for ourselves, we acquired more household mechanicals with nuts to be adjusted, filters replaced, and vulnerable parts to be protected from rust. There was no room for compromise. The manuals were brutally frank about the consequences of neglect. I doubt we could have survived the shame if our lawnmower seized up on the front lawn or if killer rust ate into the vitals of our car and released a cascade of nuts, bolts, and washers over our high class residential road.

Often, of an evening, I would flop into an armchair exhausted by ritual tasks like cleaning the cassette recorder's heads, capstan, and pinch roller, the six-weekly adjustment of the agitator brushes in the carpet cleaner, the essential monthly check on the operating temperature of the yoghurt maker, and the mandatory weekly scraping of the crumb tray under the toaster. (I wonder how many of you have read that piece of small print.)

On one such evening I recognised the nature of my illness and set about curing it with self-cognitive therapy. I now accept that all household mechanicals are disposable and, if need be, replaceable when they expire from maintenance starvation. As I've slowly shed the burden of obsession I've discovered that contentment comes to those who cultivate a few redeeming defects. People achieve maturity when they discover that while striving after perfection has a place when we're at our work or at our prayers, it has no place in our homes.

## Language barrier

Impenetrable curtain that occasionally descends between patients
and their doctors. The problem used to be medical vocabulary;
now more often it is medical vernacular.

> From a recorded conversation between a middle-aged GP
> and a young woman who had consulted him about her
> urinary symptoms.
> *GP: Are you sexually active?*
> *Patient: No. But my boyfriend is.*
> *GP (Pressing on undaunted): Does your urine burn?*
> *Patient: I've never tried to light it.*

> Query received by a doctor who writes a newspaper advice
> column:
> *Dear Doctor, The X-ray report on my Fallopian tubes says they
> are "visualised". My doctor is keeping this knowledge from me,
> and has told me nothing is wrong, but my husband and I are very
> worried. I don't know how my tubes got visualised, but would
> injections help to put it right ?*

## Lapsus linguae politicus medicalis

Medicated version of a common infection. Endemic in solemn
medical institutions.

At a GMC meeting the president responded to what I thought
was an eloquent plea by saying: "I'm not quite sure what to make
of your suggestion, O'Donnell. I suspect you want us to take it
with a dose of salts." I had to freeze my smile in mid-dawn. I had
thought it was a shaft of wit until he embarked on an elaborate
and embarrassing apology for his lingual lapse.

Medical politicians are more prone to slips of the tongue than
other doctors because they spend more time talking than thinking.
And because their audiences rarely listen, their verbal lapses often
pass unnoticed. We are therefore lucky that the journalist Paul
Vaughan misspent a year or two of his youth working as the
BMA's press officer and sometimes whiled away the hours
recording the lingual lapses of the BMA's Great and Good.

Some of the lapses illuminated, in a Freudian way, the speaker's
true intention. A member of the BMA Ethical Committee (as

opposed presumably to its unethical committees) summed up a dull but worthy speech: "Dr X has hit the nail on his head." Within minutes, another member suggested the committee was "going at present through a bad phrase."

Most of the slips were uncontaminated by Freudian association, just accidents befalling those who, eager to make their point, bulldozed their way through the language. Such a one was the London GP who said things like, "Let's accept this as more gist to our mill," or "It's time to get our teeth into something concrete." He once warned a committee: "We should, as the saying goes, fear the Danes when they bring gifts", thus confirming, said Paul, that all words were Greek to him.

## Latin
For centuries the language doctors used for cabalistic utterance.

The tradition ended in the 1990s when the editor of the *BMJ* banished Latin from its pages for the pragmatic reason that, unlike his predecessors, he had never been taught it. There had been warnings of its demise. Back in 1986 a prospective medical student at Manchester confessed at her interview that the only Latin she knew was *coitus interruptus*.

The loss of Latin robbed doctors of one of the great mystical tools of their trade. My GP father dispensed his own medicines and I remember him handing out potent looking bottles of black fluid labelled *Mistura Tussis Nigricans* which I doubt would have been one tenth as effective if labelled Black Cough Mixture. This mystical power wasn't confined to prescribing. Latin helped doctors treat patients with description rather than prescription. A patient told he had *pruritis ani* could enjoy a satisfaction he might have been denied if told he had an itchy bottom.

In the end the *BMJ* decision was not as catastrophic as many doctors feared. Other cabalistic languages were available. *BMJ* contributors continued to rely on the enigmatic vocabulary of psychspeak (qv) and, with the ingenuity for which our profession is renowned, identified another one ripe for exploitation, the language of abbreviation (qv).

As you can no longer say in the *BMJ*, *omnia mutantur nos et mutamur in illis.*

## Laughed out of court

The only possible response, you'd think, to some US medical lawsuits. Sadly it isn't.

When I was in California in 2002 I caught the announcement of the finalists for an annual award for the most frivolous yet successful medical lawsuit of year. The front runners included:

Kathleen Robertson of Austin, Texas, broke her ankle when she tripped over a toddler who was running amok in a furniture store. A jury awarded her $780,000 despite the fact that the misbehaving toddler was her own son.

Carl Truman of Los Angeles, aged nineteen, won $74,000 and medical expenses when his neighbour ran over his hand with a Honda Accord. The accident happened when Mr Truman failed to notice there was someone at the wheel when he tried to steal the hub caps.

Kara Walton of Claymont, Delaware, was awarded $12,000 and dental expenses after she fell from a window in the ladies room of a local nightclub and knocked out two front teeth. The accident happened while Ms Walton was trying to climb in through the window to avoid paying the $3.50 cover charge.

Terrence Dickson of Bristol, Pennsylvania, burgled a house, then tried to leave via the garage but couldn't open the garage's automatic door. When the door leading back to the house slammed behind him, the security lock snapped in. The family was on holiday so Mr Dickson had to survive for eight days on a case of Pepsi and a sack of dry dog food he found in the garage. When he sued the homeowner, claiming the experience had caused him undue mental anguish, the jury awarded him $500,000.

I don't know who won the award that year. I left the country before the result was announced. Nor did I discover what prize was on offer. I would have suggested a trip to the cleaners with a lawyer of your choice.

## Lay lines

Geographical determinants of gender. Neatly summarised by Robert Herrick in 1630.

> *Who to the North, or South, doth set*
> *His Bed, Male children shall beget.*

## Learning lessons

Expensive method of self education favoured by the Department of Health.

In February 2009, Radio Four news broadcast the latest instalment in a continuing saga:

*The chief executive of London's Royal Free Hospital, where a new computerised medical records system was on trial, says it has left a £10 million hole in his budget and it now takes four times longer than previously to book in outpatients. The Department of Health says it is learning lessons.*

Learning lessons won't necessarily solve the problem. The Department of Health, especially when it grapples with information technology, has a nasty habit of learning the wrong lesson. Mark Twain described the process in *Pudd'nhead Wilson's New Calendar,* written, would you believe, in Guildford.

*We should be careful to get out of an experience only the wisdom that is in it – and stop there; lest we be like the cat that sits down on a hot stove-lid. She will never sit on a hot stove-lid again, and that is well; but also she will never sit down on a cold one any more.*

## Learning opportunity

Medical euphemism for misadventure.

In the mid-1960s, an Australian anaesthetist, regarded by his colleagues as something of a philosopher, defined the three essentials of anaesthetic practice.

- Always check the oxygen supply.
- Always identify the patient and the operation.
- Hate all surgeons and hate the slow bastards most.

Around the same time, a British anaesthetist Brian Lewis was in the early days of his career. One night, a casualty officer got him out of bed to help with a patient who'd tripped when leaving a pub and broken his wrist. The casualty doctor wanted to reduce the fracture under anaesthetic and, because it was a busy night, asked Lewis "to get the patient under" while he attended to another in the room next door. The patient with the broken wrist was Polish and his name Slobachanski (Lewis's notion of a pseudonym when he later wrote about the case).

Lewis and a nurse found their patient in the waiting area, sitting on a bench clutching his right arm. They confirmed he was Mr Slobachanski and had a signed consent form in his notes. Lewis checked the spare oxygen cylinder before they helped their patient onto the operating table and, as he started the anaesthetic, he completed the Australian triad of "essentials" by directing acerbic thoughts at the casualty officer who'd got him out of bed.

When the casualty officer arrived, his patient was well anaesthetised. Yet when he picked up the right arm he discovered the wrist was perfectly normal. He and Lewis put the X-ray on the viewing box and it clearly showed a fractured wrist. Their puzzlement turned to concern when they examined the other wrist and found that that too was normal. Their concern dissolved into panic when a man closely resembling the patient walked into the room, more than slightly inebriated and his right arm in a sling. He'd just returned from the lavatory, he said, and wondered what they were doing to his brother who'd come to take him home.

The man's perception was so blunted by alcohol that doctors and nurse were able to persuade him that his brother had fallen asleep. They then whisked him into another room, anaesthetised him, and reduced his fracture. Later, when both brothers had recovered from their anaesthetic, they were despatched by prepaid taxi to North London with a carefully worded letter for their GP.

At nine o'clock the following morning Brian Lewis rang his medical insurance company for advice. Yet he never heard a word of complaint from either brother. For the rest of his career, however, he got many complaints from patients who thought he took the process of identification to obsessional lengths.

## Lecture

A ritual that, once upon a time, allowed the notes of a teacher to become the notes of a student without passing through the minds of either. Now recognised as an academic period set aside for rest and recovery, or for diversionary entertainment.

In many medical schools, according to Peter Medawar, the most reliable place of refuge from harassment is a lecture theatre. In *Advice to a Young Scientist,* he wrote, "no sleep is so deeply refreshing as that which, during lectures, Morpheus invites us so insistently to enjoy." Physiologists, he wrote, are impressed by the speed with which the ravages of a short night or a long operating session can be repaired by a nod off during a lecture.

Journalist Philippa Pigache described how the students of B F Skinner, the behavioural psychologist, experimented on him during his lectures. They rewarded him when he moved to a certain position on the rostrum by offering rapt attention but whenever he moved away from the desired spot they shuffled, coughed and fidgeted. Eventually they had the arch-conditioner pinned to a corner of the platform below the desk.

When Donald Longmore, physiologist and medical inventor, arrived to give an evening lecture to a local medical society, he discovered that the membership consisted entirely of old men. He'd been asked to discuss the engineering problems involved in designing an artificial heart but first had to dine with the members who joyfully demolished vast quantities of food and drink.

During the lecture, by Longmore's own account, each member of the audience nodded off in turn and, when he finished, the silence was so deafening that it woke the chairman who immediately rose to his feet and said: "I'm sure you'll all join me in expressing our thanks in the usual manner to Dr Barnes Wallis for his fascinating talk on the dambusting bomb." Whereupon Longmore received polite applause and everyone went home.

## Legacy doctors

Doctors in private practice who specialise in acquiring bequests.

Some fifty years ago when a revered legacy doctor fell ill, I was hired to look after his Regular List – patients he visited at the same time each week, each fortnight, or each month. All had been on the list for at least a year, many for ten years, and one had had a weekly bedside consultation for the previous twenty-two years. Most were women whose tycoon husbands had dispatched themselves to an early grave accumulating the wealth their widows now frittered away on frivolities: expensive hairdressers, expensive boxes of chocolates, expensive flower arrangements, and expensive regular visits from an expensive private doctor.

My biggest problem was trying to discover the topics on which I was expected to converse during the hour allotted to each. I quickly discovered that the one thing Regular Visits didn't want was any form of clinical examination... other than the doctor holding their wrist in pulse-taking mode while they told him long rambling self-centred stories. The condition their doctor was treating was, of course, loneliness, though I was never sure whether he was treating it or exploiting it.

Legacy doctors create these profitable Regular Visits by the early establishment of an Agreed Illness. This illness must not be too incapacitating to interfere with the pleasures of a well-upholstered life, yet serious enough to need regular attention. It must also offer the possibility of an occasional spectacular 'attack' that demands dramatic medical intervention and sympathetic clucking from sycophantic friends.

The ideal Agreed Illness has to be specific both to patient and doctor. The patient, when talking to impressionable friends, has to be able to say: "My liver (kidney/womb/metabolism) is unique, you know. Every doctor, and I've seen the very best my dear, has been quite baffled by my X-rays." But unless she can add, "Indeed they're so complicated that only dear Dr Handholder can understand them", dual specificity had not been established and the patient could, after a minor tiff, take her profitable illness – and her legacy – elsewhere. (See Harley Street.)

All in all, legacy seeking is an arduous business and best left to experts. Serendipitous opportunities arise in general practice but need delicate handling. Dr Laurence Knott, a GP in Enfield, had a ninety-six-year-old patient who owned a collection of antique furniture his doctor admired and secretly coveted.

During one home visit, the conversation took a hopeful turn.

"D'ye see that writing desk, doctor?"

"I do."

"Do you like it?"

"Yes. It's very beautiful."

"I believe you doctors like antique furniture, don't you?"

"This one certainly does."

"Well I was thinking… "

"Yes… "

"When I die… "

"Yes… "

"You ought to buy it. I'm told it's worth a lot of money."

## Legal niceties

Civilised exchanges that occur when members of the learned professions engage in discourse.

Two characteristic exchanges were recorded in the *Massachusetts Bar Association Journal*:

*Lawyer: Do you recall the time you examined the body?*
*Doctor:  The autopsy started around 8.30 pm.*
*Lawyer: And Mr Dennington was dead at the time?*
*Doctor: No, he was sitting on the table wondering why I was doing an autopsy.*

A few years later in another court.

*Lawyer: Before you began your autopsy, did you check if the victim was breathing?*
*Doctor: No.*
*Lawyer: Did you check if he had a pulse?*
*Doctor: No.*
*Lawyer: Did you check if he had brain activity?*
*Doctor: No.*
*Lawyer: But why not?*
*Doctor: Because part of his brain was sitting in a laboratory dish on top my desk.*

*(Pause)*
*Lawyer: But is it still not possible he could still have been alive,
nonetheless?*
*Doctor: Well, yes, it is possible he was alive. But he would have
been fit only to study law.*

## Leisure Centre

Euphemism for Aggression Centre. Site of much unhealthy
activity.

There was one in the town where once lived. One day, when I
eavesdropped in its dressing rooms, I heard little talk of having
fun but much discussion of how to get 'psyched up'. Small
wonder that the games themselves, from squash to basket ball,
were heavily beset with accusations of cheating, actual cheating,
and angry and aggressive exchanges between players.

Our local sportspersons were no more intemperate than
others; their attitudes, like their tracksuits, came off a production
line. They knew, because they've been told it so often, that the
only object of sport was to win. There was so much competitive
activity I was reliably informed that you couldn't get in the
swimming pool and just splash around because everyone was
swimming 'programmed lengths'.

My reliable informant, a local doctor, said that when he went
for what he hoped would be relaxing swim, he'd barely entered
the water when an aggressive Thirty Something dived in behind
him, then surfaced and shouted: "How long are you going to be
blocking this lane, grandad?"

To which he replied, God bless him, "Until my bladder's
empty, young man."

He was then left in peace to enjoy five minutes of contented
dog-paddling.

## Lèse majesté

In law, an offence against the dignity of a reigning sovereign.

Hospitals, ever fearful of the law, impose rigorous restrictions
to protect royal visitors from anything unsavoury. A Surrey
hospital, recently granted a royal visit, locked the public lavatories
in the main hall for fear a lowborn subject might exit unwittingly
from Ladies or Gents into the royal presence.

Occasionally during a royal visit a chief executive will graciously invite a senior doctor or nurse to act as hospital guide. The essential attribute they need is not grandiloquence but the facility to bend the truth without denying it.

The role-model is Dr William Whewell, the 19th century scientist and polymath who became Master of Trinity College, Cambridge. Gwen Raverat in *Period Piece: A Cambridge Childhood*, refers to a day when Queen Victoria visited the university and Dr Whewell showed her round his college.

When they reached Trinity bridge, they paused and looked over the side. In those days the River Cam was polluted by a sewer and pieces of lavatory paper drifted in the water.

"What are those papers floating down the river?" asked the queen.

"Those, ma'am," said the slick-witted Dr Whewell, "are notices that bathing is forbidden."

## Libidinal shift

Phenomenon that Freud associated with penis envy. Dr Fred Charatan, a retired geriatrician living in Florida, offers a more useful definition: the shift of appetite in old age from the genitals to the alimentary tract.

This change in libidinal desire, says Dr Fred, is an oft-ignored cause of obesity in old age. As we grow older, eating and drinking grow more gratifying and the insidious increase in weight not only restricts mobility but subverts the motivation to take regular exercise. He exemplifies the condition with a tale about Rome's Licinius Lucullus, still commemorated, in the form of an adjective, for his dedication to self-indulgence. One evening a friend, who saw his cooks preparing a particularly extravagant meal, asked who were the special guests he had invited. "Tonight," came the reply, "Lucullus will dine with Lucullus."

## Lingual strangulation

Impediment that occurs when self-importance determines a speaker's vocabulary and syntax.

Often strikes when people are over-impressed by pomp and ceremony and feel compelled to 'pomp-up' their own performance.

A definitive case was recorded during the making of the BBC Television documentary *Royal Family* in 1969. During the ceremony when the new American Ambassador to London, Walter Annenberg, presented his credentials to the queen, television cameras captured his reply when she asked him how he was settling into the embassy.

*Your majesty will not be cognisant with the fact that at this point in actuality, have unscheduled logistical and transportation deferments, so that predicted levels of re-furbishment items, why, er, at this time we have a shortfall in our present, er, what we would normally, er, acceptable re-furbishment levels.*

## Life after death
Achieved, without benefit of medics or clerics, by actors and television pundits you once knew.

Thanks to repeats of ancient programmes and black and white films, old friends whose memorial services I attended years ago, seem to live on. Indeed their work evokes their presence so powerfully I sometimes feel that, if I picked up the phone and dialled their old number, we could share the same sort of gossip we once did.

I got the feeling strongly the other evening watching Leonard Rossiter play the indestructible Reginald Perrin – maybe because he brought to the character his own delight in the way people use words. He once told me how, when he was searching for a theatrical digs in Glasgow and was unsure of the address, he knocked tentatively on what he hoped was the right door.

A formidable woman appeared.

"Excuse me," said Len, "but are you Mrs McKay?"

"Indeed I am not," said the woman. "Quite the reverse."

## Listening
One of the 'key communication skills' (qv) taught to medical students and postgraduates.

They are told, unsurprisingly, that they should listen to their patients, and are taught techniques to show that they are listening.

They are less often taught a lesson actors learn early in their training: real listening means attending to the meaning of the words you hear and monitoring the audience response to the words you speak, even when they are words you have heard or spoken a hundred times before. Each patient is a new audience with a different level of attention or response, so doctors, like actors in a long running play, must beware of settling for a routine trot through the role.

Like actors, they must also learn not just to pay attention but to respond, and to respond naturally in their own individual way. I once talked to an ageing actor who'd just done a spell in a TV soap . He'd enjoyed it because he was surrounded by people who knew their craft – with one exception. This was an actor still in his twenties who had appeared in over 200 episodes of soaps but, maybe because that was the sum of his experience, had one glaring defect. The others found him impossible to play to because they got nothing back. Dead eyes, said my chum. That's all you got. Dead eyes.

As he spoke, I remembered times in my own career when I saw a patient who needed to be understood glancing desperately around the room as if seeking for someone who could provide the response that clearly wasn't coming from me.

## Literalism
Interpretative disorder which compels the brain to accept only the literal meaning of a word.

First described by the comedy mastermind Denis Norden who was himself a literalist. One evening on Radio Four's *My Word* he offered what is now recognised as the definitive account of the disease.

*On being confronted with the headline* Public borrowing down, *my instinctive response was "What a strange thing for members of the public to be borrowing. Just shows how many people must be stuffing their own duvets." And when I turned to the Arts Page and found a story headed* Hockney draws large crowds, *my immediate thought was, "Well, I suppose it must make a change from drawing swimming pools."*

For those condemned to take words at their face value the commonest hazards, said Denis, were Public Notices, ranging from Neighbourhood Watch, – *for which the cinema inside my head never fails to screen a picture of local people popping round to see what time it is* – to a sign once seen on London's Northern Line trains: Passengers Alight Both Ends.

Non-literalists can have great sport mimicking the disorder. When Willy Rushton stayed in one of those American hotels where the pretension to luxury is never quite matched by the achievement, he found a room service menu that proclaimed: *We are proud to serve breakfast at any time.* So he rang the kitchen ordered "Bacon and eggs in the Early Renaissance".

In 1993, when a medical journal publicised the condition, a literalist doctor wrote approvingly of the sensible advice pharmacists print on the labels of drugs dispensed for old people, *Keep away from small children.*

And Dr Ramindra Seth, a GP in Nottingham, posed a question non-literalists found difficult to answer. Why did farmers talk about cows being in calf when to his eye it was clearly the calf that was in the cow?

Other readers identified environmental features most of us take for granted but could be hazardous for literalists. The public car park at Wareham in Dorset, for instance, is dangerous territory for female literalists. The wall above one door bears the traditional sign *Ladies*. But alongside it is another: *Have you paid and displayed?*

Julian Churcher, a South West London GP offered evidence that Literalism is not an exclusively British disease with a charming example. A 'temporary resident form' completed by a French visitor applying for NHS treatment included the entry:

Name of Doctor at home: *Docteur.*

## Literality

Form of word blindness in which victims grow blind to the literal meaning of just one word.

A condition so infectious it entraps sufferers and their colleagues in a world from which they find it difficult to escape, as in this exchange on Radio Three.

"He literally brought the house down,"said Paul Crossley.

"Yes," responded Michael Berkeley. "It was exciting to see the way he set that hall alight."

## Literary companions

A wise person's alternative to counsellors.

Enduring friends who sit on your shelves waiting to comfort you in sickness and in health. Ruth Holland tells us why they are so valuable:

*In literature, time and distance mean nothing; you can meet the dead just as happily as the living, and they will take you into their confidence, tell you their jokes, give you the benefit of their opinions and experience, and ask for nothing in return but your eye on the book.*

## Literary fever

Symptom that occurs when a book we read while we're ill gets irretrievably entwined with the illness.

Was the nauseous claustrophobia between the decks of a sailing ship in *Rites of Passage* created by William Golding or by the salmonella demanding their own rights of passage through my intestines? As the narrative grew more febrile in the closing chapters of *The Poet*, was it the influenza virus or Michael Connolly who raised my temperature? And I'll never know whether the depression that descended during the *The Power and the Glory* was imposed by Graham Greene or by the streptococci colonising my tonsils.

One combination of book and illness has such a powerful grip on my psyche that the merest mention of Baroness Orczy floods my nostrils with a strange medicinal smell that once emanated from the school infirmary, or was it from the school matron?

Differential diagnosis: Literary fever should not be confused with the nausea induced by a couple of contemporary authors whom it would be too expensive for me to name.

## Little old lady

Demeaning label male doctors affix to a woman of any size who looks as though she might qualify for a pension.

The phrase fits all sizes because it is a measure not of physical but of social stature: an acceptable label for NHS patients but not for, say, the late Queen Mother of whom it was a literal description.

Its use as a status indicator grew during the post-war years when middle class families could no longer afford living-in servants and used the services of local journeymen and women whom they patronised as if they were personal possessions. In the 1950s when I went into practice in affluent suburban Surrey, well-heeled patients would say, "I have a little woman in the village who cleans the carpets for me – real little treasure she is" or "We have a lovely little man who comes and does the garden."

Confirmation of the etymology came on the day a rather grand patient asked me, "Do you know our little man who looks after the boiler? Mr Wilson. Real treasure. Lives in one of those flats over Woolworths?"

Joe Wilson was one of my patients. Six feet tall and weighing around fourteen stone. But, like Joe, I knew his place. On the social scale that is. Little.

## Lohengrin effect

In the beginning comes the word. And, in medicine, the power of the word is enhanced by the Lohengrin effect.

Lohengrin arrives on a swan just in time to save Elsa. He becomes her hero and promises to become her husband provided she doesn't ask him his name. Yet, hardly has the last bar of the wedding march faded when Elsa, displaying the sort of boneheadedness without which operas would have no plots, asks the forbidden question and Lohengrin catches the next swan back up the Scheldt.

This phenomenon of people losing their power once they are named recurs in fables ancient and modern from Rumpelstiltskin, through Turandot, to Last Tango in Paris. In the hands of a doctor, it can be powerful medicine.

"Is this throat of mine serious?" asks the patient.

"No," says the doctor. "Just pharyngitis."

"Good," says the patient. The evil has lost its power. It has a name.

A Southampton GP, Dr KB Thomas investigated the power in a study of 200 patients who were unwell but in whom he could make no definite diagnosis. (Other studies have shown that GPs make 'no definite diagnosis' in 40 to 60 per cent of patients they see in their surgeries.) He divided these patients randomly into two groups. To the first he gave a firm diagnosis – a name – and told them confidently they would be better in a few days. To the second he gave no name but just said, "I cannot be certain what is the matter with you."

Two weeks, later 64 per cent of those in the first group were better, but only 39 per cent in the second.

Another GP, Simon R. Barton from Cornwall, described how the Lohengrin effect influences doctors and the way they practice: a patient diagnosed by a GP as having chilblains can be diagnosed by a hospital doctor as having Perniosis.

The difference has significant implications for patients. Chilblains have been described in British textbooks for over a century. They are a common, self-limiting disorder, managed by most GPs in a ten minute consultation. In a hospital, wrote Dr Barton, "the same condition warrants blood tests, a skin biopsy, presumably multiple consultations and a fancy name."

Meanwhile in another part of the forest, when chilblains occurred in women who exercised horses in cold weather in Virginia, USA, they were reported as a new disease – Equestrian cold panniculitis – and subjected to a battery of investigations to determine the pathology of what was only a new name. That is the power of the Lohengrin effect.

## Long sentence

Punishment imposed on doctors foolish enough to look for information in memoranda they receive from colleagues.

The usual stretch is seventy-three words, as in this specimen written by a London specialist in community medicine:

*When I have completed my enquiries with the medical and supporting services I intend to get the Authority's approval to put this on a formal basis and will then be sending copies of what I have finally decided is the best approach to the Area so that these discussions can be put on a formal basis, in order that a composite multi-disciplinary report covering all aspects of this proposed move can be prepared.*

An American physician Dr Edmund J Simpson discovered this example in a psychiatric report:

*Her spontaneous replies from unconscious sources within her indicate that the therapeutic goal of reorienting a portion of herself that has been so frantically and anxiously dependent upon outside sources of support has been responding to, accepting and depending upon internal sources of wisdom and strength and that this has lessened the panic coming from this source, and has also given the self a means of internal influence upon the formerly uncontrollable anxiety.*

It conforms to the traditional length of seventy-three words but Dr Simpson wondered if it really was a sentence. "Every time I look for a verb I get a headache."

Doctors foolish enough to seek information in NHS management documents are usually given a longer stretch. Here is a 252-worder created by an 'Operational Executive' at the Queen's Medical Centre in Nottingham when replying to a doctor who inquired about the meaning of a phrase in another document.

*'Soft Money' is any money received by or payable to any employee of the Trust, anyone holding an Honorary Contract from the Trust, (or the agent of either of them) or any Trust Fund which is used or intended to be used for the benefit of the Trust, University Hospital or any of the Trust's employees, honorary contract holders, patients or any undergraduate or postgraduate student at University Hospital, which has been received in good faith and not stolen from the Trust, and which is not held in an account opened by the Trust in accordance with Standing Financial Instructions (Section 7) and reported in the Trust's Annual Accounts, nor held in an account opened by the Special Trustees for Nottingham University Hospitals in accordance with their Standing Financial Instructions and reported in their Annual Accounts nor in the case of an honorary contract holder paid into an account in the name of his or her employer and which has been received by or is payable to, such person or Trust fund as a result of that employee or Honorary Contract Holder  acting (actually or ostensibly) under or in connection with his or her Contract of Employment or Honorary Contract with the Trust and which has been given or is paid or payable in return for service rendered or to be rendered by the Trust or that person in his or her capacity as such employee or Honorary Contract holder or for the benefit of the Trust, its patients, staff Trainee or students.*

## Lost in translation

The sense of humanity that disappears when we subject complexities of human behaviour to text book explanation. (See Reductionist snobbery.)

It's tempting to argue that novelists offer more perceptive insights into human behaviour than the authors of medical textbooks, but that's not always true. What is true is that novelists usually write more readably and are more likely to clothe an interesting thought in a memorable image.

Take, for instance, this thought about health and ageing that Edith Wharton offers in *A Backward Glance*.

*In spite of illness, in spite even of the arch-enemy sorrow, one can remain alive long past the usual date of disintegration if one is unafraid of change, insatiable of intellectual curiosity, interested in big things and happy in small ways.*

A medical textbook author, following the traditions of the genre, might express the same thought thus:

*Elderly persons, even those who have had a debilitating illness or significant depressive symptoms, may exceed their expected longevity if they are prepared to:*

- *Readily accept change in their own circumstances and in the world around them.*
- *Keep mentally active by:*
  *a) taking an interest in the political and social issues of their time,*
  *b) drawing pleasure from the minutiae of their own existence.*

I reckon I know which version a reader is more likely to remember.

## Lovesickness

Obsessive mental state explored by poets, novelists, painters, and composers; ill-understood by psychiatrists; largely ignored by neuroscientists.

A multiple choice quiz in a Sunday newspaper posed the question: *Are you really in love?* The points awarded for each answer seemed to encourage the 'Don't know's, so I was pleased that, unlike an agony aunt, the omnipotent intelligence behind the quiz didn't recommend those in doubt to consult their GP. In matters of the heart – save those that involve it as a pump – doctors are notoriously bad advisers.

When I was a GP, a patient did once ask me, "Is it really love, doctor?" but he turned out to have fallen in love with himself and sought advice only because the affair wasn't going too well. A year or two later when a young woman asked, "Am I in love, doctor?" I muttered a couple of platitudes before I realised that the last thing she wanted was an answer. So I said she probably knew better than I did. She responded with an enigmatic smile, not unlike that of the *Mona Lisa,* and we spoke no more of the matter.

Though medical textbooks have little to say about this common affliction, poets and lyricists are a rich source of diagnostic symptoms. When I was at the susceptible age the symptoms fell into three groups:

Pyrexia – *Sighing like furnace.*
Incipient deafness – *There were bells all around and I never heard them ringing.*
Forgetfulness – *I left my heart in San Francisco.*

That is the nearest I've come to understanding the condition. Lovesickness is one of a handful of afflictions – another is eczema – about which I know less and less the older I grow.

There was a time I thought the diagnosis easy. Thanks to a prepubertal diet of Hollywood films, I cruised into adolescence convinced that, though I might not know what love was, I would recognise it when it hit me. When Miss Right entered and our gazes locked across a crowded room, music would swell in the background. It pains me to recall how many attractive young women I ignored because, when we met, my attentive ears caught not one hint of violins.

Later personal experience taught me that lovesickness, as opposed to loving someone, is a self-limiting condition. Now, from the embitterment of old age the only diagnostic advice I'd give is that offered by Dorothy Parker:

By the time you swear you're his,
Shivering and sighing
And he vows his passion is
Infinite, undying –
Lady, make a note of this:
One of you is lying.

## Lucy's disease
An affliction of proud, lonely people. The eponym, suggested by Richard Asher, derives from Wordsworth's *Lucy.*

*She dwelt among the untrodden ways*
*Beside the springs of Dove,*
*A maid whom there were none to praise*
*And very few to love.*

When Asher defined the syndrome he described how great an event a medical consultation could be in the lives of lonely people, satisfying the need we all have to be noticed. An elderly person, he wrote, may be too proud to complain of loneliness but suffers no loss of pride in complaining of symptoms.

*A child cries, "Look at my sand castle"; a lonely old person cries, "Look at my stomach". The child says, "I got two goals this afternoon"; the lonely old person says, "I got two giddy turns this afternoon".*

Consultations with lonely people are often acts of deception practised in private between consenting adults. Both doctor and patient sustain the illusion that what is being sought is medical advice when the true substance of the transaction is companionship. As Asher explained:

*Lonely people miss not only companionship, but also the advice and criticism that go with it. Under the guise of seeking advice about health, a lonely lady may be seeking advice about family affairs. Ostensibly she is asking for advice about her bad heart, but* au fond *she seeks advice about her bad nephew.*

## Lucky guesswork
Phrase used by doctors who haven't learned from their mistakes to dismiss a form of wisdom possessed by those who have.

As Jane Austin wrote in *Emma*, "Depend upon it, a lucky guess is never merely luck, there is always some talent in it."

## Lump scale
In the age of the Caring Professional a useful measure for predicting which patients may respond to words rather than action.

Best explained by comparing cases from opposite ends of the scale.

At one end is a cultured person with a slight blemish on the back of a hand. Such persons may enjoy a session with a doctor who explores their social background, disentangles the psychodynamics of anxiety and conflict in their work and family, and whose conversation conjures a vision of the Renaissance.

At the opposite end is an equally cultured person whose lump is the size of a golf ball, red and angry-looking, with sinuous blood vessels throbbing across its surface. Such persons may grow fractious as the Renaissance doctor explores the complexities of their family life and start to look over the physician's shoulder seeking a gruff surgeon with a sharp knife.

## Mace
Gilded reproduction of outdated weapon of war much favoured by medical institutions.

Rarely put to useful purpose, though Michael Heseltine once swung the House of Commons mace around his head and burned off excess energy when he might otherwise have done something dangerous, like sitting down and thinking.

Anthony Clare told me that, when the college of psychiatrists was being founded, the longest and most heated discussion was over whether this new, exciting, and different college should have a mace. In the end, according to Anthony, the pro-macers won because the anti-macers could not rebut the argument proposed by one speaker that "a mace will help to open doors".

## Malaproposis.
Form of dysphasia that enables patients to demonstrate to their doctors that the *mot juste* is not always the *mot évidente*.

A patient of Eric Webb, a GP in Milton Keynes.
*I've just put in for my infidelity allowance.*

A patient of Andrew Marshall, a GP in Doncaster.
*I'm worried about the wife. She's becoming very confused and forgetful. I wonder is she getting Oldtimer's Disease.*

From Tom Madden's notes made in a South London general practice in the 1950s and 60s.

*I've brought the baby to be humanised.*
*I can't conceive. I've been serialised.*
*Bowels are all right now. I've been taking some apéritifs.*

## Malignant growth
Inexorable proliferation of senior managers in the NHS.

When Thatcherite neocons created an artificial 'internal market' in the NHS in 1989, we were told that competition would improve efficiency, cut bureaucracy, and ensure 'value for money'.

At the time there were 500 senior NHS managers. Five years later there were over 20,000.

In the late 1990s the number of senior managers increased by a further 48 per cent while the number of nurses increased by less than 8 per cent and the number of beds fell by 25 per cent.

In January 2003, thanks to rigorous Blairite pursuit of the neocon policy, the neolabs pulled off a remarkable achievement. The number of NHS administrators outnumbered the number of NHS beds. The Queen Elizabeth Hospital in Birmingham made a stab at an entry in the Guinness Book of Records by employing 1,300 administrators to manage its 1,000 beds. This heroic achievement was driven by the need to monitor the internal market (qv).

In 2004 a leaked cabinet document revealed that the cost of hospital administration, £3 billion in 1997 when the neolabs came to power, had risen to £5 billion. The same years had seen an increase only a 2 per cent in the number of treatments and a fall in hospital "productivity" – whatever that may mean – of 15 to 20 per cent.

The malignancy lies not in the administrators but in the growth. Most hospital managers are as dedicated and hard working as most doctors and nurses. The internal market ensures that most are employed not to manage the care of patients but to manage one another.

## Maliloquence
Rhetorical flourish that frees an excuse from any suggestion of
guilt or responsibility. Essential skill for NHS managers.

> Hospital Trust chairman replying to critic at public
> meeting: "We are not running a two-tier system. We are
> merely prioritising our admission protocols on the basis
> of different parameters."

> When local doctors complained that Bath's Royal United
> Hospital had raised its prices after budgets had been set, a
> hospital spokesman told reporters: "The adjustment arises
> from a more robust pricing methodology to address
> historic inconsistencies. Translated into English, this
> becomes: "We are correcting the mistake we made when
> we fixed the original prices."

## Mammon
Medical icon. Replaced Hippocrates some time ago.

> Nadine Cool of Wisconsin sued her psychiatrist, Dr
> Kenneth Olson, for malpractice, claiming he had
> convinced her that she had some 120 personalities –
> including Satan, angels who talked to God, and a duck –
> then charged her insurance company $300,000 for group
> therapy.

Dr Albert V Harmon's seminal work *Large Fees and How to Get
Them,* published in Chicago in 1911, is packed with helpful hints.

> ***Ways of getting additional fees from patients who have
> already paid well for the original treatment.***
> *It is a well-understood fact among physicians that the average man
> of fifty or over takes more interest and pride in his sexual virility
> than in any phase of his physical system. Where men of ordinary
> means will haggle over a $250 fee for being successfully treated for
> some annoying, really dangerous ailment, they will pay $1,000 or
> more cheerfully on anything that seems like a reasonable assurance
> of having their sexual power restored to its pristine vigour.*

*While conducting your examination pay no attention to the sexual organs at first, but, when nearing the end of the examination, say casually: "How long have you been in that condition, Mr. X?" This is a random shot, but it will strike home ninety-nine times out of a hundred. You have got your human fly stuck on a gummed trap from which he couldn't extricate himself if he would, and he doesn't want to.*

## Managerial revolution

Initiative governments launch every few years to solve NHS problems that don't exist by creating problems that do.

Invariably heralded as the final solution to NHS woes in stirring Arcanian (qv) prose.

*Today's main need is to provide management with the financial information necessary to control performance and to assist the multidisciplinary planning function. Apart from the characteristics of health care, a number of arguments support this ground-up approach to our work. The main purpose is to achieve health delivery services that will become the building blocks on which more streamlined higher organisation levels can be based.*

That uplifting message came not from the Cameron/Clegg coalition of 2010 but from the Heath government of 1972.

And, come to think of it, that too was going to transform the NHS by making it more efficient, more businesslike, more responsive to consumers, etcetera, etcetera, etcetera…

## Man in the street

Also known as The Common Man.

Patricians in the patronising professions – Law, Politics, and Medicine – will often tell you that their social and political judgements are in harmony with the views of this mythical creature, though I suspect only judges believe that omnibuses still travel across Clapham Common.

The delusion so comforts those who cling to it they never seem to wonder why it so often turns out to be untrue. Nor do they appreciate that those whom they patronise learned long ago how to ignore the insult and fight back. The best riposte I know dates from the early 1960s and came from a wine waiter at the Garrick club whose name was Barker – servants in those days were assumed to have only surnames.

One election night when the members were congregated around the bar, drinking champagne and awaiting the results, a bibulous High Tory announced: "What we really need to know is how the common man voted." So he called over Barker.

"Now Barker," he said. "This evening you represent the common man. So tell us how you voted."

Barker replied with quiet dignity: "I didn't like to presume, sir, so I voted Labour."

## Manufactured diseases

Diseases created in pharmaceutical marketing departments.

As the supply of useful drugs from research departments slowed, and new drugs grew increasingly expensive to develop, pharmaceutical companies realised that creating new diseases for old drugs could be more profitable than seeking new drugs for old diseases.

Long standing behavioural problems were given portentous names. Shyness became Social Anxiety Disorder; impotence became Erectile Dysfunction; premenstrual tension became Premenstrual Dysphoric Disorder; and the success of Viagra prompted the discovery of a profitable new market, Female Sexual Dysfunction.

The aim of 'disease mongering' is to convince people with ill-defined functional disorders, or common behavioural traits, that they suffer from a medical condition that needs long term treatment with a drug that just happens to be available. As a sceptical New York physician put it: "These guys have found yet another way to divide the world into two groups: those who've got a disease that needs drug treatment, and those who've yet to discover they've got one."

The game is played world wide but is at its most intense in the US, where stakes are higher and regulation more relaxed. Christopher Lane, a London-born professor of English at Chicago's Northwestern University, analyses the US game in his book, *Shyness: How Normal Behavior Became a Sickness.*

In the 1980s doctors regarded shyness as a social impediment; only in rare extreme cases was it labelled a social phobia. Yet by 1994 it had become a common condition, Social Anxiety Disorder, which acronymises conveniently into SAD.

Lane claims that GlaxoSmithKline decided to promote it as "a severe medical condition" to boost sales of its antidepressant Paxil. In 1999, the company received approval to market it for SAD and launched a national promotional campaign. In the US, prescription drugs can be advertised publicly to encourage people to get a prescription from their doctors, and Paxil posters in bus shelters across the country showed solitary despondent individuals captioned *Imagine being allergic to people...* The campaign was a huge financial success.

Disease mongering has been particularly successful with psychoactive drugs. (See Customised disease.) Marcia Angell, former editor of the *New England Journal of Medicine*, described how children became vulnerable targets:

*We are now in the midst of an apparent epidemic of bipolar disease in children (which seems to be replacing attention-deficit hyperactivity disorder as the most publicized condition in childhood), with a forty-fold increase in the diagnosis between 1994 and 2003. These children are often treated with multiple drugs off-label\* many of which, whatever their other properties, are sedating, and nearly all of which have potentially serious side effects.*

\* i.e approved for use only in another disease.

## Marital detumescence
Waning enthusiasm demonstrated by a simple experiment.

If you put a bean in a jar after each coition in the first year of a marriage, and remove a bean from the jar after each coition in subsequent years, you will never empty the jar.

Dr William H James called this phenomenon "the de Vries effect" after reading in Peter de Vries's *Witch's Milk*:

*Sex in marriage is like a medicine. Three times a day for the first week. Then once a day for another week. Then once every three or four days until the condition has cleared up.*

## Market traders
Designated role for nurses and doctors in the 'modernised' NHS revered by NeoLab and NeoCon visionaries.

We grumpy old farts aged over eighty, who remember pre-NHS Britain, grow a bit testy when Johnny-cum-latelies insist that the 'market system' is the only route to efficient health services.

The Oxford historian Charles Webster, Senior Research Fellow at All Souls, defined our reasons in a lecture to the Royal College of Physicians when the 'internal market' (qv) was first mooted. Britain's health services before the war, he said, "contained many of the elements of the market system towards which there is now a reversion" and "had demonstrated that the market system was a failure." The remarkable improvements in health care produced by the NHS were "achieved by methods contrary to market principles and which rejected the purchaser/provider split."

I grew up in a GP's household in pre-NHS days and was a student when the NHS was launched with the altruistic passion that young men and women brought home from the war; I worked as a GP and later as a journalist through those long years when the NHS was said to be on the point of collapse but managed somehow to muddle through; then in the 1980s – the decade in which we legitimised greed – I watched the altruism seep away as the wartime survivors retired and handed over to the market traders.

When the post-war government introduced its National Health Service Bill, it captured the spirit of the time. A friend, demobbed that year from the RAF, told me: "It may sound terribly pious, but the NHS did seem to sum up all the things we were told we were fighting for: a fair deal for everyone, with the strong helping the weak as they had done during the blitz, as we had done in the desert and in Europe." My memory of the spirit of the times accords with his. True, we had black marketeers and conmen who emerged from their bunkers once the fighting was over but there was an unselfconscious altruism around that needed little fuelling with political or religious slogans.

It's sad that those of us who experienced that time are now so muted, apologetic even. Sounding "terribly pious" is a grievous sin in a society that expects you to hunger after 'lifestyle', when to be too overtly concerned with the welfare of others can earn you the pejorative label 'wet', and when, if we have a government crisis, the lights burn late not in Whitehall but in the offices of Saatchi and Saatchi.

These days, those who would dismantle the NHS show more energy than those who would preserve it. In 1948 no one needed to explain that caring for the sick involved considerations that didn't encumber market traders. There is evidence that the sort of altruism that stirred the post-war politicians does still exist. But today's politicians, like the rest of us, seem frightened to acknowledge it. Surely there are ways, other than war, to rekindle the spirit that made 1948 a good time to be alive.

## Marriage guidance
Introductory advice on the art of compromise.

Once provided by GPs with variable results. Results improved in the 1940s when trained professionals took over. Yet in 2011 BBC Radio Four reported that Britain's most consulted guides were the same as in the 1930s... women's magazines.

One of my friends confessed that back in the 1970s, when she'd been married for four years, she read in a magazine, "Are you taking your marriage for granted? Are you putting enough effort into keeping your marriage fresh?"

Because her answers to both questions were ambivalent, she decided to take the article's advice: "Every so often, surprise your husband by greeting him when he gets home from work in the same way you would greet him if he were arriving to take you on your first date – put on a dressy frock and spend some time on your hair and make-up."

They were so hard up that the only 'dressy frock' she had was the 'going-away dress' she'd worn on her wedding day. So she put it on, put the recommended effort into hair and make-up, and waited carefully posed in an armchair for her husband to come home.

When he walked into the room, he took one look at her and said: "Oh Gawd. Don't tell me we're going out somewhere."

One of the troubles with guidance, as every GP learns, is that it doesn't necessarily lead in the right direction.

## Massage
Traditional treatment deployed with increasing enthusiasm in the modernised NHS. Still used to treat patients but more often used to treat numbers.

Hospitals use it to treat statistics designed to meet targets impossible to achieve: waiting lists, waiting times, staffing levels... that nature of thing.

Pharmaceutical companies, medical suppliers, management consultants and other private contractors use it to treat data that could help them market their products or services. (See Absolute risk.)

Political apparatchiks use it to firm up meaningless anecdotal snippets into meaningful 'evidence' that can be used by spokespersons. (See Smoothsayer.)

## Masturbation

Disease that in the second half of the 19th century, and the first half of the 20th, was assumed to occur only in males and threatened to destroy the youth of Britain.

Dr William Acton described the symptoms in his monumental work *The Function and Disorders of the Reproductive Organs, in Childhood, Youth, Adult Age, and Advanced Life, Considered in their Physiological, Social and Moral Relations* published in 1857:

*The frame is stunted and weak, the muscles underdeveloped, the eye is sunken and heavy, the complexion is sallow, pasty, or covered with spots of acne, the hands are damp and cold, and the skin moist. The boy shuns the society of others, creeps about alone, joins with repugnance in the amusements of his schoolfellows. He cannot look anyone in the face, and becomes careless in dress and uncleanly in person. His intellect has become sluggish and enfeebled, and if his evil habits are persisted in, he may end in becoming a drivelling idiot or a peevish valetudinarian.*

In 1908 the printer Horace Cox refused to print the first edition of Baden-Powell's *Scouting for Boys* until some "far too explicit" paragraphs were removed. One passage to which he objected was:

*The result of self-abuse is always - mind you, always - that the boy after a time becomes weak and nervous and shy, he gets headaches and probably palpitations of the heart, and if he carries on too far he very often goes out of his mind and becomes an idiot. A very large number of the lunatics in our asylums have made themselves mad by indulging in this vice although at one time they were sensible, cheery boys like any one of you.*

Another deleted sentence ran:

*Remember too that several awful diseases come from indulgence – one especially that rots away the insides of men's mouths, their noses, and eyes, etc.*

The saddest deletion was that of wholesome advice offered to boys who felt the urge coming on: *Just wash your parts in cold water and cool them down.*

The version Cox eventually printed was so enigmatic that many a boy scout must have wondered what was the dangerous activity against which he was being warned:

*This 'beastliness' is not a man's vice; men have nothing but contempt for a fellow who gives way to it.*

The high incidence of the disease still caused concern in the second half of the 20th century. In May 1974 Patrick K Fitzgerald wrote in the *Irish Medical Times*:

*I feel that the major cause of masturbation is bad genital hygiene. In the United States masturbation is rare. This I believe is due to two factors: a) circumcision of all males at birth; b) a high standard of genital and general hygiene.*

Dr Fitzgerald made his claim that the disease was rare in the United States eighteen years after the death of Dr Kinsey.

## Matthew dictum, The

Unfortunate fact of life for those condemned to publish or to perish. Enunciated in the King James Bible, Matthew 13:12:

*For whosoever hath, to him shall be given, and he shall have more abundance: but whosoever hath not, from him shall be taken away even that he hath.*

In 1982, two US psychologists D P Peters and S J Ceci resubmitted twelve scientific papers from prestigious institutions to the journals that had published them during the previous three years. They made cosmetic changes to disguise the papers but did not change the content. They did, however, change the names of the authors and institutions, creating fictitious names and unpretentious institutions that did not have the prestigious ring of the originals.

Only three journals recognised the papers as ones they had already published. Eight of the nine undetected papers were rejected by the journals that had previously published them. Not one was rejected because it added nothing new.

Clearly, when it comes to getting published, the hath nots need more help than the haths.

Luckily help is available. Just before Peter and Ceci published their results, J. Scott Armstrong working at the University of Pennsylvania found evidence, while reviewing scientific journals, of the existence of an 'author's formula': a set of rules authors can use to improve the chances of their manuscripts being accepted. His formula offers six rules based on the evidence he collected.

- Do not choose an important problem.
- Do not challenge existing beliefs.
- Do not obtain surprising results.
- Do not use simple methods.
- Do not provide full disclosure.
- Do not write clearly.

The secret, it seems, is one that any experienced journal reader would have guessed: avoid doing any thing positive or anything that might frighten the horses.

## Medical Agenda
1. (*Obsolete.*) A list of things to be done.
2. Any complex medical problem that defies simple management. Once labelled an agenda, it no longer needs to be solved, analysed, or even examined, merely addressed (qv).

## Medical committee
A group in which politely diffident doctors are manipulated by politically ambitious ones.

The purpose of medical committees is to seek consensus. They achieve this when the politely diffident accept that the only way they'll get out of the room is to endorse the views of the politically ambitious.

## Medical committee games
Diversions used by the politely diffident to insulate themselves from mind numbing proceedings.

In my early committee-sitting days I relied on a game devised by Jeremy Bullmore when chairman of J Walter Thompson. It's called Inventaproverb and you play it by creating a saying that, though meaningless, sounds wise and aphoristic.

You then have to drag it sententiously into the discussion, scoring a point if other committee members accept it as relevant or even thoughtful.

Bullmore's original creation, which is difficult to surpass, was *Somebody has to bury the undertaker.* I had reasonable success with *The patient who sees the doctor is not always the patient the doctor sees,* and scored many a point with *Success is merely failure in reverse.* Both these offer double value because you can use them straight or inverted.

I also found I could score points with a less-well crafted inventions by prefacing them with the phrase, *I think it was Churchill who said…"* (With later generations, I replaced Churchill with Nelson Mandela.) But the secret of winning points with Inventaproverb is getting the tone of voice right. (See Medical committeespiel.)

An equally rewarding game is Interrogative Blocking which can halt even the most intransigent of bores. The question should sound relevant but be unanswerable. The Lifemanship guru Stephen Potter recommended: *Yes, but that isn't really what we're discussing, is it?*

If you want to get your own back on a truly painful bore, you can't beat a form of Interrogative Blocking called the Transferred Question, which incites arguments between others and allows you to sit back and enjoy the squabble you've created. Here are a couple of templates that have served me well:

*Personally I don't feel strongly about this but I don't understand how you can ignore what Professor Bumbler just told us?*

*Surely what George is saying, chairman, is that your report ducks the issue?*

Vengeful players who seek to cause serious damage use statements camouflaged as questions to introduce uncertain – or, even better, invented – data: *Surely it was established some time ago that the normal is 49.87?* or *Isn't he the chap who caused all the trouble at Birmingham?*

In the Double Whammy version of this ploy, you wait for someone to question the data you've introduced, then snap back with an Interrogative Block: *Do you really not care what these figures mean in terms of broken lives?* or *Doesn't it worry you that the operating theatres could be unsafe?*

## Medical Committeespiel

Blend of language and intonation that committee persons know will carry them to the top. The art of making the right sort of noise… literally.

Experienced spielers know that, if they keep rhubarbing away in an unrelenting monotone, their audience will soon become hypnotised by the sound of the words and lose grasp of their meaning. I once heard a GMC president finish off a protracted monologue with the sentence: "Of course, I'm just talking out loud." And, because the words made the right sort of noise, those who sat round the table nodded in agreement as if they were in the presence of profundity.

## Medical diary game

Display ritual popular with the medical Great and Good.

In the real world when we try to fix a date with friends we look in our diaries and say something like: "Can't manage the 7th and the 9th, could manage the 15th but I'll have to rearrange something. Apart from that I'm free."

Very Important Doctors (VIDs) turn this simple transaction into an impressive ritual akin to a male peacock's sexual display of his feathers. At the end of a meeting of VIDs, the chairman will intone the traditional antiphon. "We need to discuss this again. I think we should check our diaries." Each player then takes out a pocket diary and flicks through closely written pages. Once the pages have been flicked all eyes turn towards the chairman who, using his diary as a prayer book, launches the liturgy.

"Can't manage the 7th. Meeting of the Government Strategy Group. On the 9th there's the College council. On the 12th we have the Royal Commission inaugural meeting. You on that, Roger? Oh. I thought you would be. And the day after that, of course, there's the Department's Working Party…" and so on, and so on. Once the chairman has played his hand others follow with talk of Task Forces, BMA committees, Strategic Frameworks, and Steering Groups whose very existence is unknown to normal medical folk.

I encountered the Diary Game at the first committee meeting of my stint as rebel in residence on the GMC. As the chairman intoned his opening move, I realised I had come naked to the conference table. My diary contained only two entries: *Collect Lucy from Brownies* and an exclamatory shopping reminder *New underpants !!!!!* When it came to my turn, I just mumbled the days I could or couldn't manage, which rather pleased the chairman because it confirmed his suspicions about me.

And so I managed down the years until one afternoon, emboldened by lunch with Robert Robinson and exhilarated by wine, I toddled off to a GMC meeting. That day, as occasionally happens, the Diary Game was the first, rather than the last, item on the agenda. After the others had made their moves I decided to play a hand. "Can't manage Friday," I heard myself say. "Long weekend with the Devonshires. Tuesday p.m. I have an audition at the National Theatre, and all day Thursday I'm helping Prince Charles write a lecture on Alternative Medicine."

To my everlasting chagrin, and I still sense it as I write, not one eyebrow flickered. The chairman just said, "Seems its going to be Wednesday then. Shall we make it 2 p.m."

## Medical identity
Something patients find easier to define than their doctors.

Much of the healing that goes on in general practice derives from the fact that a problem aired and put into words is easier to countenance. Sometimes the results achieved by allowing patients to sort out their troubles just by airing them in our presence tempts us to inflate the part we have played in the process. Richard Asher offers a useful deflationary tale.

*A father, thanking me for giving some psychological treatment to his son, said: "I think it's done him a lot of good being able to tell all his troubles to someone. When I was his age I used to tell all my troubles to a large rubber duck, and it seemed a great help. I suppose you're much the same sort of thing."*

## Medical pronunciation
That which distinguishes a genuine doctor from any other well-known brand of person.

Ruth Holland described some of the elements in a *BMJ* article. Patients, she wrote, are prescribed "cheemotherapy" but not advised to take their prescriptions to the "cheemist". They may also suffer from "enkephalitis". That, say doctors stuffily, is correct. But, says Ruth, it's not what the rest of us say, nor does the *Oxford English Dictionary:* "c before e, i, y, is soft". And if they're so correct, how many doctors go to the kinema on their night off?

"I suppose," wrote Ruth, "we must just accept it for what it is: a professional oddity, a sign that you belong, like a BMA car park sticker, or a verbal equivalent of the Masonic handshake."

The clinical physiologist Dr Kenneth John Collins offered me another example of pronunciation's diagnostic power. Emphasising that true research involves constant re-questioning of received truth he had noticed that, just from the way they pronounced the word, he could distinguish the genuine *re*-search worker from those who just report research.

## Medicated folklore

Apocryphal tales that fulfil a human need once satisfied by mediaeval fables: bizarre events alleged to have involved a friend or a patient – or a patient of a friend – which doctors insist on telling you while insisting even more vehemently that they are true.

Back in the 1970s I described in a medical journal how in just one month I'd been solemnly assured by readers that the same incident, with slight variations, had occurred in Bilston, Croydon, Exeter, and Liverpool. Thirty years later, I received reports of the original 'Bilston incident' re-occurring in Windsor, Harrogate, and Lancaster all within the space of six weeks.

In this tale the 'friend of a friend' to whom "it really did happen" is a tennis player who, when he serves, tucks the spare ball into the pocket of his shorts. At the end of a match he forgets to remove it and when he's in the bar notices a girl looking suspiciously at the bulge in his shorts. Somewhat embarrassed, he explains: "It's only a tennis ball".

To which she replies: "That must be very painful. Last year I had a tennis elbow."

Another tale I've heard only twice – so far. The first time was in Los Angeles where the teller was a psychiatrist who claimed a local surgeon had overheard the conversation.

The second time was in Atlanta where a cardiologist who buttonholed me at a party claimed that one of his colleagues had spotted a former patient, a tall young Southern Belle, in a smart store in the Lennox shopping mall and had overheard this exchange.

"I'm not worried about the colour or the style, I just want shoes with the lowest heels you got."

"To go with what madam?'"

"A short, fat, and very wealthy gentleman."

## Medicelebrities
Doctors whose reputation owes more to publicity than to achievement.

### Christiaan Barnard
Surgeon who on 3 December 1967 became an 'international celebrity' by performing a singularly unsuccessful operation.

The first patient to receive a transplanted heart, fifty-three-year-old Louis Washkansky, died of pneumonia eighteen days later. When his condition started to deteriorate, Barnard was out of the country, jetting round the world on a publicity tour.

The man who established heart transplantation as an effective treatment was the American surgeon Norman Shumway and, despite the setbacks caused by the precipitate action of Barnard and others, he and his team at the Stanford Medical Center in California eventually made it an acceptable operation.

Shumway and Richard Lower, his colleague at Stanford, had been the first people to transplant a dog's heart successfully and then devoted eight years to intensive research into ways of preventing, detecting, and treating tissue rejection. Shumway decided his team would not operate on a human until a dog with a transplanted heart had survived for at least a year. Barnard came to Stanford during the experimental programme and learned the operative technique which makes no great demands on surgeons. Observers at Stanford think he then went back to South Africa and "jumped the gun".

Because he wanted to avoid publicity Shumway was reluctant to criticise Barnard at the time of the disastrous South African operation but when I interviewed him nine years later he suggested that the best way to decide whether a team was ready to operate on a human was to ask it to produce an animal that had lived for six months after a heart transplant. "That condition was not fulfilled in South Africa," he said. "They never had any animal that lived more than a few hours."

A special issue of the *South African Medical Journal* appeared within days of Barnard's 'breakthrough' and was wholly devoted to the 'miracle'. Even the ads joined in with celebratory messages. "Well done, Chris!" cried the suppliers of the ligatures.

The main article signed by Barnard and his team was headed *Successful Human Heart Transplant*; the front page carried an announcement, edged in black, of the death of Louis Washkansky. The combination echoed the ancient medical jest that the operation was a success but the patient died.

## Alexander Fleming

Doctor who won international renown for failing to recognise he'd discovered the first 'miracle drug'.

Ten years later Howard Florey and his co-workers at Oxford realised the drug's potential and developed it's use as a treatment. Yet Fleming readily accepted all the glory.

Though Fleming did literally discover the existence of penicillin, he seems not to have understood its significance. When the now famous mould contaminated a bacterial culture at St Mary's Hospital, London, he gave it a name, noted that it seemed to produce an agent that killed bacteria, showed it was non-toxic to animals, used it in just a few cases but without much success as a local antiseptic, suggested it might be injected locally, then turned his mind to more interesting things.

His record of these events remained virtually unnoticed for ten years until it was found in a library by a young chemist working in the department of pathology at Oxford University. Ernst Chain, a Jew born in Berlin, had fled to England when Hitler came to power and it was he and his professor, Howard Florey, who turned penicillin from a laboratory curiosity into the first 'miracle drug'.

One reason Fleming got all the glory was that he had that most valuable of medical advisers, a spin doctor. The newspaper magnate Lord Beaverbrook was closely associated with St Mary's, the hospital was hungry for publicity, war-stressed Britain needed a hero, and Fleming, unlike Florey, was happy to cooperate with journalists.

Though he'd played no part in the Oxford work, Fleming allowed himself to be portrayed as a hero who had spent those ten wasted years in a long struggle to harness his discovery and once claimed, "I would have produced penicillin in 1929 if I'd had the luck to have a tame refugee Jew chemist at my right hand."

He even allowed journalists to suggest that he had produced large quantities of penicillin at St Mary's for use there or at Oxford under his direction. As the *Dictionary of National Biography* records in its 1981 biography of Florey, *Such distortions, continuing uncorrected for many years, created a general impression that only Fleming's name should be associated with penicillin.*

## Edward Jenner

An impostor who claimed in 1796 to be the 'originator' of small pox vaccination.

The first known vaccination was performed nearly a quarter of a century earlier by a Dorset farmer, Benjamin Jesty. The event is commemorated on a tombstone in the cemetery at St Nicholas in Worth Matravers on the Isle of Purbeck in Dorset.

*Sacred to the memory of Benjamin Jesty (of Downshay)*
*who departed this life April 16, 1816 aged 79 years.*
*He was born in Yetminster in this County,*
*and was an upright honest man*
*particularly noted for having been the first Person (known)*
*that introduced the Cow Pox by Inoculation,*
*and who from his great strength of mind made the Experiment from the*
*(Cow) on his Wife and two Sons in the Year 1774.*

Celebrating the centenary of Jesty's experiment, Bryan Brooke, Professor of Surgery at St George's Hospital London wrote:

*It seems to me that Jenner must have heard what Jesty did; but there was never a mention, never an acknowledgement by him, nor is there by those who write today about the history of vaccination. Can it be a conspiracy of silence by the medical profession – starting possibly with Jenner – because the first known vaccinator was not a medical man?*

## Medicine and the Media

Topic popular with organisers of medical meetings when scientific subjects lose their pulling power.

High on my list of resistible invitations are those to symposia that have the phrase, or anything resembling it, in the title. The rubric is depressingly predictable: a day – or, God defend us, sometimes two – of polite exchange of grudge and prejudice topped off with a moment of consensual high mindedness. Then the journalists rejoin the world where *Jogging cures cancer says Top Doc,* and the doctors with a mission to explain go off to meetings held *in camera* because that's the way their meetings always have been held.

One problem is that Medicine and Media are blanket words and, like blankets of another kind, cover multifarious activities. When used in tandem they describe a territory so broad it invites folk to range across it, scavenge in selected areas, then shape their scavengings to fit any theory they wish to promote.

Over the years, I've decided that when doctors ask me how to 'deal with' importuning journalists, television producers, and folk of similar ilk, the only useful advice I can offer is that, like other people, they have to learn to live in a world in which the media exist. They need to judge, as they do with patients, whether the individual with whom they are dealing is trustworthy or manipulative, and use their clinical shrewdness to assess the motives behind any promises being made. The notion of cosy consensus, though the *raison d'etre* of the public relations business, does not appeal to journalists; nor come to think of it to ambitious competitive doctors.

Doctors should remember that journalism, by its nature, is arbitrary, over-influenced by fashion, and unfair. Medical reporting is just as arbitrary as any other sort. Those who practice it can quote a host of instances. David Loshak claimed he cemented his tenure as medical reporter on the *Daily Telegraph* by writing regular uplifting stories about the hospital where his news editor's mother had received kindly treatment. Joan Shenton devised a Channel 4 series on the victims of drug injury after she suffered disastrous side-effects from a drug she took on holiday. And I readily admit I once won an award for something I wrote after walking absent-mindedly into the wrong meeting and sitting next to a man who had a good story to tell.

## Medico-legal brief
Paradoxical title of un-brief document, consisting of prose devised by lawyers to ensure that doctors who need to understand it have to employ other lawyers to translate it.

This letter to a Harrogate GP, Dr Michael Matthews, offers a fine example of the prose.

*We are not enclosing at this stage Mrs X's letter of consent on confidentiality, since if she is not capable you will no doubt say so, and any consent given by her would in any event not be valid if she is capable, no doubt you will merely advise us that you do not see any objection, in which case we respectfully suggest this would not involve the divulgence of any confidence, otherwise, you may wish in any event to advise on your next visit or consultation with her, in which case you will no doubt seek her approval generally as appropriate.*

And that, mark you, is only one sentence in a long, long document.

## Mediquotes
Penetrating insights into current events provided by media medical correspondents.

When a Saudi Arabian court sentenced a British nurse to repetitive flogging, *The Times* medical correspondent told us what we would never have guessed without his expertise. *The punishment will be as much psychological as physical. She will know that, even after she has lived through any particular session, the whole process will be repeated again many times. The sentence will inevitably bring on severe depression.*

An anonymous doctor (traditionally introduced as A N Expert) told Radio Four's *Today* programme: *They are suffering from starvation due to lack of food.*

From the News on Radio Two we learned: *The grass pollen count issued by the Asthma Research Council at 10 a.m. today was nil – which Dr Anderson says is very low.*

## Memorable achievements
Less common in the lives of real people than in ceremonial speeches, introductions of visiting speakers, obituaries, and hospital newsletters.

The prouder the boast the greater the need for close examination. I suggest you apply this golden rule of scepticism to a triumphal claim Dr J S Randhawa of Wythenshawe discovered in a newsletter from South Manchester's Old Age Psychiatry Service:

*The results* [of a survey] *again indicate that 100 per cent of memory clinic patients are either satisfied or very satisfied with the service provided.*

## Metaphoresis.

Addiction to extravagant images that develops in doctors who don't listen to the words that they write.

John Gardner in *Clinics in Obstetrics and Gynaecology: Contraception: As the concept of wrongful life swims upon the precarious seas of judicial reasoning, one wonders whether it will serve forth a veritable Pandora's box of litigation to become a fish bone in the throat of obstetric practice.*

Anonymous US physician displaying his bejewelled prose in *Res Medica: The neurologist with all of his knowledge of minutest anatomy was for years, "like the man who stood on the bridge at midnight," not dreaming the dreams of a Longfellow but soliloquising after the manner of the cynic on the vanity of all earthly things when the voice of the syphilographer first cried out from the darkness "Fear not for I am always with you."*

Simon Chapman in *British Medical Journal: Since then he has served as a bipartisan consultant to several governments, furthering his reputation as a creative egg cracker in medico-political cake baking. And the cake of long waiting lists and spiralling costs needs the cracking of an emu sized egg...*

Letter from a GP to a surgeon: *Many thanks for seeing this over-stretched record producer who has been burning the candle at both ends and has now developed rectal bleeding.*

## Metaphoretic dysphasia.

Using metaphor to disguise lack of substance. A common ingredient of High Falution (qv).

In December 2008, Professor Peter Rubin wrote in the *BMJ*:

*The GMC as regulator has to walk the tightrope between maintaining standards and moving with the times. It's not easy, but it's important to walk the tightrope, not stand still on it.*

Quite so. Unless, of course, your name is Blondel and you're carrying a balancing pole.

But hang on a minute. A tightrope is stretched between two points. So the metaphor poses immediate questions. In which direction does the GMC have to walk: towards maintaining standards and away from moving with the times, or vice versa? If the GMC can't stand still, what we readers want to know is which end is it aiming at. Professor Rubin doesn't tell us. He raises the question but the answer gets lost in the metaphor.

It's possible, of course, that the professor's 'ear' betrayed him when he was groping for another cliché. "Treading a fine line," perhaps. That would make a sort of sense, treading the delicate border between "maintaining standards" and "moving with the times". But it would destroy the conclusion he draws from the metaphor. Treading a fine line doesn't become dangerous if you stand still. Indeed it's rather sensible to do so – preferably often and for long spells. It gives you time to think.

## Milestones

Events that mark our progress along the road to oblivion.

The textbook ones are pretty obvious. The ages at which we crawl, stand, walk, start school, come of age, marry, become parents. More depressing are the middle-age ones we observe never in ourselves but in our contemporaries. Most have to do with flesh sagging rather than melting and doubts metamorphosing into opinionated certainty.

Post-pension milestones receive less attention. You will search textbooks in vain for mention of the age at which bottles of wine hold less than they used to or the age at which the only follies we regret are the ones we didn't indulge when we had the opportunity. Nor will you find the milestones defined by the American comedian George Burns:

*First you forget names, then you forget faces. Next you forget to pull your zipper up and finally you forget to pull it down.*

## Miraculous

Adjective journalists reach for when a sick people stage a recovery; the adjective when they don't is 'scandalous'.

Local newspapers, an occasional national tabloid, and sofa-sitters on televised magazine programmes, still describe someone who has had routine cardiac surgery as a 'heart miracle patient'.

The implication is that surgical survival rates are still the same as they were when the idea of anyone operating on the heart was one of the wonders of the world. (Just as the equally common accolade 'Miracle cancer survivor' implies that the diagnosis of any form of cancer is an immediate death sentence.)

Like one of the characters in Robertson Davies's *Fifth Business* I wonder why, when life itself is such a miracle, we make so much fuss about "potty little reversals of what we pompously assume to be the natural order".

## Misadventure proneness

A tendency to suffer minor but bizarre misfortune.

A disability with which I'm well-acquainted. Funny things really do happen to me on the way to the theatre. Denis Norden, who knows about these things, tells me it's a well recognised syndrome and I should be grateful for being blessed with it.

In the early 1970s I suffered a discomfiting episode in the artistes' ablutions at Lime Grove television studios.

I'd spent a week in New York at a medical conference which finished on Friday afternoon and had to be in Lime Grove on Saturday morning to talk about it on that week's recording of *Inside Medicine*. The overnight flight from New York was delayed for four hours and, on the plane, I was surrounded by noisy children and got little sleep. Luckily I'd written my script and cabled it to London so all I'd have to do would be read it off an Autocue.

I went straight from Heathrow to the studio, unaware that I was suffering the additive effects of jet lag and fatigue. I'm told I arrived, unshaven and red-eyed, and chattering enthusiastically about everything except American medicine. Even the producer Karl Sabbagh, a man of notorious tranquillity, was mildly disturbed to see me load a cup of black coffee with lump after lump of BBC sugar without first removing the wrappers. Karl suggested I didn't just shave but took a refreshing shower in the hope that when I read the Autocue I might look as if I knew what I was saying.

The Lime Grove ablutions were built in an age when showering carried no sybaritic overtones and existed only to protect schoolboys from ungodliness. I hung up my clothes, stepped gingerly across the duck-boards, and put my spectacles on the top of the cubicle. Then, still buoyant on jet-lagged euphoria, I stood beneath the steaming spray, singing loudly and tunelessly. As I turned off the shower, I heard a slithering sound as my spectacles slipped down the gap between cubicle and wall.

Luckily, I had sunglasses fitted with my prescription so I put them on and rejoined the production team. Karl accepted the news about my spectacles with his natural stoicism and sent the BBC janitorial squad to retrieve them. Meanwhile, I'm told, I treated the company to another monologue of unrelated sentences and stirred more unwrapped sugar into black coffee.

After half an hour, the janitor returned to say his lads had dismantled the cubicle. My spectacles had disappeared into the fabric of the building and, in his opinion, were likely to be recovered only by archeologists as yet unborn. The programme was about to start and now I couldn't read the Autocue. "You'll have to wear your dark glasses," said Karl. "If disgraced government ministers can do it, so can you." Quick as a jet-lagged flash, I came up with a more acceptable solution. Four people in the room wore glasses. Why not borrow a pair? I tried each in turn and found a pair through which I could read. The only drawback was they belonged to Michael Reinhold, the main presenter.

This was no time for quibbling. Karl gave us our orders. The American item began with some film. After the other Michael introduced it, he and I would swap specs while the film ran. I would then read my script from the Autocue and during a second piece of film, we would re-swap glasses. Later I would look down at my desk and shuffle my papers, keeping my tinted lenses away from the camera.

Miraculously the plan worked, despite the fact that we were sitting at opposite ends of a large studio and discovered that when two semi-blind men rush towards one another waving their specs, the recipient may have difficulty locating the hand of the donor. I'm told our blind man's square dance was more entertaining than anything the viewers saw, though Mrs Reinhold claimed to have been deeply affected when she recognised the same spectacles appearing throughout the programme with only the face behind them changing.

For writers and GPs, misadventure proneness is, as Denis said, less a disability than a blessing. The secret of enjoying both jobs is not to intervene but to sit back comfortably and watch… and, if the flames threaten to fade, throw another log on the fire.

## Mischief
Revivifying activity for those who seek to grow old disgracefully.

On the eve of my eightieth birthday I received an email from a contemporary who lives in New York.

> Yesterday I went downtown and popped into Joe's to collect a book.
> I was there only about five minutes but, when I came out, there was a cop writing out a parking ticket.
> I said to him, 'Come on, man, how about giving an old guy a break?'
> He ignored me and continued writing the ticket.
> So I called him a Nazi.
> He glared at me and wrote another ticket for having worn tires.
> So I called him a doughnut-eating pig.
> He stayed silent, finished the ticket, put it on the windshield with the first, then started a third for having a crack in the headlight.
> When all three tickets were in place, I walked away.
> I'd come downtown on the bus, and the car he was putting the tickets on had a bumper sticker saying 'I love Sarah Palin'.
> I try to have a little fun each day. It's important to my health.

## Mistakes
What doctors are not allowed to make yet from which they're supposed to learn.

The case for getting things wrong was well put by the American physician Lewis Thomas in his book *The Medusa and the Snail*:

*Mistakes are at the very base of human thought, embedded there, feeding the structure like root nodules. If we were not provided with the knack of being wrong, we could never get anything useful done. We think our way along by choosing between right and wrong alternatives, and the wrong choices have to be made as frequently as the right ones. We get along in life this way. We are built to make mistakes, coded for error.*

*We learn, as we say, by "trial and error" not by "trial and triumph". The old phrase puts it that way because that is, in real life, the way it is done.*

## Mixed-sex wards

Blemish on the NHS which nurses, doctors, administrators and politicians have tried desperately to remove but have never quite succeeded.

Fifteen years of failure have taken their toll. In 2011, two anaesthetists on a postnatal round found this notice on a ward door:

*Please be aware that in the maternity unit our policy*
*is to care for boys and girls in adjacent cots.*
*If you have any concerns regarding this*
*please will you discuss your concerns with the nurse in charge.*

## Modernising the NHS

Striving earnestly to fix that which does not need fixing while not fixing that which does.

The process involves turning relatively simple human activities into complex procedures that need elaborate managerial planning, outcome targeting, quality frameworks… etcetera etcetera. It's a huge drain on NHS resources because the task is usually delegated to cash hungry management consultants and supported by doctors in need of flattery, publicity, or a leg up the Honours List.

On 17 April 2009 a consultant physician, Professor Tony Waldron, wrote to the *The Times*:

*So, a former director-general of the BBC, a former chairman of John Lewis, a vice-admiral, an author, and the chief executive of a chain of US private clinics are going to sort out the NHS. It seems that the less qualified one is for a job, the more likely one is to be given it by the government. Those who work, or have recently worked, in the NHS know perfectly well what is wrong with it. Why doesn't anyone ask them? Or is the Government frightened of the likely answers?*

## Modesty

Becoming quality still found in the ritual of consultation.

In *Maybe the Moon*, Armistead Maupin, the gentle chronicler of San Francisco, writes of Aunt Edie who, whenever she visited her gynaecologist, took a special bag to put over her head during cervical examinations.

On this side of the Atlantic, a woman in her early thirties, attending a GP for an insurance examination, asked if he would also do a cervical smear. He agreed to do one and, after asking all the questions that insurance companies deem essential, ushered her into the examination room and told her to take off her clothes and lie on the couch under the blanket.

He closed the door and waited outside to give her time to undress. After a generous pause, he knocked on the door, waited for a response, went into the room, performed a full physical examination and took the cervical smear.

As the woman pulled the blanket back over herself, he asked: 'Do you have any questions?'

"Just one, doctor. Why did you knock?"

## Moment of truth

The discomfiting pause in conversation that invites intervention. Exploited by television interviewers and GPs who know that the longer the silence lasts, the more the interviewee feels the need to break it by adding a remark. And that remark is often the most revealing of the interview.

Intolerance of over-stretched silence develops at an early age. When my son was aged eleven, I took him to a matinee at a West End theatre and, in the interval, he needed to visit the Gents. The tiny room had a two-berth urinal where my son stood silently alongside a tall severe-looking man who wore a black jacket and pin-striped trousers. As the silence stretched, my son clearly felt the need to say something companionable to someone engaged in the same manly act. Eventually he looked up at the unsmiling face alongside and said: "Cartwright can hit the ceiling."

## Monologophobia

Debilitating condition that afflicts people who want to write but don't quite know how.

Theodore Bernstein of *The New York Times* defined the typical patient as someone "who would prefer to walk naked in front of Sachs Fifth Avenue than to use the same word twice in four lines of copy".

A French physician, Dr Peter Mark Roget, sought to ameliorate the symptoms with a treatment called Thesaurus. He hoped his dictionary would supply writers with alternative words but sadly its content – a doleful compendium of clapped out phrases – encourages them to substitute one cliché for another. Roget's progeny have now become part of word processing programmes and the combination of Roget and computers encourages the notion that words are interchangeable packets of digitised characters. This has bizarre side effects.

Sherrill Babcock, a Los Angeles attorney, was blocked from joining an online service when a software filter used to censor 'offensive' words refused to accept her surname. The Moderator for Member Services (sic) apologised twice for the inconvenience, telling Ms Babcock: "Unfortunately, the letters that form the word 'Cock' is (*sic*) unacceptable and will not be recognised by our system." When the site refused to modify the software, Ms Babcock got herself onto it by changing her cyberspace name to one acceptable to the software. She chose the name Babpenis.

Tim Richardson reported this happening in *The Register* to highlight the problems facing anyone hoping to spread the news that, thanks to a prickly referee and a mishit penalty, Arsenal won their game against Scunthorpe.

## Mortality

Concept that confuses the unthinking, many of them journalists.

A *Guardian* columnist, criticising the self-help leaflets available in GPs' surgeries, wrote: *Most failed to mention the importance of rehabilitation, which evidence shows reduces the risk of dying by 25 per cent.*

Encouraging news in an official press release from the Edinburgh Science Festival: *Teetotallers run a greater risk of dying than drinkers who consume in moderation, say researchers.*

A woman asked by her South London GP what had been the cause of her father's death: *I don't know really, but I know it wasn't anything serious.*

Rachel Simhon wrote in the *Daily Express*: *According to the study, men can cut their risk of dying by 36 per cent for every 100 orgasms they have a year.*
There could be duller ways of achieving immortality.

## Mother Nature
Malevolent old bat whom some worship as a benevolent matriarch.

Natural is a useful word if you want to sell health foods, but a dangerous one if you want to stay healthy. Natural foods and remedies have no intrinsic advantages over unnatural ones, indeed can be more dangerous. When I was a child I got a tuberculous gland in my neck because I drank natural cow's milk. If I'd had milk subjected to the nasty unnatural process of pasteurisation, I would have been spared a painful operation and my parents a great deal of worry.

Nature has no bias. It is neither for us nor against us. Natural laws can be defined as clearly – and work as inexorably – in the spread of an epidemic as in the birth of a healthy baby. Thousands of people are killed by 'natural disasters', most people die of 'natural causes' and doctors spend much of their time trying to repair bodies and minds that have been visited by a malevolent Mother Nature.

When I consulted a list 'natural therapies' issued by The British Foundation of Natural Therapies the first on their list was acupuncture. I'd be grateful if some barefoot philologist could tell me what is natural about having those needles stuck into you.

Insights into the inherent injustice of Nature are granted not just to doctors but to all who work at the sharp end of life. The *Police Review* published the story of PC Francis of the Cheshire

Constabulary who stopped his Panda car when he saw a cat stalking a baby sparrow. He got out of the car and chased the cat away. Aglow with satisfaction at a job well done, he got back in the car and, as he drove off, ran over the sparrow.

## Münchhausen

Baron Karl Friedrich Hieronymus Freiherr von Münchhausen, an 18th century teller of tall tales, won his place in European literature thanks to Rudolf Raspe's political satire *The Surprising Adventures of Baron Münchhausen.*

He won his eponymous place in medical literature in 1951 when the London physician Richard Asher used the name to label the behaviour of disparate individuals behaving in disparate ways who had only one thing in common: they were intensely irritating to doctors and nurses.

Those of us attracted to Richard Asher's lectures by his impish sense of irony heard him explain how he purloined the Baron's name to illustrate his proposition that if you took a collection of symptoms, called it a syndrome, and gave it a memorable name, doctors would start diagnosing it. He stuck the Münchhausen label on a tiny collection of individuals who went from hospital to hospital telling dramatic and untruthful tales that deceived ingenuous doctors.

Their tales were plausible enough for the storytellers to be admitted and they sometimes ended up on an operating table, their abdomens becoming scoreboards where the number of scars recorded the number of surgeons deceived. They nearly always discharged themselves against advice after quarrelling violently with doctors and nurses.

Asher stressed that Münchhausen Syndrome was a descriptive not a diagnostic label – and a description of behaviour, not of motive. Individuals had different reasons for embarking on a voyages of deception. These included:

- Wanting to be the centre of interest and attention. Walter Mitty fantasy in which, instead of playing the surgeon, they assumed the equally dramatic role of patient.
- A grudge against doctors and hospitals which could be satisfied by frustrating or deceiving them.

- Wanting to get drugs.
- Trying to hide from the police and seeking refuge in a hospital by swallowing objects such as nails and chains, enlarging or infecting wounds, or warming up thermometers.
- A desire to get free board and lodging for the night.

Asher suspected these scanty motives were supplemented by some "strange twist of personality" but warned us against accepting a description as a diagnosis or a disease.

Yet, in my professional lifetime, I've seen what started as bizarre behaviour being impishly upgraded by Asher to a syndrome, and more recently upgraded to a disease.

We have medicalised so many aspects of our lives we should refrain from the reckless creation of new diseases... and of 'proxies' of non-diseases. But that is another kettle of fishy tales.

# N

## Name badges
Labels issued to hospital staff to prevent them from stealing one another's working clothes.

Also issued at medical school reunions. A futile gesture. For the first thirty or forty years physical changes rarely hinder recognition of old friends. When physical change becomes so great that people need a label to help identification, their vision is no longer sharp enough to read the names on the badges.

## Nasty turns
Sometimes called 'funny turns'.

Peculiarly British symptom. Usually described with pride – "Had another of those nasty turns last Friday" – possibly because of the Music Hall tradition that the nasty turns of today are the stars of tomorrow.

A hospital doctor writing to Quentin Shaw, a Telford GP, described one of his patients as: "The lady with funny terns." When Dr Shaw consulted his aunt, a keen bird watcher, she explained that the syndrome is well recognised. Arctic terns and common terns are sometimes difficult to distinguish and when ornithologists are unsure they call the bird a comic tern.

## National illness service
Favourite butt of health campaigners.

"What we have in this country…" the MP, concerned doctor, or caring spokesperson pauses for a moment, "is not a National Health Service but a National Illness Service." The speaker smiles triumphantly and the audience erupts into applause.

Yet what's so wrong with an illness service? It's certainly more useful than some of the crazier edifices erected in the name of health. Caring for sick and disadvantaged individuals has always been doctors' main contribution to society. Politicians, epidemiologists, and some medical researchers deal with the health of communities; front-line doctors and nurses generally concern themselves with the illnesses of individuals.

Sick people appreciate the virtues of an illness service. As a patient I've been happy to let others pursue the fantasies of the WHO definition of health (qv) while I settled for a mundane 'patch up' job from the kindly doctors who removed my gangrenous appendix, zapped the malevolent bacteria that invaded my lungs, restored the blood supply to my heart, replaced my opaque lenses and may one day have to replace my worn-out hip joints.

They may not be advancing the concept of Health, as considered by deep thinkers at week-end seminars in country houses, but in these islands the patching up is done by skilled people, many of whom show concern about our plight as individuals.

Until we've actually built the New Jerusalem, I remain grateful for the skill and understanding we can find in our imperfect but, by no means, incompetent 'illness service'. To use the phrase as a pejorative is to demean the useful service our profession has rendered to the human race since a caveman first removed a thorn from another caveman's foot.

## Natural

Highly effective marketing 'concept': not man-made, therefore wholesome.

Doctors don't see Mother Nature (qv) as a benevolent old lady. Indeed they spend most of their time trying to protect people from the ravages of our often hostile natural environment and, when protection fails, trying to repair the damage.

Yet the mythology lives on and 'natural' was the great selling adjective of the late 20th century, its inclusion in an advertisement or on a label guaranteed to improve sales.

Its 21st century successor, equally illogical, seems to be 'herbal.' Every hotel bathroom I visit is stocked with herbal soap, herbal shampoo, and herbal 'shower gel'. (Gel is another word that titillates today's marketeers). I reckon I achieved the ultimate reward when my bathroom contained not only a neatly packaged *Potter & Moore Herbal Bath-cap* but a *Potter & Moore Herbal Mending Kit.*

## Natural childbirth

Doctor-free parturition. Phrase coined in the 1920s and 30s by campaigners who wanted to free women from the need for analgesia during labour. Since then has been annexed by groups promoting any unusual way of conducting childbirth.

In *The Cynic's Dictionary*, Russell Ash asks:

*What could be more natural than a woman giving birth while naked, supported by a hairy French doctor, singing "La Marseillaise" and dropping the baby into a plastic paddling pool full of dirty, tepid salt water?*

As is the way with enthusiastic campaigners, promoters of unusual methods attribute failure not to the process – nor, heaven forbid, to themselves – but to their patients. When French women started to complain that the Lamaze method of 'painless childbirth' had in fact been unbearably painful, a French obstetrician claimed in *Le Monde* that such a thing was impossible. If a woman suffered pain, she had started her training too late or had not trained hard enough.

## Negativism

A not uncommon professional quirk that makes it not unusual for medical writers not to accentuate the positive.

Often found in letters to GPs from consultants who think a double negative adds dignity to their prose. As in this fine specimen created by an orthopaedic surgeon:

*The fact that there is no evidence to believe that they are due to tuberculosis or mental illness would not necessarily lead me to conclude that they are not due to these things, but it would lead me to conclude that there was no reason to believe that these causes were responsible for the pain and disability.*

More pernicious is the use of negativism by medical writers more concerned with sounding 'scientific' than being understood. In 2005 the authors of a paper in the *Canadian Medical Association Journal (CMAJ)* offered their 'interpretation' (*sic*) of the result of a drug trial:

*Our results did not support the research hypothesis that placebo was non-inferior to amoxicillin and that rates of clinical resolution would not be substantially worse in the placebo group than the treatment group.*

For readers seeking information, a thoughtful *CMAJ* editor added a translation on the contents page: *The results showed a higher rate of cure in the group receiving amoxicillin.*

Unfortunately no translation was included with an example from the *Journal of the American Medical Association* which Richard Lehmann drew to my attention: *The six-month rate of expulsion of an IUD after immediate insertion was higher than but not inferior to that after delayed insertion.*

If there be sense in that sentence, I find it just beyond my reach.

A British GP Dougal Jeffries stumbled upon a rare syntactical specimen while browsing through the *BMJ:* not just a double but a quadruple negative: *Having thrown out the motion to rescind last year's decision to stop opposing fundholding, the conference…*

"A particularly fine example," said Dr Jeffries, "because it contained no 'not's or 'no's, just four negative transitive verbs."

## Neurotic/psychotic

Distinction drawn by doctors. A neurotic dreams of a castle in Spain, a psychotic lives in one, and a psychiatrist is the person who collects the rent.

Or, as the distinguished American psychiatrist Karl Menninger put it: *Neurotic means he is not as sensible as I am, and psychotic means he's even worse than my brother-in-law.*

## New Age medicine
Paradoxical label for hotchpotch of Old Age superstitions that lost much of their power when our ancestors grew confident enough to question the dogmatic utterance of priests and shamans.

## New scientists
Those who hold the future of biological science in their hands.

I'm indebted to a teacher writing in a pharmaceutical journal for a selection of answers submitted in recent GCSE biology examinations.

- Lead can make you sterile. It is an anti-knocking agent.
- A major disease associated with smoking is death.
- A sexually transmitted disease is gonorrhoea, the penis becomes inflammable.
- A 20 metre tree can break wind for up to 200 metres.
- Cows produce large amounts of methane, so the problem could be solved by fitting them with catalytic converters.
- A drone bee comes from an unfertilised egg and therefore has no father. It has to have a mother in order to get laid.
- The largest mammals are found in the sea because there is nowhere else to put them.
- Once sperm is ejaculated, it is upwardly mobile.

## Newsflash
Sparks that fly when the news desk reaches for the medical dictionary.

*Minister rapped over organs – New Scientist.*

*National Organiser Lawrence Kirwan is now recuperating from an operation for hernia and hopes to be back in harness in early November – The Journalist.* (Official organ of the National Union of Journalists.)

*A psychiatrist for the defendant said that he was suffering from a psychiatric condition known as ambivalence – Oxford Times.*

## Next man
Measuring tool used to calculate the level of concern that will allow caring persons to air their sensitivity without actually having to do anything.

"I'm as concerned as the next man, but I can't see how we can help."

## Nightfall
Mystical fading of the light that ushers in the hours of medical eccentricity.

> Dr K R Sumner of Castle Donington had a 3 a.m. phone call from a young woman who asked if he could visit her boyfriend who had chest pain. Dr Sumner asked a few quick questions about the symptoms and, wondering if the man was grey and sweating, asked "What does he look like?" Back came the answer: "Quite short and very blond."

> Thomas Hunter was a kindly erudite man, a former Rhodes Scholar at my college in Cambridge who became dean of the medical school at the University of Virginia in Charlottesville. One night when he was dean he was awakened at 4 a.m. by his bedside telephone.
> "Your dog is barking and keeping me awake," said an angry woman's voice. The dean accepted her rebuke in his usual gentle way, then hung up.
> The following morning, again at 4 a.m., the woman's telephone rang. "Madam," said Dr Hunter, "I have no dog."

## Nightingale
Once the *Nom de guerre* of any nurse trained at St Thomas' Hospital in London – a logical consequence of being taught in the Nightingale school founded by Florence herself.

Until the 1960s, St Thomas' medical students perceived the school as the home of an exclusive religious order for the daughters of top drawer families. In the immediate post-war years, Nightingales were still warned against fraternising with medical students, though by the time I arrived in 1949 the warning was about as effective as today's warnings on cigarette packets.

The Nightingale tradition produced a rather special type of nurse who tended to handle crises in a smooth professional way that combined practical efficiency with aloof disdain for anything or anyone except her patient.

I got a sharp reminder of that quality when I read about Gaston Palewski, who at one time was De Gaulle's *chef de cabinet*, and, at another, the lover of Nancy Mitford in whose novels he makes an occasional lightly disguised appearance.

Palewski was, in the jargon of the times, a 'womaniser' who fancied himself as a playboy. One evening he met an attractive young St Thomas' nurse at a party and, after an hour or so of skilful 'chatting up', offered to drive her home. She responded in a way that every St Thomas' person will recognise and admire.

Smiling oh so politely, she said: "Thank you so much, but I'm very tired. So I think I'll walk."

## Night starvation
Disease endemic in Britain in the 1930s and immediately after World War Two. Its incidence declined with the disappearance of the advertising that created it.

A recurring figure in magazine advertisements of the 1930s and 40s was the all-wise family doctor who appeared in a strip cartoon advertising Horlicks. In the first frame of the strip, tragedy would strike at the heart of middle-class life: young Daphne's backhand would deteriorate, Daddy would lose his temper with his secretary, Mummy would grow tired and irritable, or Grandpa would stumble over the agenda at the golf club committee. Some kindly friend would then suggest they saw a doctor. In the next frame a serious-faced GP would diagnose "Night starvation" and prescribe a cup of calming Horlicks to be taken at bed time.

The final frame, usually labelled *A month later*, would show Daphne winning the tournament, Daddy voted 'Boss of the Year' by the typing pool, Mummy being lauded by members of the Women's Institute for organising the fete, or Grandpa driving himself in as the newly elected golf club president. And above each proud visage would float the bubble: *Thinks… Thanks to Horlicks.*

The campaign was so successful that Ovaltine, another bedtime drink, fought back by founding a children's club, the Ovalteenies, of which my sister and I were enthusiastic members. Our club song *'We are the Ovalteenies, little girls and boys'* blared out regularly from Radio Luxembourg and so worried Horlicks that they organised a competition for a song of their own.

That competition was bitterly remembered in our household because a grave miscarriage of justice denied the prize to the schoolgirl who was later to become my wife. Her entry (set to a traditional Welsh air) began:

> *Men of Horlicks Lead the Nation.*
> *Save us all from night starvation...*

## Nominal aphasia

Socially disturbing affliction sometimes known as "name blindness". A common affliction of US presidents even before the arrival George W Bush.

Gerald Ford toasted the Egyptian president Anwar Sadat as "the distinguished President of Israel" and Jimmy Carter, when delivering fulsome praise of Senator Hubert Humphrey, repeatedly called him Hubert Horatio Hornblower.

A more engaging condition when it occurs in old people.

Dr M A A Rahman, a research fellow in rheumatology at London's University College Hospital, writing in *Hospital Doctor*, reported a delightful case he saw in the early 1980s.

A patient, whom he described as "a charming lady" told him proudly that her abdominal scar was the relic of a hysterectomy performed by Sir Geoffrey Howe. Noting Dr Rahman's reaction she said: "Oh, I'm sorry, have I made a mistake? Is he not a Sir?"

"It's not that," said the good doctor. "It's just that Sir Geoffrey Howe is the Chancellor of the Exchequer."

The lady beamed back. "Fancy that. Hasn't he done well?"

## Nominal hypertrophy

Under-publicised feature of practising medicine in a multi-ethnic society.

Letter from a hospital to a GP: *An interesting problem arose this afternoon in that the Abdul Malik who came to the clinic was the father of the Abdul Malik whom you referred. In contrast, the notes brought from Records were for the Abdul Malik who is the son of Abdul Malik whom you referred. Various Abdul Maliks were sent round to the Record office to make an appointment for the correct Abdul Malik who will attend with Abdul Malik, an interpreter, at an appropriate clinic.*

From another hospital letter: *The patient, Muhammad Rahman Mubarraq bin Ali Bellamchi, says he is an artist and came to this country to make a name for himself.*

## Non-cognitive dissonance

The confident denial of incongruity I first recognised when a BBC radio announcer solemnly announced that we were about to hear the Grimethorpe Colliery Band playing *In a monastery garden*.

Non-cognitive dissonance was the source of some of my happiest memories of general practice, such as the morning when a woman confided, "I think my daughter may have kleptomania. Is there anything she can take for it?"

No surprise then that I felt I was back in my GP surgery when I read Matthew Norman's report in the *Guardian* of the apology offered by a man arrested in Wisconsin for boarding a bus while wearing no trousers.

"I'm sorry," he told the court, "but I thought it was Monday."

## Non-disposables

Ill-chosen gifts that doctors receive from patients.

Swift use of the obvious repository is hedged around with moral reservations. Not everyone can face the guilt of throwing away something that, though unwanted, is fresh-minted, unused, and emblematic of commendable emotions such as kindness, gratitude and generosity.

Other methods of disposal pose not moral but pragmatic hazards. Charity shops put gifts on display where they may catch the eye of the passing donor. And handing them on to those in greater need is no less hazardous. Grateful recipients tend to flaunt the precious gift they received from their doctor and sometimes do so in the presence of the donor or the donor's family.

Some gifts have an endogenous indisposability. One fine spring morning I received an elaborately wrapped parcel which, as I opened it, started to play a tinkly version of *Jingle Bells*. When I tore away the final wrapping, I discovered not a musical box but a pair of socks: not any old socks, mark you, but, to quote the label, *Superior men's musical socks with flashing lights*.

They were forwarded by the Birmingham GP who had received them. He suggested that I run a competition for the least likely present a GP had received from a patient, and the socks could act as a benchmark. Each of them not only contained a musical box and lights but was decorated with embroidered pictures of Santa Claus, a reindeer, a smiling Christmas tree wearing a pair of red wellies, and what looked like a duck-billed platypus with a congenital deformity.

They'd been haunting the GP's consulting room since the previous December. Every time he put them in the waste bin, he said, the surgery cleaner put them back on his desk, and when he hid them in a drawer, *Jingle Bells* would occasionally self-start in the middle of a consultation. By mid-March the tune had become painfully unseasonal and, in the hope of their humane disposal, he sent them to me. Clearly he thought that, as a third party, I would be free of moral reservations. And he was right.

But the socks were not to be thwarted. Next morning, as they left my house in the 'non-recycling' wheelie bin, they burst into song. The refuse collector stopped in mid-stride, lifted the lid, and extracted them. He listened for a moment then, as he swung them to make the lights flash more rapidly, his frown transmuted into a smile of pure delight. He put them in his pocket and chuckled contentedly as he wheeled the bin down the path.

I had a reassuring feeling that the socks had found a good home.

## Non-medicinal leeches
Private contractors and consultants who attach themselves to the NHS and feed greedily on its lifeblood.

Medicinal leeches (*Hirudo medicinalis*) have two suckers. The non-medicinal variety survives with only one; it assumes the NHS will be the other.

Apart from this anatomical peculiarity, it behaves like other leeches, attaching itself to its host until surfeited, then falling off to digest the riches it has imbibed. When the haemorrhagic mess it leaves behind has been cleared up, it may try to reattach itself, sometimes in a new disguised form.

Back in 1997, when politicians, neocon and neolab, fell hopelessly in love with these creatures, a merchant banker charged with developing private finance for public services invited a public health doctor, Allyson Pollock, to meet him. To do so, she had to step from one culture into another.

*We ate in the bank's private dining room with a prime view over the Thames. Black-coated waiters, who seemed to outnumber us by about two to one, served a lunch that lasted almost three hours. When I wryly observed that he might like to try our hospital canteen at St George's Hospital in south London, he laughed heartily. He explained how using the PFI (Private Finance Initiative) would 'take the fat' out of the NHS and introduce new efficiencies, and enthused about the savings to be made from cutting the number of hospital support staff. I could not help thinking of the rows of terraced houses in the impoverished community of Tooting from which St George's mainly female, mainly black, ancillary workforce is drawn.*

## Nordic diagnosis
Crucial skill for itinerant physicians.

My heart sank when I heard a distinguished Norwegian professor being introduced at an international medical meeting as a Swede... just about the greatest insult you can offer a Norwegian. According to my Scandinavian friends, there are two infallible diagnostic rules. When you see a group of smiling and cheerful Swedes, you know they're Danes. Just as when you see a bunch of gloomy Norwegians you know they're Swedes.

## Nose
A versatile organ, its activities not confined to running, sniffing, sneezing and snorting.

Self-important people claim it serves a dual social purpose: its anatomical design encourages irritating people to get up one's own, and prevents stupid people from seeing what goes on under theirs.

## Note taking
Doctors' habit of doodling while a patient talks.

Wise doctors discover that if they write too much, they miss most of what is being said and all of what is being implied. Yet patients are reassured to see their words being noted, so doctors will often jot reminders to themselves to call at the bank or collect something from the cleaners.

Even when relevant, the notes are often uninformative. I once worked with a psychiatrist who after an hour-long, probing, in-depth etc. interview with a patient, wrote: "Jolly little woman."

Doctors who specialise in diseases of the rich make extensive notes to enable them to pick up the conversation where they last laid it down – such as "Handicap 18" or "Daughter starts next term at Benenden" or "Shrub outside bedroom window is *Acer Talmatum Dissectum Atropurpureum.*"

## Nursery rhymes
A neglected opportunity for health educators.

Nursery rhymes contain relics not just of folklore and ancient incantations but of past reform campaigns. Though the meaning of many is forgotten, their jingling rhythm has helped them survive. We should tap into this oral tradition and encourage children to dance around school playgrounds singing such songs as:

> *Jack and Jill*
> *Went down the pub*
> *And sank ten pints of lager.*
> *Jack fell down*
> *And broke his crown*
> *And Jill's completely gaga.*

## Nursing auxiliaries
Persons with minimal training hired to walk around hospitals with stethoscopes draped across their necks to give the impression that the place is properly staffed.

## Obsequies
Rites of passage from this world. Susceptible to variation.

My father once went to the funeral of a patient and old friend who'd been a stalwart member of the Irish community. The requiem mass included a panegyric in which the deceased was near canonised in a stirring oration by his life-long drinking companion. At the end of it, the great man's widow turned round, scanning the congregation in search of my father. Once she'd spotted him, she called in a loud voice: "Wasn't it well worth you letting him die so he could have that said of him?"

A Sussex cemetery, 1995. A surgeon, struck down in his prime, had just been buried. The last shovelfuls of earth filled the grave and the friends and family of the deceased shuffled towards their cars. Suddenly an eerie sound filled the air. The mourners turned their heads and, when they realised it came from the grave, their alarm threatened to turn to terror. Then the deceased's registrar announced: "Don't worry. It's just his bleeper."
A week later the widow opened a letter from the hospital administration rebuking her husband for "unauthorised absence from duty."

## Obstetrical record
An award once held by the actress Lucille Ball's husband.
While Lucille was under contract to Harry Cohn at Columbia Pictures, she was loaned to Paramount for a De Mille picture *The Greatest Show on Earth* but then discovered she was pregnant. De Mille sent a message to her husband: "Congratulations. You're the only man who's ever screwed his wife, Cecil B. De Mille, Paramount Pictures, and Harry Cohn all at the same time."

## Obvious

What learned journals put a lot of effort into explaining.

*Excessive sleep is characteristic of hypersomnia* – New England Journal of Medicine.

*Accurate sexual information, given by a variety of sources including schools, parents and family planning services has resulted in... the acquisition of information that is more accurate* – Annual Review of Nursing Research.

*Patients with chronic disease consult their general practitioner frequently, and patients with more than one chronic disease consult even more frequently* – British Journal of General Practice.

*Distance to school and car ownership are greatest determinants of car travel to school* – British Medical Journal.

*Patients' unwillingness to take warfarin seemed to be a major factor in limiting the number who would eventually take it* – British Medical Journal.

*Surprisingly (sic), 36 per cent were stated to be alive up to one hour before death* – The Practitioner.

And not only journals.

The General Medical Council's *Recommendations on Basic Medical Education* offered an authoritative definition of one of the standard measurements: *The overall length of the pre-registration year is, as it has been since 1953, twelve months.*

Clare Wilkie, a GP in Brixton, received a report on one of her patients from her 'local community team' which dressed up the obvious in Decorated Municipal Gothic (qv): *A full Functional Analysis was done... and sought to bear a hypothesis as to the function of his attempts at masturbating. The conclusion of the assessment, or the analysis of meaning, of this behaviour was that it appeared to serve the function of self-stimulation.*

## Oculogenic confusion
Common interpretative dysfunction. Many people see only what they want to see. (Compare Audiogenic confusion.)

> Margaret Barker, a consultant paediatrician in Dorchester, found a page in the *The Sarum Link* dominated by the headline: *Harvest of the Sewers*. Expecting to learn of some new biological method of reclaiming valuable essences from effluent, she read the article only to discover it was about dedicated embroiderers refurbishing shabby hassocks in Salisbury Cathedral.

> An anthology of items from the *Lancet* column *In England Now* includes the case of a professor who, when walking from hospital to university with the chest piece of his stethoscope dangling from his hip pocket, was stopped by a respectful boy scout. "Excuse me, sir," said the young Samaritan, " but your catheter is hanging out."

> A characteristic case was reported by a geriatrician who encouraged a new patient to talk to him about her life. When he asked her what she watched on television, she said: "I like the boxing best. It can be lovely. But I'd like it better if they didn't take their teeth out at the end of every round."

## Off his trolley
Hospital slang for: "He has fallen out of his new improved NHS bed."

## Officiously to keep alive
Phrase from a sentence that casuists use to protect themselves from difficult decisions about euthanasia: *Thou shalt not kill; but need'st not strive officiously to keep alive.*

Often quoted as the 'correct' medical attitude by teachers who don't realise it comes from Arthur Hugh Clough's satirical re-working of the ten commandments to suit 'market forces'.

Other commandments include:

*Do not adultery commit;*
*Advantage rarely comes of it.*

*Thou shalt not steal; an empty feat,*
*When it's so lucrative to cheat:*

*Thou shalt not covet; but tradition*
*Approves all forms of competition.*

## Old fogey

Honourable state under attack from misguided euphemists.

For the past ten years or so, persons determined to iron-out our language have declared it ageist to use 'old' or 'elderly', as a noun or adjective. Their preferred euphemism is 'older', as in older person or older people. Their campaign has seriously affected editors of medical journals and denizens of the Department of Health who created a *National Framework for Older People*. Wales even has an Older People's Commissioner.

After an epidemic of 'older' in the *BMJ*, I wrote, on behalf of the euphemised, to complain. I pointed out that while sentences such as 'I am older than you' were acceptable, the word older, in the absence of a comparative object, got its meaning from its place in the progression old, older, oldest.

Older therefore meant older than old but not as old as oldest. I might well be frailer than I thought but I resented the journal labelling me as being older than old.

'Older people' is not just grammatically unsound but is every bit as patronising as 'senior citizen.' Ironically it also is a symptom of an attitude that one of its proponents condemns as "the solid core of ageism within the English healthcare system."

As it happens, though I'm happy to be called old or elderly, I prefer being called an old fogey, a title that confers an air of benignity I feel compelled to live up to, much to the benefit of those around me.

It also looks good in the box that self-consciously 'user friendly' forms invite you to fill after you've entered your name: *Please tell us your preferred form of address.*

## Old Mother Hubbards

Small epiphanies hoarded in cupboards.

Every so often, life grants us a glimpse of the actual world in which patients and their doctors try to support one another, as opposed to the unreal world which is the subject of reports in medical journals, practice audits, ongoing studies etcetera, etcetera.

Such a moment came to a London neurologist when he visited his elderly mother.

After washing his hands in her bathroom he had an inquisitive root around in the cabinet above the basin. Among the multitude of medicinal objects crammed therein, he found many vintage specimens but the most revealing was a bottle carefully labelled: *Could be aspirin.*

## Old scores

Carefully calculated debts that ambitious academics never forget.

Soon after the biochemist Arthur Kornberg received his Nobel prize he was invited to give a guest lecture at a medical school. A local professor with whom he'd worked when both were at the start of their careers introduced him to the audience with an extravagant flattering eulogy: "Great man of our time", "One of the truly great minds of the 20th century", that sort of thing. The introduction concluded: "Arthur, you have brought great distinction to yourself and to your profession so maybe the time has come to admit you were wrong that evening thirty years ago when you criticised my wholly justified opinion about…"

When I became editor of *World Medicine* I became a natural target for the sort of doctor who gives paranoia a bad name. I had to acquire a new diagnostic skill to detect doctors who approached me ostensibly offering me articles or information but really wanting to pay off old scores. For sixteen years, I carried in my head a list of people whose motives needed closer scrutiny than that normally applied to contributors. (I never wrote the list down for I believe that editors can grow too sceptical and we all know that paranoid people do occasionally have something to be frightened of. I remember when I was a young GP taking a psychiatrist on a domiciliary visit to an old woman who complained that the man next door was spying on her. As she told her story, the psychiatrist strolled to the window and found himself under surveillance from her neighbour crouched behind a telescope at an upstairs window.)

At times during my sixteen years as an editor I thought, when in depressive mood, that far too much grudge-harbouring went on in medicine. Then I reminded myself that I was a potential ally for the harbourers and that dermatologists probably thought there was a lot of skin about, and chiropodists a lot of feet.

## Omniscience

Gift granted to only a few in medicine and always self-awarded.

Despite the claims of GPs, the true generalists of medicine are the medical know-alls.

Dr Knowall, nearly always male, will explain within minutes of meeting you, why his practice is the envy of the world and, regardless of his specialty, why GPs are so badly organised and hospitals staffed by craven fools.

And that's just for starters. He will soon explain why any authority you care to mention is run by idiots, how the railways should be reorganised, how the government should have handled the banking crisis, how, were he in charge, the NHS would run smoothly and efficiently, and how, if people had only listened, the Dome could have been a spectacular success and Arsenal could have topped the premier league.

At a medical conference some years ago I spent the coffee break in the company of such a one and, by the time he paused to draw breath, all those who knew him better than I did had left for the next session. As I set off to follow he said: "No, no, don't go that way. You'll have to cross the yard in the rain. I'll show you a better route."

We descended to the basement in a service lift and wandered though a warren of cellars linked by a bewildering series of passages. After five minutes it was clear we were lost. He didn't admit it but blamed our predicament on others: "They've changed it all round since I was last here." After another five minutes the two of us stood beneath a courtyard grating shouting, "Is there anybody there?'"

Luckily a passing porter heard us and came down and rescued us. Yet Dr Knowall remained unabashed. Within ten minutes of our return to the meeting, he was on his feet telling a speaker exactly what was wrong with his data.

As Bill Clinton said: "Denial ain't just a river in Egypt."

## One of the Old School

A doctor proud to be an alumnus of what Charles Dickens defined in *Bleak House* as *any school that seems never to have been young.*

When I was a student, in the mid-20th century, teaching hospital Old Schoolers were called 'characters' and revered by students until, I hope, experience taught them better.

One of my contemporaries, the physiologist and medical inventor, Donald Longmore described his first ward round at Guy's Hospital.

*"Why are lumps in the breast like barmaids?" The surgical knight was presenting the first patient. The answer was: "Because they are rarely innocent and have to be taken out to be proved so."*

*The second patient in this staged show came with an abdominal X-ray showing a large pessary in place so we could be told that this was the front wheel of the menstrual cycle. Next came a large lady with a vaginal discharge. She was told, with a slap on the back, that without it she would squeak when she walked.*

In the heyday of the 'characters', indelibly recorded by Richard Gordon, Old Schoolers often referred to patients as 'teaching material.'

A few years ago I met a doctor who qualified in the 1950s and did his first house job in Leeds.

One day his boss, accompanied by houseman, two registrars and retinue of students, surrounded the bed of a cheery golden-haired woman who worked behind the bar in a local pub.

Without introducing himself, indeed without so much as a glance in his patient's direction, the consultant launched into his spiel.

"Here we have woman of fifty-seven who has been treated by our venereologists for seven – or is it eight? – separate infections with gonorrhoea… though there may, of course, have been more. She now has arthritis and the question we have to discuss is whether her present condition has any connection with her previous profligate life."

His idea of a discussion was to interrogate his students across the bed as if it were empty and, when he had finished, the round moved on without one word spoken to the patient.

Later the houseman returned to visit the woman. She was still fuming.

"Isn't your boss a rude old buggger?" she said. "Fancy revealing my age in front of all those students."

## Operatic doctors

Minor characters with deplorable professional standards who drift on stage during operas to keep the story going.

Such is the concern these days about doctors' competence, I suspect some authoritative body is already devising a code of behaviour to which operatic doctors must conform at peril of losing their licence to sing.

Consider, for instance, the ethical behaviour of the doctor in the last act of *La Boheme* who accepts Musetta's earrings as pre-payment for a visit. That action alone warrants a complaint to the GMC. Few would blame him for not making it to the garret before the final curtain: that could happen to any busy GP. But when he hands Musetta a 'cordial' for Mimi to take before he gets there, he is committing a Red Card offence, prescribing for a patient he hasn't seen.

The only claim he could make in his defence is that he knew she was a soprano – he may have heard her belting out her reprise of '*Che gelida manina*' across the rooftops of Paris – and it was just another routine case of operatic terminal phthisis.

Even more worrying is the doctor in Verdi's *Macbeth* who seems addicted to the question mark. Once his scene gets under way, his lines, apart from four *Oh, horror!*s, are all questions to the maid: *What did she speak of in her sleep? She carries a light in her hand? How wide open are her eyes? Why does she rub her hands? What did she say? She sighs?* and *This too?* All but the first, mark you, asked while the lady in question is singing none too quietly just a few yards away. Many of his patients must have expired while he was still interrogating the servants.

Then there's the doctor who turns up in the last act of *La Traviata* who, like so many operatic doctors, is a harbinger of the imminent triumph of tuberculosis. He usually stands beside

Violetta's bed doing little save gazing down on her while chanting a few unconvincing lies, *Then we must take heart... Convalescence is not far away...* that sort of thing. Only once, in a Kent Opera production, has he convinced me he was fully qualified, maybe because the director was Jonathan Miller.

Miller, a real doctor, managed to turn the operatic GP into the genuine article. The doctor didn't stand by the bed but sat on the side of it and put his hand on Violetta's wrist, not just to take her pulse but to establish human contact while he offered words that he and she knew were only words. Her acknowledgement of their real meaning *Doctors are allowed a pious fib* was a painfully accurate echo of a moment familiar to clinicians. This doctor was so real that a scene that often feels like a time filler allowing the audience, and Violetta, to draw breath before a melodic shuffling off of the coils, became one of the most poignant moments of the evening.

But he was an exception. Most operatic doctors offer wholly unacceptable role models. I trust a working party of high minded persons is already rewriting librettos to replace each dangerous individual with a responsible caring team. *La Boheme*, for instance, would end on a more rewarding note if Rudolf (tenor) didn't tear out his hair over the dead Mimi (soprano) but sought closure with the help of an appropriately trained bereavement counsellor (cornetto).

## Ophthalmologist
An unromantic doctor who gazes into your eyes and sees only anatomical detail.

When my cousin-in-law was on a course at Moorfields Eye Hospital in London, he asked a new patient, "Have your eyes ever been checked?"
"No," she replied demurely. "They've always been blue."

In a front garden at the residential end of Esher High Street, a large signboard announces: *Combined Ophthalmological and Dental Practice.*
Designed, no doubt, to provide for those seeking an eye for a tooth or vice versa.

## Opportune infection
A propitious illness that temporarily confines the body but leaves the mind active.

These useful afflictions can help you catch up on books you would never finish, maybe never start, if you were up and about. The removal of my appendix allowed me to get through *Dr Zhivago*. A lingering chest infection saw me through Harold Wilson's memoirs. And without sundry enabling diseases I doubt I'd ever have read *Cosima Wagner's Diaries*, Ivan Illich's *Medical Nemesis* or, of course, *War and Peace* (though I did skip the philosophical bits).

I might even have managed Proust's *Remembrance of Things Past* if it hadn't been for an early recovery.

## Optimism
A healing quality.

With so many doctors revelling in the role of Dr Killjoy (see Prophet of Doom), it's not surprising that patients turn to 'alternative medicine' in search of the homely optimism they once found in their GPs' surgeries. In the distant days of *Dr Finlay's Casebook*, viewers warmed more readily to dear old Dr Cameron than to finger-wagging Dr Snoddie.

Optimism has always been powerful therapy and I have often seen optimistic doctors help patients fight off – even overcome – the effects of serious disease. It also enhances a doctor's reputation. When optimists' patients die, relatives say: "The doctors were marvellous. They did all that was humanly possible but the disease beat them in the end." Their reputation always outshines that of the medical pessimists whose patients never die despite their efforts; even worse, they occasionally survive despite their efforts. The world is full of gleeful old fogeys eager to describe how they outwitted their pessimistic doctors. They wave their walking sticks and tell us proudly how, maybe forty years before, some gloomy killjoy gave them only six months to live.

Optimism I'm convinced is an essential component of that ephemeral quality possessed by doctors whom patients feel better for seeing no matter what treatment they prescribe. Such doctors are often assumed to be endowed with gifts denied to their colder hearted colleagues. Seventy years of casual doctor watching have persuaded me that the 'gift' is largely a matter of self knowledge.

Doctors at ease with themselves are more likely to engender ease in their patients. Given a little self knowledge, today's gloomy denouncers of cream cakes, crisps, and adventurous sports could transmogrify into the genial GPs of yesteryear.

## Ordinary people

Those who suffer the misfortune of not being doctors. Also known in medical circles as the General Public, the Laity, or Patients.

An odd choice of phrase by a profession whose members learn early in their careers that once you get to know ordinary people they become extraordinary individuals. Not only is the adjective patronising, "You are ordinary, ergo we are not", but it derives from the mind-set that nurtures racism, sexism, ageism and all the other 'isms' with which we typecast groups too bothersome to treat as individuals.

So what are we to make of the claim by NICE (the National Institute for Clinical Excellence) that its Citizens Council "is made up of thirty ordinary members of the public, reflecting the age, gender, socioeconomic status and ethnicity of the people of England and Wales"? I would like, as NICE might put it, to see the evidence on which the claim is founded. I've calculated that I would need nineteen of NICE's ordinaries to reflect "the age, gender… etc." of just the members of my extended family.

Such claims give succour to those who use 'public consultation' as a euphemism for 'public relations.' Pollsters in search of useful opinion, like epidemiologists in search of hard evidence, prefer to count their samples not in tens but in thousands. The reality is that NICE can draw on the opinion of thirty disparate individuals. This opinion may be helpful but the notion that it reflects the opinion of 'ordinary' people is, to put it politely, fanciful.

Meanwhile I fear that, with the exponential growth of models, supermodels, Big Brother housemates, X-factor rejects, publicity seeking politicians and sports people, not to mention the battalions of all-purpose celebrities, there could soon be a national shortage of real people. My fear was reinforced when I read that British Airways, in search of 'real people' for an advertising campaign, had to ask for help from a social anthropologist.

## Organ transplantation

Grafting an organ onto a city to attract medical tourists.

One afternoon, transiting through Basle airport I saw a large banner: *Welcome to Basle Liver Week* and assumed that local farmers were promoting one of their products; on my way back it might be Basle Cheese Week. Only when I spoke to a porter did I discover I'd happened upon an international medical symposium.

How far should cities debase themselves to attract visiting doctors and their wallets? Clearly the liver was a winner for Basle which lies at the confluence of three countries – France, Germany and Switzerland – where doctors are none too poor and citizens hold their livers in high regard. On a spectrum of organ acceptability, Basle Liver Week would come at the desirable end whereas Basle Rectum Week might lie, if you'll pardon the expression, at the other extreme.

In between would lie some tricky decisions for city fathers. Would the Royal Borough, for instance, be prepared to stage a Kensington Kidney Week? And once the news gets out that an Organ Week can attract medical largesse, might we hope for an Orpington Ovary Week, a Burton-on-Trent Bladder Week or, given a none too finely tuned sense of local pride, an Andover Anus Week?

## Orgasm

Standard unit for measuring efficiency of earth moving equipment.

A subject on which, not for the first time, the late Rob Buckman had the last word.

*Physiologists in New Jersey have shown that different species of animals have orgasms with different frequencies. They occur least often in rattlesnakes, ants, and the virus of German measles, and most often in laughing hyenas and New Yorkers.*

## Orthopaedic surgeons

1. Surgical carpenters.

When Terence Millin, one of the 20th century's great innovative surgeons, switched from orthopaedic surgery to urology he claimed: "I ceased to be a hewer of wood and became a drawer of water."

2. Surgeons regarded by many of their colleagues as "not as other men".

In 1990 Dr John S Fox and colleagues proposed a theory in the *BMJ* that orthopaedic surgeons are really gorillas. Previous reports in that journal supported the belief that orthopaedic surgeons were men of enormous build and great strength, if perhaps a little slow.

To test their theory, Dr Fox and his team first measured the innermost glove size of a selection of orthopaedic surgeons and general surgeons and found the orthopaedic had larger hands. They then measured the glove sizes of locally available gorillas and found they were closer to those of orthopaedic than of general surgeons.

Sadly, the finding fell short of statistical significance because of the low numbers involved. As the authors explained: "Live gorillas' glove size is a difficult variable to measure."

## Out of hours commitment
NHS managerial euphemism for night calls.

When the general practitioners' newspaper *Pulse* ran a competition for the most outrageous night call, one of the winners was a GP who had been called at 1 a.m. by a woman with asthma who had no inhaler. The GP visited, supplied a new inhaler, and made sure the attack had settled. "Thank you, doctor," she said as she saw him to the door. "My own inhaler is in my daughter's bedroom and I didn't want to wake her."

Night calls can be justified for reasons other than the seriousness of the illness. A young GP told me how one night he was summoned to a seedy terraced house in the poorest part of town to see a small boy with a mild infestation with scabies. Having recently attended a course on Doctor/Patient Communication he addressed the mother in what he hoped were firm yet kindly tones. "You're supposed to call your doctor at night only if it's a matter of life or death."

"I know that," said the mother. "But it is. My husband works nights and he's always complaining that I don't look after the kid properly. If I called you in the daytime he'd be here. And if he heard you say the kid had scabies, he'd murder me."

## Overflow
Displaced patients parked wherever there's room in a hospital.

As recorded in the minutes of a hospital management meeting: *Mr X said that he and the surgeons were unhappy that the urological patients were overflowing into general surgical beds.*

## Overseas meetings
One way to encourage doctors to show an interest in science.

Well attended when the organisers hold the meeting at an exotic destination and invite 'accompanying persons'. If you accept the scientific sessions as a penance you have to endure to enjoy a subsidised holiday, a well-chosen venue can offer unexpected 'learning opportunities'.

When the BMA held its Annual Scientific Meeting in Cairo, I found the surroundings more instructive than the science. One evening, I managed to escape from the conference hotel and wandered around the pyramids at Giza. After dark the pyramidal shadows thrown by the moon become a meeting place for lovers and I like to think that for 4,000 years young Egyptians have been whispering to each other: "See you down the pyramids tonight".

It couldn't happen at home. We would fence off the area and allow visitors no closer than a bungaloid Heritage Centre with audio-visual theatre and souvenir shop. Despite the touts and baksheesh hunters, the pyramids retain their majesty and on the evening I was there even transcended a *Son et Lumiere* commentary of such banality that the Sphinx was hard put to remain inscrutable.

The Egyptians, like the British, draw on their history when naming hotel conference rooms. On my way back to the penitential stool the following morning I tried to telephone one of the speakers. As I started to explain my mission, a husky female voice interrupted: "You're speaking to Nefertiti. I think you really want Cleopatra."

After three days of listening to BMA Speak(qv), I would have settled for either. Preferably down the pyramids in the moonlight.

# P

## Parish pomp

Preferred ceremonial style for Pooterish medical events such as foundation stone laying (qv). *De rigeur* when the BMA feels the need for divine guidance.

I first encountered it when, as an ingenue journalist, I watched a flock of BMA grandees assemble in the centre of Harrogate the day before their Annual Representative Meeting. A grey wind, heavy with mist from the Dales, meandered down the Ripon road and gave a playful tug at the academic finery outside the Royal Hall whence eighty or more Representatives, most in cap and gown but a few swathed in exotic doctoral silk, were to process to their ecumenical service at St Peter's Church.

Questions meandered through my mind. Did the finery escalate with status? Was the BMA Secretary's robe signifying an honorary MD (Manchester) intentionally more gaudy than the humble gown of an MB (Cantab) earned by examination? And what was the High Office held by the distinguished looking party enwrapped in the most resplendent robe of all. I recognised it as the one bestowed on Licentiates of the Apothecaries' Hall in Dublin where, 'twas said, degrees were available in exchange for cases of fine wine? He must have held very high office indeed because a medical plebeian who turned up in silk more regal than that worn by the BMA's top brass would surely be banned from the procession or perhaps compelled to follow it in one of those limousines with darkened windows.

A solemn character, dressed like an undertaker in morning suit and a shiny topper, stepped into the road in front of the traffic lights. In lieu of a religious icon, he held aloft an attenuated staff of Aesculapius. The doctors lined up hurriedly behind him like a company of *Dad's Army* trying to get into 'column of three' while the traffic lights were on red. Then as the lights turned green, the procession stepped bravely forward to tackle the angina-inducing slope of Parliament Street.

There was a minor panic when the lights reverted to red and cut off the rear of the procession but the quick-thinking Dublin apothecary grabbed the undertaker by the coat tails and brought him to a halt. In the confusion Aesculapius took a nasty toss and the undertaker had to dust him down on a dangling sleeve of the Secretary's doctoral silk. Meanwhile those in each half of the divided column stood self-consciously waiting for the lights to change and pretended not to hear the impertinent comments of pedestrians and motorists: "Where's your handbag, Dearie?", "Give us a twirl, love", "Get back on the bloody pavement"...

Yet, when the lights once again turned green and the reconstituted column moved off, I almost envied them. Once into their stride, they seemed so confident, so secure: born to process and put their trust in an ecumenical God. A sermon from the Archbishop of York would set them up nicely for another year of points of order, referrals back, amendments to amendments, and hours of thank-you-for-the-loan-of-the-hall style oratory; his words would make me only more confusedly agnostic.

## Partner

Front runner in the hunt for a neutral name for the other half in a permanent or semi-permanent human relationship.

Confusing when used by general practitioners. Recently when a GP introduced me to his partner, it took some delicate conversational probing to determine whether they shared a bed or an NHS list. Just to add to the confusion, it turned out they shared both.

What term should we use? Lover suggests that the relationship is based only on sex and 'live-in' boyfriend or girlfriend has too tabloid a ring. The only acceptable phrase I've encountered came from a Californian who introduced me to "the woman who shares my American Express card".

Frank Giles, a former editor of the *Sunday Times*, became an old hand at this naming game. On one overseas trip he and his wife, Lady Katharine Sackville (as an earl's daughter, she retained her title) received an invitation from the British consul addressed to Mr and Mrs Giles. Aware of the weight placed on diplomatic protocol he rang his hostess and explained with diffidence that his wife wasn't exactly Mrs Giles. "That's all right," came the cheery response. "Bring her along anyway. We're not at all stuffy about that sort of thing."

## Passage of time
Nature's way of dealing with the moralising doctor.

Browsing through the notes of a sedate and respectable old woman, Mike Ebdy a Preston GP, found a letter a hospital consultant wrote about her in 1963.

*I saw this couple last Friday and I must say I am very sorry for the husband. He seems an incredibly charitable person who is prepared to let his wife have two years fling, in order to sow a few wild oats and then, he hopes, settle down happily to married life. I think, in actual fact, that once she has tasted the Christine Keeler type of existence she will want to go on with it, and I told him this. I do not think that there is anything wrong with this girl, she is just a nymphomaniac who wants a damned good spanking and I gather he is taking her up to xxxx next week, where she is to going to live with her father. The one hope is that she has a sister-in-law up there whom she both respects and fears and I have told the husband to go and see this sister-in-law, tell her the whole story and get her to give this girl absolute hell. It is just possible that being really ticked off by somebody whom she respects might make her realise what a cheap little hussy she is.*

After reading the letter, Dr Ebdy says he treated his patient with greater respect, even with awe.

## Patent medicines
Household remedies still available on chemists' shelves throughout the pharmaceutical revolution in the second half of the 20th century.

Their appeal relied more on nostalgia – 'the treatment mother gave me' – than on pharmacology and well into the 1980s middle-aged shoppers could create a litany of childhood just by reading the labels on the shelves: *Ellimans Universal Embrocation, Scott's Emulsion, Iron Jelloids, Andrew's Liver Salts, Veno's Lightning Cough Cure, Dr J Collis Browne's Chlorodyne, Potter's Catarrh Pastilles, Milk of Magnesia, Beecham's Pills (Worth a guinea a box), Lofthouse's Original Fisherman's Friend…*

Even the descriptive words and phrases came from the pre-pharmaceutical years: rubbing oils, camphor, balsam, teething jelly, children's cooling powders, capsicum and eucalyptus, iron tonic and syrup of figs ...

Read out loud, they sound like lines from a Betjeman poem evoking sun-kissed days when Len Hutton was at the Oval, Henry Hall was on the wireless, the Wizard and the Hotspur were on the counter in the corner shop, and Robert Donat, Jean Harlow, and Will Hay were on the silver screen.

My favourite label was: *Morris Evans Oil. Traverses the globe from Ffestiniog to Patagonia.*

Despite the lack of an apostrophe the oil was Morris's own creation and the bottle carried a portrait of the creator and his autograph, *None genuine without signature.* (As a child I used to wonder how, if you bought a non-genuine unsigned bottle, you would know it was a fake?)

Morris recommended his oil not just for the traditional rheumatics, sciatica, lumbago, gout, neuritis, stiffness, muscular pains, sprains, and backache,' but for insect bites, burns, scalds, cuts, earache, stiff neck, sore throat, swellings, weak chest, tender feet, and sunburn.

*Just apply the oil*, said the label. *Don't rub.*

Goodness knows what it would have cured if you rubbed.

Then, as now, alternative medicine was sold largely by endorsement. These quotations come from the leaflet still enclosed with each bottle of *Dr J Collis Browne's Chlorodyne* in the 1980s.

Edward Whymper, Esq, the celebrated mountaineer, writes on February 16, 1897: *I always carry Dr J Collis Browne's Chlorodyne with me on my travels, and have used it effectively on others on Mont Blanc.*

*During my fifteen years' active service in South Africa, I found your medicine of the greatest value to myself and comrades –* Troop Sgt A E Rogers et al, Kitchener's Fighting Scouts.

*Gaunter and gaunter grew the soldiers of the Queen. Hunger and sickness played havoc with those fine regiments but somehow the RAMC managed to patch the men up with chlorodyne and quinine –* Cassel's History of the Boer War.

## Pathography

Autobiography that exploits the experience of illness while teaching us little.

Ideal medium for those who feel compelled to talk about their illness but have run out of ears to bend. Bruce Charlton defined it in an article in *Theoretical Medicine*:

*You know the sort of thing: someone, perhaps a celebrity, writes, or has ghost-written, a book about a real or self-diagnosed illness, and then tours the talk shows and lecture circuit as an expert on victimhood. Luckily, expert victimhood is perfectly compatible with a life of wealthy hedonism.*

Charlton argued that pathography's success relies heavily on our reluctance to criticise those who have suffered. As a result it's not the illness but the readers who are exploited. Ruth Holland spoke up on their behalf:

*It must be one of Nature's jokes that those most eager to talk about themselves are the ones with the least interesting things to tell. Nothing brings on the yawns more quickly than earnest self-revelation, and there's a lot of it about these days, when we're all being urged to dig into the unconscious, bare the soul and generally let it all hang out. Most people's souls, like their bodies, are best kept decently covered.*

It will be sad if this fashionable genre drives out those honest accounts of illness 'from the inside' that can teach a lot to doctors and bolster the confidence of patients.

## Patients

The awkward squad of health care systems.

Ill-assorted bunch of quirky individuals whose idiosyncrasies disrupt well-ordered professional lives. Put on this earth to thwart the plans of clear-thinking, well-meaning nurses, doctors, and health administrators.

Yet clinicians who have learned their craft, and find their work rewarding, would wish patients to be nothing else.

## Pattern recognition

The first step towards a diagnosis.

Doctors are at their best when they recognise patterns in the way other people behave and in what they say. Doctors are at their worst when they try to impose patterns of their own making. Within that imposition, I suspect, lie the seeds of medicine's oft criticised paternalism or, as I prefer, parentalism. (The sexes are equally guilty.)

One evening during the second act of *Schwanda the Bagpiper* – a detail of quite stunning irrelevance – I got a nasty pain in my belly. At that stage of my life I must have seen and diagnosed over forty cases of acute appendicitis and, in doing so, had created in my mind a picture of what the pain must feel like and of the way it moved. When I got the pain myself it was so unlike my picture that, at first, I didn't recognise it. Only when I described it to my doctor did I find I was using the words that patients used to me. Till then I had not been, as I thought, recognising the entity but the patient's description of it.

Pattern recognition has other limitations.

When one of Britain's brightest young physicians attended a conference in Rio she became the darling of the conference – if such an accolade exists – not just because of her striking looks but because of her fluency in Portuguese.

One night when she and her husband were returning from a restaurant in an open taxi it suddenly started to rain.

The driver's response was to accelerate like a madman.

The physician kept shouting at him in his own language: "Stop! You're ruining my clothes. What's the hurry? We have all night. Stop, st-o-o-op!"

But the driver didn't even turn his head, just kept going.

When they reached the hotel she jumped angrily from the cab and harangued the driver.

He listened politely and, when she'd finished, shrugged his shoulders and said: "I'm sorry, madam, I thought you were making love."

## Peerage

The ultimate prize for those who practice the black art of medical politics: admission to an old people's day centre attached to the Palace of Westminster where attendees receive a handsome daily allowance, free notepaper, subsidised meals, and an opportunity for group discussion with other patients.

Irreverent doctors refer to the process as being 'lorded' though the patients themselves prefer the spelling 'lauded.'

## Perseverance fatigue

Weariness induced by attempts to correct those who know everything.

The playwright Michael Frayn was approached at the BAFTA awards by a man who said: "I very much enjoyed your play about Joe Egg." Frayn explained politely that the play was written by Peter Nichols and that the pair were often confused.

"Oh no," said the man emphatically, "I know Nichols and I'm talking about your play."

The gentle Frayn turned his attention elsewhere but some months later at another party found himself alongside the same man. "Do you remember when we met at the BAFTA awards," said Frayn, "you confused me with Peter Nichols?" The man stared at him sternly and barked: "I've never been to the BAFTA awards."

## Personal physician

One who so cossets fee-paying patients they become rewardingly dependant on their doctor.

Sir Walter Farquhar (1738-1819) was a revered proponent of this style of practice. When one of his patients wanted to take the waters at Bath but feared separation from the only doctor who really understood her, Farquhar assured her he had a "wholly reliable" colleague in that city and gave her a letter of introduction which set out the details of her case.

During her journey, the woman realised that, though Sir Waiter had been her doctor for years and had assured her that her condition was one of the most complicated with which he had ever had to deal, he had never told her exactly what it was. The answer clearly lay in the letter so, despite the protests of her travelling companion, she steamed it open. It read: *Dear Davis. Keep the old lady for three weeks then send her back*.

## Perspective

Repository in which we are encouraged to keep other people's problems.

When I was young, perspective was a device used by artists to create a three-dimensional image on a two-dimensional surface. It has since become a device used by politicians to turn a three-dimensional problem into a two-dimensional soundbite: "Of course I have every sympathy with the sick and underprivileged but we must keep their problems in perspective."

## Philosophies of care
Fashionable nostrums prescribed in the New Improved NHS in lieu of money for real treatment. (See Platitudes.)

Often displayed in prominent positions in wards and clinics. A typical specimen is a notice outside a Sheffield paediatric ward:

> *The philosophy of care in this ward aims to deliver holistic individualised family centred care meeting the needs of both the hospitalised child and their* (sic) *families.*

Even when the notices are free of grammatical solecism, who the hell are they aimed at? We patients, burdened with pains and aches, and even more frightening intimations of mortality, have little intellectual space left in which to ponder insubstantialities such as "philosophies of care."

If, as most of us believe in our naiveté, the doctors and nurses are trying to do their best for us, we'd prefer to read that message in their actions than in ill-constructed statements on the wall. And if they start telling us too loudly just how clever they are, we may begin to wonder if they feel as insecure as we do.

I suspect the exercise is designed to impress any passing manager who's recently been on a Ongoing Communications course and whose space between the ears is so stuffed with Mission statements, Business plans, Protocols, and Paradigms it has become a nous-free area.

Most NHS 'Mission statements' are smug and platitudinous and have that bragging tone clinically associated with insecurity.

Why did St Thomas' Hospital in London suddenly feel the need, with the coming of the internal market, to emblazon a slogan across its facade: *Serving the community 24 hrs a day.* It had been doing that for 900 years. What Business School edict demanded that the 'news' should now be shouted at every passer-by?

The claim isn't even unique; most hospitals (well, at least for the time being) could shout the same if they weren't too busy bawling platitudinous slogans of their own.

## Placebo

A substance guaranteed to be inert and to have no therapeutic effect, yet thought by some to be the most effective medication known to science.

Subjected to more clinical trials than any other drug, it always seems to do better than expected. And the range of conditions that it helps appears to be limitless.

David Colquhoun, research professor at University College London, suggests that placebos get more credit than they deserve: their effect may be small and transient.

*The reason that so many people think that ineffective treatments work is probably regression to the mean. Echinacea (a herbal remedy) cures your cold in only seven days when otherwise it would have taken a week. Most people (if they have any sense at all) would take homeopathic pills only for minor, self-limiting conditions. The condition goes away and the pill gets the credit. That doesn't need any placebo effect whatsoever.*

## Planet

Word that, when used by non-astronomers, confirms a diagnosis of hyperbolitis.

On the opening morning of the London 2012 Olympic Games, a woman presenting BBC Radio Four's *Today* declared in authoritative tones, "This morning Danny Boyle [producer of the opening extravaganza to be performed that evening] is the most anxious man on the planet." Later news items revealed that men in Syria that morning were sheltering with their terrified families in the cellars of houses shelled by tanks, and men in South Sudan were compelled to watch their children perish from starvation.

The *Today* announcement was the precursor of an epidemic that would sweep through the *BBC* commentariat over the following two weeks when hyperbolic  interviewers spread the disease by grabbing exhausted athletes on the edge of the track and subjecting them to heavily infected questions such as, "Isn't this the most amazing, wonderful, unforgettable moment you will ever have in your  lifetime ?"

Few of the athletes were able to resist the infection so my heart went out to a young man from Sheffield. When a hyped-up interviewer asked, "What thoughts were going through your mind as you stood on that winner's podium, with this huge crowd singing our national anthem?" he replied, "I was trying to remember the words".

## Platitudes

Cheap medicaments over-prescribed in a self-consciously 'consumer friendly' NHS. Sometimes called Mission Statements.

Produced in bulk at the Department of Health and embossed on letterheads and title pages of portentous documents. Reported side effects include nausea and occasional vomiting. Detectable with a simple diagnostic test: "If the converse is absurd, platitude is present."

First appeared in the 1980s and 90s in the titles of government white papers:

*Promoting better health – 1987.*

*Working for patients – 1989.*

They soon infected the letterheads of NHS Trusts:

*Putting Patients First* – Green Park Healthcare Trust.

Only one let the light shine in:

*Advancing learning and knoledge (sic) through teaching and research* – St George's Hospital Medical School.

In 1998, Peter Moore, a GP in Torquay received a note from the Royal Devon and Exeter Healthcare Trust. It's simple message that a patient had died was enhanced by the mission statement on the letterhead, *Working together for your well-being.*

In a munificent gesture, Jennifer Caddy, when a consultant anaesthetist at Pontefract General Infirmary, created an all-purpose mission statement for any medical institution unable to think one up for itself: *Committed to Commitment.*

## Pleasure

Concept that makes doctors uncomfortable.

In an article in the *Journal of Medical Ethics*, R P Bentall proposed that happiness be classified as a psychiatric disorder. Future editions of diagnostic manuals, he suggested, should call it: "Major affective disorder, pleasant type." His review of the way happiness was treated in medical texts revealed it was statistically abnormal, associated with a range of cognitive abnormalities, and probably reflected abnormal functioning of the central nervous system. (See Euphoria.)

## Political correctness

Absurd code imposed on decent people by the sort of person who has no idea of how to behave in a golf club, officers' mess, or ancient medical school.

Ne'er a day goes by, it seems, without some retired officer, or other natural born *Telegraph* reader, sounding off about the iniquities of political correctness. Yet many of the sounders-off have their own form of correctness – they call it 'the done thing' – and come from backgrounds that impose rigorous codes of correct behaviour.

When I did my National Service, young doctors commissioned into the RAMC received half an hour's instruction on the rituals of the Officers' Mess where even passing the port in the wrong direction was a sin that dare not speak its name. And golf clubs can be hazardous places if you don't know the local rules.

A woman fell foul of Little Aston golf club when her husband had a heart attack on the course. As soon as she heard, she rushed to his side and went with him to hospital in the ambulance. The club reacted with a sharp letter from the committee pointing out she had broken the weekend rule that bans women from the "confines of the club" and "circumstances notwithstanding, we would like to remind you not to park in the main car park."

When I was a clinical student at St Thomas' Hospital (1949-52), conformity was a necessary virtue. Eccentricity was tolerated only if it emerged in gentlemanly form. Active dissent led to a drying up of sources of privilege and patronage. I wonder how much of the conformity was part of a St Thomas' tradition and how much was brought back by ex-service students from their officers' messes. Its observance certainly involved service-like detail. I remember how students who didn't wear a black tie for the full period between King George VI's death and his interment were subjected to unostentatious yet pointed ostracism. One person's 'good manners' is another person's 'political correctness'.

Like all rules of etiquette, the edicts of political correctness, if applied unthinkingly and without imagination, can be ridiculous and extremely irritating. Yet on the whole I find today's social ambience less irksome than it was when we were all expected to know our place and when the social crime that dare not speak its name was being too big for your boots – a phrase most often used, in my experience, by people who were too small for theirs. Those were the days when mediocrity ruled, OK.

## Political discretion
Quality demanded of medical MPs.

When young Dr David Owen was elected as MP for Plymouth Sutton in 1966, he was determined to continue his day job as a doctor at St Thomas' Hospital directly across the Thames from the Houses of Parliament. He harboured an ambition to become a professor of psychiatry and may have thought that attendance at the House of Commons would provide some useful field work.

He also discovered he was unable to shrug off his medical identity during the short walk across Westminster Bridge. The Palace of Westminster had no 'company doctor' and MPs struck down suddenly by illness had to rely on the skills, often rusty, of their medically qualified colleagues. In an emergency, the choice of doctor was made by the police and, as Owen points out in his autobiography *Time to Declare*, they first called the doctors whom they judged to have the greatest knowledge. "In my early years I was near the top of their list. As the years passed they wisely dropped me to the bottom."

He soon discovered that dealing with an emergency north of the Thames posed problems not encountered by doctors working in the well-equipped hospital to the south. In the Palace of Westminster the doctor had no skilled and experienced colleagues near at hand and had to conduct a medical examination in a tiny room that contained an examination couch and little else. Owen's response to the challenge was pragmatic. If he were certain of the diagnosis, he sent the ailing MP to St Thomas'; if he were uncertain, he sent the patient to Westminster Hospital and so protected himself from the mockery of his St Thomas' colleagues.

One day he was called to see an MP who had collapsed in the Chamber and arranged for him to be carried to the medical room and placed on the couch. Owen stayed with him for a while until, confident his patient was stable, he slipped out for half an hour, asking the young policeman on duty to keep an eye on the sick MP till he returned. As promised, he was back within thirty minutes and returned at regular intervals over the next few hours.

The young policeman grew concerned that a seemingly comatose MP was being left untreated in the room and called his Superintendent. When Owen arrived on his next visit, both policemen enquired politely whether it might not be wise to call an ambulance and send the MP to hospital. Owen replied, equally politely, that it would not and continued his regular visits until the MP was well enough to go home.

As Owen writes in his autobiography: 'I am not sure the young policeman ever realised the diagnosis. The MP was, quite simply, drunk.'

## Pollutant
Any chemical that threatens the fantasy of a wholesome natural environment.

Forty-three of the fifty classmates of fourteen-year-old Nathan Zolmer voted to ban Dihydrogen Monoxide – a chemical definition of water – after he reported its many dangers. DHMO, he pointed out, is a major component of acid rain, has been found in cancerous tumours, accelerates the corrosion of metals and, when withdrawn from those who've developed a dependency on it, causes certain death.

## Pooterography
Form of medical autobiography that can dull the lustre on a glittering career.

For aged specimens of *Genus Medicopoliticus* the final folly can be a lapse into autobiography. The flattery of sycophants eager to win preferment convinces them of their importance and encourages a belief that the world is eager to hear every word they are prepared to commit to paper, word processor or, Lord protect us, dictating machine.

A few, because of what they have achieved, have an interesting tale to tell but, as is the way with the professions, most have taken the easy route to the top, conforming with convention and keeping their thoughts zipped up in public. Because they cannot break the habits of a lifetime they lapse into bland recital of every tedious detail of their lives yet leave out any 'spicy' bits that we might like to read but they think 'impolitic' to reveal.

As a result their acquaintances are lumbered with huge volumes even heavier than the prose within, near impossible to read, and none too easy to get rid of. They can't be gifted to charity shops or libraries because of the embarrassing messages the authors inscribe on the flyleaves and not everyone has a shelf sturdy enough to support them. Many are interred in the back of cupboards, I have seen one in use as a doorstop, and 'twas rumoured, in the 1970s, that a crusty old surgeon, gifted a volume of pooterography by one of his rivals, kept it alongside the WC in his bathroom where, every morning, he put a page or two to practical and satisfying use.

## Positive health
1. Ill-defined entity marketed on urban High Streets where health food shops, sports couturiers, and 'work-out' parlours proliferate with an exuberance that indicates real money is changing hands.

The concept of 'positive health' is popular with middle-aged spreaders who like dressing up in track suits. Yet the phrase is as meaningless as a line in a patent medicine advertisement. Individuals have only a tiny degree of control over their own health compared with the influence of heredity, culture, environment, and chance.

I prefer the spiritual approach Dr Somerset Maugham prescribed in *The Moon and Sixpence*.

*I forget who it was recommended men for their soul's good to do each day two things they disliked... it is a precept that I have followed scrupulously; for every day I have got up and I have gone to bed.*

As for the WHO fantasy that health is "A state of complete physical, mental, and social well-being" (see Health), I've found it a pretty sound rule that once people start wondering whether they're perfectly healthy, they're well on the way to feeling ill.

Doctors don't exist to sustain fantasy. They're in the business of make do and mend. If I sound grouchily dogmatic, it could be because every time I look at that WHO definition I get a severe attack of negative health.

2. Occupational therapy for the obsessional.

The *Guardian* reported that the Japanese have invented an "intelligent toilet" which automatically measures "indices of health and disease" in the stool and urine and, if the user inserts a finger into a device built into its side, gives an instant record of pulse rate and blood pressure.

A spokesman for the research team said:

*It is our dream that some day people's homes will be linked via communications lines to a health centre which could monitor the changes in vital signs read by the toilet.*

What's the Japanese for 'Dream on'?

## Possessive pronoun

Useful diagnostic sign.

When people talk of their illnesses and refer to 'my cardiologist' or 'my surgeon' they are most likely private patients.

NHS patients prefer a less possessive approach: 'the surgeon', 'the eye specialist' and so on.

There is, as always, a third group: the pseudo-possessives who talk private but act NHS. These are the sort of people who, when they travel up to town from Guildford, walk through the train as it arrives at Waterloo so they can be seen to alight from a first-class compartment.

## Post-traumatic stress

1. Severe anxiety disorder occurring after exposure to psychologically traumatic events. Afflicts some servicemen and women who survive a killing war.

2. Lingering anxiety after a nasty shock. Often sustained by counselling.

Uncertainty persists about who has the knowledge to make the diagnosis. In Palo Alto, California, a van driver crossed traffic lights as they were turning red and rammed into the side of a car that had already started to cross. The guilty driver pulled over, jumped from the van, ran back to the car he'd hit, and found a badly shaken woman still fixed in place by her seat belt and covered with pellets of shattered windscreen.

"Are you all right?" he asked anxiously.

"How would I know," came the angry reply. "I'm a doctor, not a lawyer."

## Precocious puberty
Puberty in other people's daughters.

## Prefabricated prose
The *lingua obscura* of the medical 'literature'.

Created in the 20th century by generations of scientists overexposed as students to Decorated Municipal Gothic (qv). Eagerly sustained by their 21st century successors.

Back in the pre-synthetic days in 1885 when William Marsden produced his historic report on cancer treatment, he wrote:

*A hospital devoted to the treatment of cancerous disease seems to me to hold out the only prospect of progress in the treatment of the malady; an institution conducted by those who recognise in medicine and surgery but one art. The records of such an institution are sure, in time, to narrow the field of incurable malignant disease.*

Like most of his contemporaries, Marsden expressed himself clearly, choosing simple words to convey his meaning. Today a lesser Marsden would feel compelled to write:

*It would seem to the author that only a specialist centre organised on the basis of concentrating its resources solely to address the treatment of the malignant disease process could offer a potential for realistic measurable improvements in treatment outcome.*

*Furthermore, such an institution would be a de facto resource centre under the direct line management of personnel sensitive to the proposition that the multifaceted disciplines of medicine and surgery are each essentially manifestations of the same single entity. Aside from this consideration, the accumulation of follow-up data by such a resource centre would establish new parameters that could be a major determinant of success in reducing the incidence of those manifestations of the malignant disease process which are, at present, regarded as being wholly resistant to therapy.*

You may recognise the style because I didn't invent it. I spread a month's supply of medical journals across a table then used phrases plucked from the open pages to encode Marsden's original message.

## Premarital check-up
In Eastern tradition, concerned with virginity and potential fecundity; in Western tradition, the concerns are less physical than fiscal.

A Californian surgeon was much smitten by a night-club singer but, before asking her to marry him, hired a detective agency to "run a check" on her.

The agency reported: "The young lady has an excellent reputation. Her past is without a blemish and she has many friends of good social standing. The only scandal associated with her is that she has often been seen recently in the company of a surgeon of questionable character."

## Pre-menstrual tension
Mounting anxiety in a mother awaiting her daughter's first period.

As expressed by a mother speaking to a paediatrician at St Christopher's Hospital for Children in Boston: "She's twelve years old but I don't think it's the you know what. She ain't a virgin yet."

## Pre-nuptial advice
In 2011 I discovered to my amazement that this service was still occasionally demanded of GPs by mothers who like their advice backed by medical authority.

When I acted as a GP locum in a Yorkshire mining village during the 1950s, young women due to be married were dragged along to the GP's surgery for 'a word with the doctor'. Mother and daughter always arrived together and God help the poor GP who tried to see them separately. They would sit solemnly in front of the doctor (i.e. me… young, newly qualified, and naive) who was expected to say something significant. My trouble was that nobody had told me what it was, so with mother watching with critical suspicion, I usually confined myself to mechanistic remarks about contraception.

I'm not proud of that episode in my life. The young women – many of them more sexually experienced than I was – survived my hesitant remarks in a state of barely suppressed giggledom yet their mothers seemed oddly reassured when they left. Maybe it was because they felt they'd done their duty and it hadn't been too painful after all.

One evening a mother came on her own. "I wonder, doctor, could you have a word with the daughter," she said. "She's getting married next month and she doesn't know what she ought. I were waiting for t'dog to come on heat so I could explain… but t'dog died."

It was the lamest, three-legged excuse I've ever heard. But the underlying assumption was no more mechanistic than my own. I could understand her insecurity because I shared it.

## Prescription

Originally a device for ensuring that a patient would pay another visit to the doctor. Just as, when doctors dispensed their own medicines, a request that patients bring a specimen of urine on the next visit ensured the doctors got their bottles back.

Lost much of its power when it ceased to be handwritten. Before that Mark Twain could claim:

*He wrote a doctor's hand – the hand which from the beginning of time has been so disastrous to the pharmacist and so profitable to the undertaker.*

Yet prescribing is still regarded an essential component of the mystical process of healing. Bill Yule, a retired GP, pointed out in the *BMJ* that the only thing that distinguishes man from the lower animals is man's desire to take medicine, and anecdotal evidence suggests the prescription itself may have curative properties. Samuel Butler, in his *Notebooks*, described a man who was cured of a dangerous illness by eating his doctor's prescription which he understood was the medicine.

Carlo Levi, in *Christ stopped at Eboli*, suggested that the custom of prescribing medicine for every illness, even when it was unnecessary, was equivalent to magic, "especially when the prescription is written, as it once was, in Latin or in indecipherable handwriting." Most prescriptions, he proposed, would be just as effective if they were not taken to the pharmacist but hung on a string around the patient's neck.

In December 1999, after half a century of medical progress that included the 'pharmaceutical revolution', one of my contemporaries who'd retired from general practice had a letter from a patient pleading with him to return to work because "the new doctor's prescriptions don't work the way that yours did".

## Prestigious

Adjective invariably used in medicine to express what the *Oxford English Dictionary* gives as its first meaning: *Practising juggling or legerdemain; of the nature of or characterised by juggling or magic; cheating, deluding, deceitful; deceptive, illusory.* Hence:

> Speaker at BMA annual meeting: *It is an honour to be present on this truly prestigious occasion.*

> Press handout about a notorious medical writer: *He gave the prestigious College Day lecture at the Royal College of Physicians.*

## Preventive medicine

Deploying medical skills as a means of self defence.

Rudolf Ludwig Karl Virchow, the German pathologist, was an energetic political reformer and such an outspoken critic of Prussian conservatism that Bismarck challenged him to a duel.

When Bismarck's seconds called on him, Virchow explained: "As the challenged party, I have the choice of weapons and I choose these." He held aloft two large sausages. "One is infected with deadly germs; the other is perfectly sound. Let His Excellency decide which he wishes to eat, and I will eat the other."

When the seconds conveyed the challenge to the Chancellor he sent them back to tell Virchow he'd decided to laugh the matter off.

## Prison

Traditional 19th century treatment for mental illness.

The treatment was revived in the late 20th century and used with undiminished enthusiasm in the 21st.

## Problem area

A problem that poses no problems. Once you reclassify anything as an area, managers can discuss or 'address' it, without incurring any obligation to solve it.

I once wrote to a hospital administrator on behalf of a friend who'd received pretty shabby treatment from the department alleged to be in charge of admissions. In lieu of apology, the reply, which mysteriously transmogrified my friend into my 'client' offered a finely wrought piece of NHS Management Speak. Here, stripped of the surrounding sentences expressing phoney 'concern', is the central core of explanation:

*We recognise that this is a problem area. We have been addressing it for some time but regret that as yet we see little hope of resolving it in a manner that would meet your client's expectation.*

## Professional detachment
Stoic quality cultivated by doctors and theatrical landladies.

Theatrical digs, and their landladies, loom large in the anecdotage of actors. They also provide occasional uplifting moments for GPs. Late one evening a Manchester GP was telephoned by an actor lodging in theatrical digs. He feared that a fellow lodger might have appendicitis. When the GP entered the digs he opened the door to the kitchen to ask the number of the invalid's room. To his embarrassment he found the landlady on the floor in *flagrante delicto* with a notorious Music Hall troubadour. Completely unfazed she peered over the shoulder of her heaving lover and said: "Oh doctor, you must think me a terrible flirt."

## Professional privileges
Perks that come the way of doctors thanks to the nature of their calling.

A young woman doctor at the Bristol Royal Infirmary, who needed a car to get to work, went for her driving test. The examiner said very little during the test and, just after they'd completed it, collapsed with an acute myocardial infarction. To his great good fortune, his pupil gave him immediate cardiopulmonary resuscitation, used his car phone to call for help, and an ambulance took him to hospital.

His saviour was left with an unusual dilemma. Lack of a full driving licence was costing her a fortune in taxi fares. The Department of Transport told her that, if she hadn't resuscitated her examiner and he'd expired, she could have had an immediate re-take. Because she'd completed the test, they had to wait for his report before they could do anything.

She could hardly walk into the coronary care unit and ask a dangerously ill man if she'd passed but, in desperate mood, she petitioned the examiner's cardiologist. After a number of postponements, he eventually told her that his patient was well enough for a visit.

The examiner greeted her effusively and solemnly thanked her on behalf of his family and himself for saving his life. She moved diffidently towards the purpose of the visit. "I'm terribly sorry to bother you but I just wondered did I pass?"

The examiner responded with a kindly smile.

"I'd like to assure you, my dear, that I reached my decision before you saved my life. So I can tell you, quite without bias, that you failed."

## Professional secrecy
Long standing tradition of confidentiality whereby doctors never disclose secrets confided to them by patients, save to professional colleagues or to fellow guests at a dinner table.

## Professions
Ancient guilds wherein lurk predators from whom our Masters are eager to protect us… though not from all of them.

In 2005 Dame Janet Smith, the judge who chaired a government inquiry set up after the conviction of the serial killer Dr Harold Shipman, recommended that doctors should be regularly assessed and revalidated. Her recommendations are now being implemented and, if they don't get wedged in the traditional bureaucratic bottleneck, should give us greater protection from incompetent doctors… though not, ironically, from doctors like Harold Shipman.

When Dame Janet published her report I wondered why we needed more rigorous protection from incompetent doctors than from incompetent members of her own profession. If you Google 'revalidation' plus 'solicitors' or 'barristers' or 'judges' you get references only to lawyers who have involved themselves in the revalidation of doctors. Yet my lifetime experience suggests that incompetent doctors are responsible for no greater levels of morbidity, or even of premature mortality, than incompetent lawyers.

And as for politicians, you don't need to look too far back into political history to see how incompetent or disingenuous members of that profession can be several hundred thousand times more lethal than Dr Shipman.

If the government is serious about protecting us from the professions, it should set up a new enquiry, this time under the chairmanship of a distinguished doctor, maybe the president of a Royal College, to advise on improving professional standards in the legal and political professions.

The president would, I hope, adopt the simple practical approach that sustains clinical medicine: suggesting, for instance, that MPs be cleared by a breathalyser before being allowed to vote and that judges pass the same test before every court session. No reasonable person could argue against the proposition that people who make decisions that gravely affect the lives of others, and sometimes cause unnecessary deaths, should at least be sober when they make them. Psychiatric assessment of suitability could come later.

Such thoughts, I fear, are the stuff of which dreams are made. MPs revealed their disposition when it came to protecting the public purse from their expense claims. And, as the seasoned commentator Simon Jenkins points out, many MPs are barristers. "They regard professional reform as something applicable only to doctors, academics and journalists. They launch constant inquiries into them, but curiously none into lawyers."

## Prognosis
A guess that some doctors make with extraordinary precision. As in: "His doctors gave him six months to live."

Successful prognosticators give details only to suggestible patients and deliver them in firm dogmatic tones.

The most skilled practitioner of the art I've encountered was an obstetrician who built a profitable reputation for forecasting the sex of unborn babies. He told each pregnant woman that she was going to have a boy, but wrote girl in the notes. If his patient delivered a girl, he showed her the notes written in her presence and explained that she must have misheard.

## Prophet of Doom
Role eagerly assumed by medical crypto-sadists who delight in issuing warnings about activities they see other people enjoy. (See Masturbation.)

Whenever a new toy or game appears some doctor will be at hand, eye bright and pen primed, eager to publish the first account of the hazard it poses to health. It's an ancient medical tradition – some doctors are still uncertain whether they approve of sex – but, in the mid-20th century, doctors discovered that if they issued gloomy warnings about popular activities, not only did they get their letters in professional journals but their names in newspapers read by their patients.

They needed little further encouragement and, in the closing half of the 20th century we had grave pronouncements about Jogger's Nipple, Break-dancing Neck, Crab-eaters Lung, Swim-goggle Headache, Amusement Slide Anaphylaxis, Cyclist's Pudendum, Dog Walker's Elbow, Space Invaders' Wrist, Unicyclist's Sciatica, Jeans Folliculitis, Jogger's Kidney, Flautist's Neuropathy, and Urban Cowboy's Rhabdomyolosis – a painful nastiness in the muscles caused by riding mechanical bucking broncos in amusement arcades.

Three punctilious Swiss, Drs Itin, Heanel and Stalder reported an unusual jogging hazard: bird attacks by the European Buzzard (Buteo buteo). The three wise men from Kantonsspital Liestal described how attacks occur during the buzzard breeding season and how "the birds attacked by diving from behind and continuing to dive as long as the joggers were in motion." They didn't speculate on what might be passing through the buzzards' minds at the time.

When the *Independent on Sunday* listed some ailments that afflict 'clubbers': PVC Bottom – friction burns that manmade fibres inflict on sweating bodies, Techno Toe – lacerations caused by neighbouring toenails during dancing, and Ravers' Rash – once known as 'heat rash', they wheeled out a professor from St Mary's Hospital, London, to offer the expert opinion that a combination of amphetamines and "excessive dancing on concrete floors" could "put stress on backs and joints."

There's erudition, for you.

## Prophylactic records
Medical notes designed to avoid repeated discussion of the tedious.

I once had a patient who, whenever he entered my surgery, would hand over a note that included a neatly typed list of his symptoms, a month's record of his temperature and pulse, and a series of boxes in which ticks and crosses recorded the pattern of his bowel movements over the previous two weeks. He claimed he made the note because he didn't want to waste my time. I suspect he meant he didn't want me to waste his.

Some years ago, Leonard Peter, a GP in Pinner, encountered an altogether more valuable use of the technique. When on holiday in Corsica he met an amiable lawyer with a bandaged hand who, whenever he made a new acquaintance, handed over a note:

*Yes it was an accident. A lawn mower actually. In France.*
*I know I was stupid. Everyone has told me that already including my wife.*
*I have lost the top part of my middle finger. The other two will be okay.*
*They are just fractured.*
*I am not sure how long it will take to heal but the consultant wants to see me each week for the next few weeks.*
*I don't think it will affect my life a great deal and I still intend to play tennis and golf.*
*When an Arsenal footballer did the same thing I said at the time that I thought he must be particularly stupid. I was right.*
*Thank you again for showing sympathy. I will be more careful in the future.*

## Protective clothing
Garments patients wear when visiting their GPs.

A Glasgow GP, Richard Watson, once asked if other GPs had silent invisible arctic blizzards raging outside their consulting rooms. The Glasgow blizzard was so fierce, he said, that many of his patients were unable to leave his presence until they had perfectly rearranged their jumper, waistcoat, jacket, coat, scarf, hat and possibly even gloves. This process, said Dr Watson, sometimes took longer than the consultation and, even if he held the door open, continued at its own deliberate pace until every button was buttoned and every fold of every garment lay neatly in its place.

## Protocol
A trick 'modernisers' play to encourage doctors to abandon the principles of their profession.

When surgeon Graham Chuter did his postgraduate training at a series of hospitals, he managed to antagonise the surgical pre-assessment nurses at nearly every one. When asked to sign pre-printed analgesia prescriptions for patients he'd never seen who were coming in for joint replacements, he refused. He pointed out that the prescribing doctor had to take full responsibility for any adverse events that occurred, including those that might have been prevented had he actually seen the patients, talked to them about their medical history, maybe even examined them. The nurses' response, he says, was to "demand my name and rank in a tone accusatory of hindrance and obstruction."

In a letter to *BMA News Review* in 2011, he asked, "Should I sign just because 'that's how it works here', 'everyone else signs them', or, perhaps worst of all, because 'it's protocol'?"

To comply would have been easy. To defend himself in court or at the GMC would have been more difficult. And if he did end up in court, I doubt the protocol devisers would volunteer to take his place in the dock.

## Pseudo-empathy

Quality exuded by self consciously caring people with a firmer grip on jargon than reality.

A fine example is the closing paragraph of a letter to parents of a child attending an Oxfordshire child guidance clinic:

> *I would be happy to offer you an appointment at 3 pm on the 18th of next month in order that we may work out together a task-centred goal-orientated approach which will hopefully build up X's strength and self-confidence. Hope to see you then.*
> *Go Well.*
> *Yours sincerely,*
> *xxxxxxxxxxx (Mrs.) Psychiatric Social Worker.*

I know I've reached the age of old bufferdom but, even making allowance for the state of my cerebral arteries, I find that mixture of mumbo jargon and false mateyness so patronising that, like the doctor who showed it to me, I hope the parents had enough self respect to Go Well – and rapidly – to some other source of help and advice.

## Pseudologia fantastica
Medicalised lying and boasting.

The condition was argued in mitigation by lawyers representing a Californian judge Patrick Couwenberg, sacked after investigators discovered he had lied during his application to join the bench. He claimed he'd been a CIA operative during the Vietnam war, had been on CIA missions in Africa, had worked underground in Laos, and been awarded a Purple Heart when wounded in combat. Investigators discovered he was never in the CIA and, during the time he claimed he was, he was a social worker in Orange County, California.

Reporting the case in the *Guardian,* Duncan Campbell described Couwenberg's explanation as "poignant." His wife had typed out his application and he couldn't bear to tell her that the service career he invented when they first met was bogus.

Pseudologia fantastica affected another judge, Michael O'Brien from Chicago, who falsely claimed to be a winner of two Medals of Honour, and of a Pulitzer prize But the condition is not exclusive to judges. Professor Joseph Ellis was suspended for a year without pay by Mount Holyoke Community College in Massachusetts after he'd told his students he was a platoon commander near My Lai when, in the real world, he was teaching history at West Point.

Over the past decade, dogged researchers and disgruntled veterans' organisations have exposed what Campbell calls "dozens of tin soldiers who have strutted at the head of their veterans' parades or used a bogus war record to parlay their way into a job or a relationship."

Yet ten years before, few Americans blinked an eye when a physician Peter Dans described in the American medical journal *The Pharos* how:

*President Ronald Reagan raised cognitive dissonance to an art form. He extolled the family though he was divorced and never saw his children or grandchildren. He praised God and religion but professed none. He could say and believe that he was in a photographic unit accompanying the troops liberating concentration camps, when he never left the United States during the war.*

Maybe the US citizens who deified him at home and erected a statue of him in London's Grosvenor Square forgave those deceptions because they'd seen him playing heroes in the movies.

Some of the deceivers exposed by investigators continue to protest their innocence despite the evidence. These individuals, who carry self belief to the extreme, suffer from a different condition Pseudologia Toxophilus (see below).

## Pseudologia Toxophilus

An advanced form of Pseudologia fantastica that drives people to rewrite their personal history in a way that stretches the credulity of everyone except themselves. The name is a Latinisation of Archer Syndrome, named after Jeffrey, the noble lord, whose self-told life story proved to be his most imaginative work of fiction.

Jonathan Swift offers a memorable description of the condition in *Tale of a Tub:*

*When man's fancy gets astride of his reason; when imagination is at cuffs with the senses; and common understanding, as well as common sense, is kicked out of doors; the first proselyte he makes is himself.*

In *The Psychology of Anomalous Experience,* Professor Graham Reed describes a young woman who arrived late for her appointment looking distraught yet giving the impression of bravely fighting back tears. She asked for time to compose herself saying: "I feel a bit shaken, you see. Something just happened that rather upset me." Then after a show of decent reluctance, she explained she had caught her bus in good time and was late only because, as she got on the bus, the conductor had brutally ravished her.

Reed agreed that this was conduct unbecoming a municipal employee but unusual in mid-afternoon on a main road in the city centre, not to mention on a crowded bus. He asked if she'd reported the outrage to the police and she replied with wide-eyed sincerity that she hadn't done so because: "That would have made me late for my appointment here."

After the session, when Reed took her back to the waiting-room, he found her mother waiting for her. The mother, he discovered, had travelled with her daughter on the bus and had seen "nothing untoward".

The young woman, says Reed, was not at all disconcerted by her mother's denial of her story. The rape, she explained, had taken place as she was about to follow her mother down the stairs. And she hadn't mentioned it during the walk from the bus stop because the conductor had also tried to strangle her with his ticket-punch strap and she was temporarily unable to speak.

## Pseudo-parentalism
Attitude sometimes adopted by the young towards those they assume to be in their 'second childhood'.

As in a note received by a Surrey GP: *Dear Doctor, Could you please call and see my mother who has taken to going out on walks on her own though she's now sixty-five.*

I heard a typical case history from a doctor I met in Philadelphia. His household consisted of his wife and himself, their three adolescent daughters, and his widowed eighty-year-old mother. The family worried that the old lady rarely got out of the house so they arranged a 'date' for her with a widower who lived nearby and was also in his eighties. She was very late getting home and the whole family had to sit up to wait for her.

When she came in, her son asked anxiously: "Did you have a good time?"

"Are you kidding?" snapped his mother. "I had to slap his face three times."

"Gosh," said one of the granddaughters. "Did he try to get fresh?"

"No," said the old lady. "I thought he was dead."

## Psychogaming
Competitive sport in which players devise entertaining theories about human behaviour. The prizes go to those who use the least experimental evidence and provoke the most cries of "Oh what a clever idea".

"It was the carrots what did it," said the woman behind me on the southbound platform at Goodge Street station. "He never did anything kinky till he started eating those carrots. I reckon they put him in mind of it." An inconsiderate train rattled in, drowning the rest of her remarks and leaving my curiosity insatiate. But I recognised the game that was being played.

There's nothing new about this trivial pursuit. The more imaginative cavemen probably played it to relax after a hard day drawing bison on the wall. For those who would like an introductory manual I recommend *The Book of Life* which I found in our local library. A chapter modestly entitled "Understanding sexual attraction" contains a brilliant opening move: "Female breasts appeal to men because their shape mimics the buttocks which are obvious zones of erotic interest." How's that for instant dogma? No concessions there to perverts who might find breasts attractive because they resemble breasts, or bottoms attractive because they resemble bottoms.

No matter how outraged you are by the opening move, you feel compelled to riposte. "The female umbilicus attracts the male because it resembles the foxhole in which every man in our anxiety-ridden world would like to hide." And, once you tune in to the wavelength, profundities spill from your lips like imitation pearls popping from their moulds.

"Female legs," says the book, "are triggers to sexual response because they lead to potential delights."

"Depends on which way you're travelling," you riposte. "A foot fetishist is someone who took the wrong turning at his mother's knee."

I once initiated a lively game by proposing that Man's driving force is an unquenchable desire to eat stewed prunes and custard. The moves that followed included:

"A predilection for a blonde or brunette sexual partner is an individual's attempt to compensate for an interactional conflict at the prune/custard nexus."

"White racists are driven by a fundamentalist custardian fervour to deny the attraction of a black skin."

"Oedipus married his mother because of her wrinkles."

Those were but the first thoughts that flowed. (Gosh, could that use of 'flowed' be a custardian slip?)

## Psychspeak

Language developed by psychogamesters who want to invest their speculation about the working of the human mind with an aura of authority.

From a clinical psychologist's letter to a Weymouth GP:
*He has developed insight regarding factors which precipitated his*

*islets of verbal dyscontrol and he has begun to utilise his emotional gearbox particularly his brakes appropriately.*

From a psychiatrist's report to a GP in St Austell: *He denied any delusional material and laughed when I tried to question him about Schneiderian first rank symptoms.*
This failure to understand a simple question seemed more extraordinary when the report later revealed that the patient was a regular reader of the *Sun*.

A *BMJ* correspondent putting us right about Conan Doyles's best known creations: *Together, Holmes and Watson represent Doyle's intrapsychic conflict: Holmes is the free-spirited (albeit Victorian) id, while Watson is the stodgy stumbling superego. Doyle resolves this intrapsychic conflict by aligning Holmes (good id) and Watson (superego) against the evil Professor Moriarty (bad id) in a battle of wits (ego). Doyle's masterpiece memorializes Freud's tripartite structural theory of id (instinct), superego (conscience), and ego (intellect) so skilfully that it seems elementary.*
Quite so, my dear Watson.

## Public health advice
Not the sole property of registered practitioners.

Often more effective when delivered by workers 'on the ground', as in this tale I heard from Peter Moloney.

The new manager who took over the village pub had, to the villagers' great misfortune, come hot foot from a brewery marketing course. Among the innovations with which he tried to 'freshen the image' of the old place was a sign behind the bar that announced with grating cheeriness: *A pint, a pie, and a friendly word.*

One evening a visitor sat up at the bar and placed his order. When it arrived he put on a roguish smile and said to the buxom woman who'd brought it: "I've got the pie and the pint. How about the friendly word?"

She leaned across the bar and whispered: "Don't eat the pie."

## Public opinion
Dangerous concept that occasionally drives medical researchers up the poll.

I long ago decided that public opinion doesn't exist. What does exist is a public mood that becomes an opinion only when a decision is demanded of it, such as a vote, an answer to a pollster's question, or an irresistible urge to back one side in a televised argument or one contestant in a televised talent show.

In the mid 1970s, the Royal Society of Medicine invited me to take part in a discussion of the effect of public opinion on medical practice. "When dealing with public attitudes," wrote the organiser, "we hope you will try particularly to distinguish justifiable anxieties from uninformed fears."

The only distinction I could draw was that "uninformed fears" were what patients suffered before their doctors told them what they were going to do to them, and "justifiable anxieties" were what they suffered after they were told. But the invitation showed how the notion of 'public opinion' exists more substantially in the minds of those who seek it than in the minds of those from whom it is sought.

We're stuck with the phrase because it's a useful rhetorical prop – like 'silent majority' or 'all right thinking people' – for those who lack visible support but still want to boss us about.

To test my prejudice, I got a friend in a market research company to add an impish question to a list they were using in a series of street interviews:

*You have just given me your opinion on a number of topics to do with medicine and medical research.*
*Do you think your opinions:*
  *a) generally reflect public opinion on these matters,*
  *b) differ from public opinion on these matters, or*
  *c) you don't know.*

Though the series was too small to be statistically significant, I discovered with delight that only around 20 per cent of those surveyed thought their views reflected 'public opinion', nearly 70 per cent thought their ideas differed from it, and around 8 per cent didn't know.

I'd like to think the response told us something about British people's image of themselves. I fear it may just reveal their attitude to people with clipboards who ask them questions in the street.

## Pulling rank

Dangerous gambit for patients to try with an experienced GP. Especially one who comes from Yorkshire.

A Bradford-bred GP who'd moved South was wakened in the early hours by a phone call from a celebrated television comedian who wanted an urgent visit to his girlfriend who had a painful wrist. After asking a few questions, the GP said he didn't think the condition was urgent enough to merit a night call and suggested the young woman came round to the surgery in the morning.

"I expect a visit," said the actor. "Don't you know who I am?"

"Should I know you?" asked the GP, his Yorkshire accent growing more defined with every word.

"I am X, the comedian."

"Oh, a comedian, are we? Well, let's strike a bargain. I'll visit your woman if you can make me laugh… now."

## Pulpit

Dangerous platform from which to offer medical advice.

The most wholesome book on my shelves is a slim volume *What a man of forty-five ought to know*, written in 1901 by The Rev Sylvanus Stall, Doctor of Divinity, of Philadelphia and sent to me some years ago by a GP who clearly thought I needed it. It is one of a series of "Pure books on avoided subjects" which were translated into "several languages including Urdoo and Tegeloo."

The blurb, no doubt to boost sales, includes the phrase "conjugal relations", but the text never dwells on such unsavoury matters. The Rev Sylvanus writes as if he's prepared to put nothing on paper he would not be happy to say in the pulpit. As a result the hints he drops about "avoided subjects" are dangerously enigmatic. Readers are left unsure whether they are threatened by mild discomfort or a terrifying biblical dissolution of mind and body in retribution for the sin of enjoying life too much.

A characteristic injunction is a warning about cycling that Sylvanus embeds in a paragraph I had assumed was about healthy exercise.

*Eighteen years ago, when thirty-five years of age, the writer was among the first to adopt the bicycle as a means of recreation. For some six years I rode the high wheel, usually devoting the month of August to a tour of several hundred miles. The saddles at that time, and for years afterward, were unsanitary and injurious in their effects because of the pressure against the perineum. As the riding was at that time largely confined to young men, the results of the unsanitary saddles, rigid frames and excessive vibration were scarcely realised even by the medical profession. What these consequences have been to many men, it required the later years to disclose.*

If you think that last sentence begs more questions than it answers, try the next one:

*At this period of life, the reading of inflammatory literature may produce the same injurious results.*

And that's as far as the explanation goes.

Maybe it reads less enigmatically in Tegeloo.

## Punchbag therapy
Knocking sense into those deemed guilty of aberrant behaviour.

My interest in punitive medicine was fired by S J Perelman's suggestion that the best way to control thumb-sucking was to nail the infant's hands to the side of the cot. The traditional victims are those least likely to resist.

In the 1930s Ellia Berstock, when a medical student in Dublin, watched a Dr Murphy at The Meath Hospital treating a man rendered immobile by "hysterical paralysis." Dr Murphy cured the condition, if only temporarily, by applying a red-hot metal disc to the patient's backside. The paralysed man leaped out of bed and strutted round the ward like an automaton. He then returned to bed but made no complaint about being branded.

In 1943 researchers at the University of Cincinnati hospital kept sixteen patients in refrigerated cabinets for 122 hours at -1°C, hoping that refrigeration might cure their mental illness. The only success they could claim was that all their patients survived.

Around the same time a psychiatrist at the Verdun Hospital in Montréal injected turpentine into his patients' abdominal muscles. He hoped the huge painful abscesses that resulted would raise the white blood cell count, which they did, and thus "regularise" the mental processes, which they didn't.

In the 1940s Walter Freeman, president of the American Board of Psychiatry and Neurology, claimed to "cure" a variety of mental illnesses. After administering a local anaesthetic, he would lift his patient's eyelid and insert a gold-plated ice pick beneath the tear duct. When the pick had penetrated two inches into the brain he would give it a sharp twist and then withdraw it.

He called the operation "transorbital lobotomy" and, travelling in a specially equipped van which he called a Lobotomobile, visited twenty-three states picking at the brains of 2400 people. Researchers found little evidence that he did any good. One claimed he behaved "with a recklessness bordering on lunacy, touring the country like a travelling evangelist. In most cases, this procedure was nothing more than a gross and unwarranted mutilation carried out by a self righteous zealot."

One of Freeman's victims was Rosemary Kennedy, sister of the future US president, whom he permanently incapacitated with a lobotomy when she was aged twenty-three.

Punitive medicine was not a 20th century phenomenon. Hilton's *Rest and Pain*, "a medical classic" recommended to generations of medical students, including mine, for its "delicacy of approach to the problems of healing" was published in 1863.

Hilton was gravely concerned about masturbation – or, as he preferred, onanism – which he regarded as a source of much serious illness. He described it as "a habit very difficult to contend with in practice", assumed it afflicted only males, and recommended painting the victim's penis with a strong tincture of iodine to ensure that it blistered and became so sore that the patient could not bear to touch it.

## Pundits

Commentators assumed to speak with authority because, in front of a television camera, they look pretty, or stereotypical, or acceptably loopy.

For those who pretend to fill every twenty-four hours with twenty-four hours of 'news', punditry comes less expensive than hard slogging research. So, when the pretty, stereotypical, or acceptably loopy are unavailable, hardworking reporters are expected to plug the gap.

Despatches from 'trouble spots' used to consist of itinerant reporters answering questions from the studio, and providing the sort of information reporters are trained to collect – details of troop movements, explosions, casualties, local reaction, and such like. But now, all too often, there follows the pundit question, "So what does this mean, Nigel, for the stability of the Middle East/Northern Ireland/the Balkans /the peace process?"

It's an enquiry that might draw an informative answer from an experienced diplomat who'd spent a lifetime studying the issues and was given an hour to explain the nuances. Yet our newshound is expected to give an instant answer with the authority that 'special correspondents' bring to predicting what will happen in cabinet meetings that have yet to take place, to explaining what the Queen is saying in private to her son, or to answering questions that would have daunted Einstein: "So, in a sentence Nigel, what effect will this breakthrough in particle physics have on the man in the street?"

Yesterday's newsreader, or 'presenter', or game show host slips easily into the role of today's omniscient pundit. If a visiting Martian were to hear an interview on Radio Four's *Today* or *World at One,* he would assume that the confident person who knows all the facts and barks them out with dogmatic certainty is the interviewee and the more tentative person trying to make what is complex easier to understand is the journalist. And, as you and I know, the visiting Martian would be wrong.

Medicine, said a man on the train, has lost the voice of authority. Not so much lost it, I thought, as had it purloined. In matters medical, the new all-purpose, all-wise wielders of the voice of authority are dextrous operators of the retrospectroscope. Looking back at a medical 'blunder', they will explain exactly what the wretched nurse or doctor should have done. Yet face them with a real decision and you hear the ring of an empty vessel.

"If patients are worried by this news, Nigel, what should they do?"

"I suggest they go and see their own GP."

Even Nigel recognises that in times of stress the only useful voice of authority is the voice of experience. Yet that doesn't worry him or the Ms Nigels because they know that today's decision maker can be served up as tomorrow's scapegoat.

## Punsterism
Cognitive disorder that deludes its victims, most of them English, into thinking that punning is a form of wit.

Some puns *are* witty. The delusion at the heart of punsterism is that all puns are witty just because they are puns.

The likely causative agent is a virus that invades selected cognitive areas of the brain. If that proves to be the case, the transmission route will almost certainly be television and the most dangerous carriers will be game show hosts. Not every game show host but those who, when presented with a contestant called Woods, will say: "I'm *tree*-mendously pleased to greet you. I'm sure you'll quickly *twig* the rules and if you *branch* out bravely I'm sure you will *leaf* with a prize." They actually pronounce the italics and mark them with knowing looks lest we fail to spot the rapier flashes.

And the audience, may their Gods forgive them, encourages the perpetrator with applause.

Television news has been seriously infected. A reporter covering a solemn conference in Brighton took himself off to the aquarium and stood in front of a giant fish tank just so he could say: "The Treasury today reminded City sharks that there other fish in the sea." Then after delivering sober facts about financial regulation he wound up: "Those who monitor the sea bed of our economy will discover that the minnows have now been given greater protection against the corporate predators of the deep."

What I ask, more in hope than expectation of an answer, is the point of it all?

The most depressing feature of punsterism is the way its spread has debased a linguistic skill that was once a source of genuine wit. As when Dorothy Parker, asked for her thoughts about horticulture, replied: "You can lead a whore to culture but you cannot make her think."

## Puppy love

Disneyesque euphemism suggesting loyal, tail-wagging, slavering teenage infatuation.

A million miles removed from the reality: a confusing, debilitating, misery-making obsession that afflicts adolescents.

I was aged about fourteen when I fell in love with Little Red Riding Hood. Before any psychiatrist shouts "Eureka!" I should explain I fell in love with the golden-haired girl playing the title role in the pantomime at the Grand Theatre, Doncaster. I went with my parents and my young sister to the Saturday matinee and spent the whole weekend mentally banjaxed. I managed – just – to camouflage my distress by pretending I was tussling with difficult homework.

On Monday I plundered my life savings from an old jam jar half-filled with copper coins and, for four days, lashed out ninepence a time to stand at the back of the stalls at every performance, including the children's matinee on Wednesday. Each night on the lonely bus home I thought of my beloved being swept away from the stage door in a Rolls-Royce (Shirley Temple was getting a lot of publicity at the time) to the dazzling new 'roadhouse' on the Great North Road.

On Thursday night I summoned the courage to hang around the stage door after the performance – in truth to lurk in the shadows across the street – to catch another glimpse of my Beatrice. I almost didn't recognise her. There was no fur coat, no top-hatted stage door Johnny at her elbow. She was all on her own and wearing a gabardine mac that could have been my sister's school coat. She also looked older than she did onstage but I wasn't going to let a difference in age stand between us.

The Rolls failed to turn up so, as she walked away, I did a quick Sexton Blake and trailed her to the bus stop where she got onto a Trackless – our name for a trolley bus. I kept her under observation from the back seat and, when she got off, followed her along dismal streets, flitting Sexton-like from shadow to shadow, until she let herself into a house with a big sign in the front window: ROOMS.

I didn't sleep that night and early next morning was back on watch outside the house. She didn't emerge until midday. I trailed her onto another Trackless, climbed the stairs behind her and, with a courage I've never known since, plonked myself in the seat beside her.

For three stops I gazed unflinchingly ahead, then I turned to her and explosively declared my passion in a mixture of rehearsed poetic phrase and stumbling improvisation.

For a moment my beloved stared at me with soft grey eyes before she spoke. "Fuck off," she said.

So I did. I slunk back down the stairs and, at the next stop, hopped off the Trackless. At some point on the three mile walk home I realised I was cured.

Six months passed before I discovered I was only in temporary remission. There was this girl behind the cosmetics counter in Boots the Chemist...

## Quackery

The mainstay of traditional medicine.

As the Dublin physician and literary scholar Petr Skrabanek pointed out:

*The difference between a doctor and a quack is determined not by the nature of their practice but by the possession of a medical diploma.*

An American physician, Eugene A Stead Jr, explained why:

*We understand only about ten per cent of what patients complain of; ninety per cent of what they report you have to handle empirically. In that ninety percent of your practice, you will be practising like a quack. You will not know what you are doing...*

*I've always been an excellent quack. The only difference between me and the quacks I don't like is that I don't try to get rich off my quackery, and I try to be honest about it. There's medicine that has a basis in science and medicine that has no basis in science. I have treated a large number of people with rheumatoid arthritis, and I don't know what causes it. But I know how to arrange their lives and their way of working so that they are happier. You can call it experience if you want. But I call experience without science quackery.*

## Qualification
Mysterious process that transmutes the raffish medical student into a wise, trustworthy, and kindly physician.

I still remember the degree of startlement I suffered all of forty years ago when a figure from my past appeared as an 'expert' on my television screen. When we were students no one would trust him with the price of a drink, not to mention the address of a girlfriend. Yet there he was telling the nation why every fifteen-year-old girl should or shouldn't be on the contraceptive pill. I forget which it was but he said it with great authority.

## Quality of life
A judgement doctors consider themselves capable of making about other people's lives.

When used as a way of rationing resources, becomes a judgement of other peoples' worth. I suspect the lives some doctors would have judged of little worth would include indubitable loonies like Vincent van Gogh, hopeless drunks like Scott Fitzgerald and Dylan Thomas, and the Irish artist Christy Brown, who was born with cerebral palsy and could control only his left foot.

Peter Hillmore described in the *Observer* how when his elderly mother was ill, the surgeon told him there was nothing he could do but added that, if her "quality of life" had been better – if, say her husband had been alive – he might have come to another decision. "I am not arguing with his decision," wrote Hillmore, "but as he broke the news I wondered for a moment what right an expert in removing intestines had to be an expert on someone's quality of life."

If doctors want want to measure people's quality of life, I suggest they ask them how they rate their own. The safest definition of a person's quality of life is what he or she says it is.

## Quasi-hallucination
Bizarre mental state afflicting those who fail to seek ordinary explanations for extraordinary experiences.

On my way to speak at an international conference in Australia, I decided to break my journey in Singapore to give me time to de-lag. It was a wise decision. My plane arrived in Singapore eighteen hours late. Deprived of sleep, desperately tired, and seriously jet-lagged, I decided to have a relaxing float in the hotel pool before taking a couple of sleeping pills and going to bed. As I emerged from the pool I heard a voice say: "Didn't know *you* were here."

I have only hazy and disjointed memories of what happened next. All I remember clearly is that three hours later I was replying "on behalf of the guests" at a dinner of Singapore Chinese surgeons. I have no idea what I said but, as I sat down, I started to hallucinate. My hosts gathered round a piano and sang what sounded like Irish ballads. Hallucination was confirmed when I found myself confronted by forty Chinese faces singing: "When Irish Eyes Are Smiling.'

When I awoke next morning I was delighted to discover that sanity had reasserted itself. As I enjoyed a comforting breakfast, three of my erstwhile audience came across to my table. As we chatted I learned that Singapore medical students complete their training at the Royal College of Surgeons in Dublin where they learn the songs that students sing in local bars. There is even a riddle.

Q: What happens when a Singapore boy meets a Singapore girl at a bus stop in Dublin.

A: A group practice in Singapore.

When it comes to treatment, quasi-hallucination, like many a mystical experience, is susceptible to mundane explanation.

## Radio doctor
One who presumes to follow in the footsteps of Charles Hill who offered genial advice to warriors on the Kitchen Front in the dark days of the war: "And now for prunes, those black-coated workers in the lower bowel."

I was aware of the presumption when I took part in Britain's first medical phone-in, sitting opposite Allan Hargreaves in a tiny studio at Capital Radio. It wasn't really my sort of thing but I promised I'd do it for two weeks to get it started. To add the necessary gravitas the producers insisted I be called The Doctor

even though, in another part of the same building, I'd just done a
television series with Allan under my own name about the state
of the NHS in London.

We hammered out a protocol for dealing with callers: no
surnames, no addresses only the district from which they rang,
no treating people on air, no criticising treatment they were
already having. The last one was difficult. The audience now is
more sophisticated but, in those days, most folk who rang didn't
want my advice; they wanted me to rubbish advice they'd already
had from their GPs. I ended up mouthing platitudes worthy of
*Private Eye's A Doctor Writes…*

When we started, Capital still had the builders in and our
temporary studio was no more than a cramped corner under the
roof where we had to generate relaxed conversation while sitting
on opposite sides of a thick wooden beam under which we needed
to duck to see one another. The programme was often punctuated
by a clinking noise when unthinkingly I moved my feet and
disturbed the growing collection of empty champagne bottles
Gerald Harper discarded during his *Music for Lovers*.

A couple of days before my two weeks ended, Allan's face
appeared beneath the beam wearing a sinister grin.

"And now, doctor," he said, "we have Louise on the line who
has a problem with incontinence."

"Hello, Louise" said I, caring and avuncular. "And where are
you ringing from."

She responded in a stern Scottish accent. "From the waist
down, doctor."

I somehow managed to keep gabbling platitudes, Allan
strove valiantly to keep from giggling, and in a heroic triumph
over adversity we staggered uncertainly to the end of the
programme.

Only when I emerged into the real world of Euston Road, did
the penny drop. I went into a phone box and called an old friend
at his GP surgery in Watford. Sure enough his receptionist
answered in the accent of Louise, now more friendly than stern.
When she heard who was calling she shouted my name and
started to laugh, though not half as loud as her boss in the
background.

## Reading matter

Items hospital patients leave on their beds to entertain visiting doctors.

When I was a GP I learned a lot about patients by glancing at the books they read. Yet when I was student trailing behind consultants on hospital teaching rounds, only the physicians looked at the books. The surgeons read the patients' newspapers: the ENT men glanced at the gossip columns, the orthopaedic surgeons scanned the racing page, and an ambitious young obstetrician took an abiding interest in the Court Circular and Social Calendar.

Books are more reliable indicators of progress than temperature charts. After Norman Tebbit suffered appalling injuries in Brighton many of us heaved sighs of relief when the *Daily Mail* reported he had sent out for the complete set of *Just William* books. We knew then that he was coming along nicely.

## Real world

Parallel universe we enter when we want to behave in a way we know is selfish, irrational or morally indefensible. As in: "I have every sympathy with the sick and underprivileged but we have to live in the real world."

Most often used by those who want be known as a caring but don't want to make personal sacrifices.

In hospital management its most irritating usage is by senior officers in the Market Forces who bandy it about as if it were a new idea; as if, before the arrival of 'managerial expertise', doctors and nurses had never made realistic decisions in their work.

## Reciprocal arrangements
### 19th Century

System of barter used by the professional classes.

In the late 19th century, Sir Morell Mackenzie was London's most fashionable ENT surgeon. Proud of his position in society he was delighted to receive an urgent summons from the artist James Whistler. He was less pleased when Whistler explained that he was not the patient but would like the great man's opinion about his poodle whose bark hard turned a trifle hoarse.

Mackenzie contained his irritation, examined the dog's throat with the dexterity for which he was renowned, wrote a prescription, and departed with his fee.

The next day Whistler got a message to call on Mackenzie without delay. Fearing bad news about the poodle, he hurried to the surgeon's house.

"My dear Whistler," said Mackenzie. "So good of you to come. I was thinking of having my front door painted."

### 20th Century
Medico-political version of the axiom 'You scratch my back and I'll scratch yours.'

In the early days of the NHS, the BMA demanded a meeting with senior civil servants at the Ministry of Health to express its outrage over rumours that foreigners were visiting Britain just to get free NHS prostheses – their favourites being false teeth and glass eyes. The BMA wanted these to be supplied only to visitors from countries which had "reciprocal arrangements."

In those days, doctors' representatives were even more pompous than they are now and, according to John Carswell, a junior civil servant present at the meeting, the leader of the delegation put the case tediously and at great length until he was interrupted by the exasperated Sir Humphrey of his day.

"Thank you, doctor, for that lucid explanation," he drawled. "I shall inform the minister that the BMA's position is an eye for an eye and a tooth for a tooth."

### Recovered memories
The work of psychological upholsterers. More accurately spelled 're-covered memories', as in 're-covered sofas'.

Re-covering would have been a relatively harmless form of psychogaming (qv) if it hadn't become a rich source of 'evidence' of child abuse. Dr Harrison G Pope Jr, associate professor of psychiatry at Harvard medical school, has described how a young woman remembered during psychotherapy that her school teacher raped her when she was thirteen and that she became pregnant and had to have an abortion. There was no corroborating evidence and because she hadn't started to menstruate until she was fifteen she was extremely unlikely to have become pregnant two years before. Yet she was able to file criminal charges against the teacher, who had to spend his life savings on legal proceedings that lasted several years. The case ended only when the New Hampshire supreme court ruled that repressed and recovered memory lacked sufficient scientific foundation to be admissible.

In 1998, a working party set up by the Royal College of Psychiatrists in London concluded there was a high probability that memories 'recovered' after long spells of amnesia were false.

*Their creation seems to depend upon the conviction of the therapist or the patient that child sexual abuse underlies adult psychopathology. Memory-enhancing techniques do not improve the quality of remembering. They do increase the conviction with which memories, true or false, are held. They appear to be dangerous methods of persuasion.*

Faced with this evidence, aficionados of the therapy use an argument often used by proponents of unproven remedies: no one has disproved the possibility that repressed memories *might* exist. This objection, says Dr Pope, turns logic on its head. After 500 years of shaving their ideas with Occam's razor, "scientists have acknowledged that the burden of proof rests with whoever proposes a novel theory of causation, and not the reverse."

Repression may be a powerful motivational force in novels, movies, and television dramas. It may even be a common popular belief. But popular belief is no proof of its existence. Time was when most people thought the sun revolved around the earth until those pesky non-believers Copernicus and Galileo upset the applecart.

## Reduced mortality
What doctors achieve by withdrawing their services.

When doctors in Bogota, Columbia, went on strike and provided only emergency care for fifty-two days the death rate fell by 35 per cent.

When Los Angeles doctors went on strike the death rate fell by 18 per cent. When they returned to work the death rate returned to its previous level.

During a strike by Israeli doctors, who provided only

emergency cover, the number of patients seen fell from 65,000 to 7,000 a day and the death rate was halved. Only once before had the death rate fallen so dramatically. That happened twenty years before during another doctors' strike.

## Reductionist snobbery

An assumption that the only 'scientific' approach to researching complexity is the reductionist one.

The phrase was coined by Bill Silverman, one of the founders of American neonatal medicine who suffered vilification as a "baby killer" for promoting possibly the most significant randomised controlled trial of the 20th century. (See RLF.) Bill was also a fine provocative essayist and suggested that the reductionist approach would have led Newton to seek the source of gravity by dissecting the fallen apple and cataloguing the structures that lay within.

Reductionist snobbery influences not only our investigation of disease but the way we seek to teach one another about the complexities of our craft. Some medical educationalists assume, for instance, that you can 'teach' students complex emotional responses such as empathy and understanding by training them in 'key communication skills' (qv). These mechanistic tricks may have a palliative effect on the uncomfortable relationship some doctors have with their patients but they are the tools of spin doctors not of healing ones.

The route to empathy and understanding starts with doctors gaining some knowledge of themselves, their motives and their attitudes. Reductionism offers little help. We need what the poet Simon Armitage has described as "forms of language that go beyond the rational and the prosaic, and which mirror our fragmented, highly metaphorical and moment-to-moment perception of life itself." (See Healing Art.)

Medical educationalists who turn their hand to teaching 'communications' feel more comfortable with an analytic approach because it seems more 'scientific'. Their detailed examination of each tree while ignoring the existence of the forest is redolent of a style of music criticism still found in programme notes at concerts and recitals. Years ago, Bernard Shaw parodied it in an analysis of *Hamlet's*: "To be, or not to be: that is the question."

*Shakespeare, dispensing with the customary exordium, announces his subject at once in the infinitive, in which mood it is presently repeated after a short connecting passage in which, brief as it is, we recognise the alternative and negative forms on which so much of the significance of repetition depends. Here we reach a colon; and a pointed pository phrase, in which the accent falls decisively on the relative pronoun, brings us to the first full stop.*

## Reincarnation

Flamboyant symptom of doubt deficiency.

In some US communities belief in reincarnation is now as common as belief in alien abduction.

Roger Katz, a fifty-year-old teacher in Santa Fe, California was found in the back of a van with a naked schoolgirl. At his trial he claimed that he and the fourteen-year-old girl had met in Tibet in 640 AD when she was a mature woman and he was a teenage monk. She'd saved his life by stepping in front of him and taking in the chest an arrow intended for him. All he'd been doing in his van was repaying a "debt of love and devotion".

The Californian judge showed a sad lack of faith and sent Katz to prison.

## Refurbishment

Deploying resources on tarting up premises rather than on what takes place within them.

In the 1990s a hospital consultant took early retirement rather than move his department into the new premises that, after years of broken promises, his masters had eventually provided. "You may think I'm mad," he told me, "but after spending my entire professional life practising 20th century medicine in 19th century surroundings. I didn't want to spend the last two years in unfamiliar territory."

I assured him that if he were mad, it was a common form of loopiness and told him of the evening Sir Seymour Hicks, the actor manager, entered the lavatory at the Garrick Club and discovered that, while he'd been on tour, it had been lavishly redecorated.

As he stood at the urinal, the man in the next stall gazed around the new surroundings and said: "Impressive, isn't it?"

"Indeed," said Seymour Hicks, "but it does make the old prick look a bit shabby."

## Regular
Adjective that, when applied to health, is prone to irregular usage. Consultant gynaecologist Jonathan Scott offered examples.

> Q: Do you have your bowels open regularly?
> A: Since the operation I have them open very regularly indeed.

> Q: Do you have regular sexual intercourse?
> A: No because I only see my boyfriend every other weekend.

> Q: Do you have regular periods?
> A: No, doctor, they are always two days late.

## Relationships
Human alliances doctors seek to explain but rarely understand.

My father once had a difficult time delivering a baby in the bedroom of a Yorkshire farmhouse. After the baby had arrived safely and the mother lay comfortable and content, my father said to her: "This is the sixth child you and Harry have had. Why don't you marry him?"

"I could never do that, doctor."

"Don't you think it might be better for the children?"

"Maybe. But I could never marry him, doctor."

"Why not?"

"Because I've never really liked him."

## Religion
Collective noun for contradictory systems of belief that ensure we will never achieve a consensus on medical ethics.

The condition is nearly always inherited. Some change their religion or acquire it later in their lives and many discard it altogether, but most religious people stick to the one they inherited. As James Joyce's doppelgänger explains in *Stephen Hero*, "I was sold to Rome before I was born."

As a result, religion can become a social definition rather than a spiritual one. I wouldn't be surprised to hear someone in Northern Ireland exclaim: "You say you're an atheist but are you a Catholic atheist or a Protestant atheist?"

Historically, religion has been a crucial item in hospital documentation. Time was when every patient had to have one. Some years ago, when I took my seat at a medical dinner in Birmingham I found I was the meat in an ecumenical sandwich, parked between the city's Anglican Bishop and the Roman Catholic one. During the meal the Anglican bishop, Hugh Montefiore, told me that when he was visiting one of the male surgical wards in a local hospital, he encountered an old and deaf patient.

"Are you an Anglican?" asked His Grace.

"Eh?"

"Are you Church of England?"

"Eh? You'll have to speak up."

The Bishop raised his voice. "Are you C of E?"

"Oh no. I'm a strangulated hernia."

## Resentful prisoners

Doctors in their late thirties and early forties who feel imprisoned by their careers. Many who are good at their job extract most of the personal satisfaction from it by the time they reach their late thirties. They become bored and sometimes turn their hands to more dangerous activities like politics or management.

When I wrote about this phenomenon some years ago, I was at first surprised and then alarmed by the number of letters I received. Some came from academics who felt they'd done all the useful research they were likely to do and wondered where, outside the mainstream of medicine, they could find work that would challenge their minds and their imaginations. Most came from clinicians whose attitude towards their work had run a similar course: excitement, enthusiasm, and involvement in the early days; boredom entering insidiously, and at first un-noticed, as they reached their late thirties; eventual acknowledgement of the boredom and a depressing feeling of imprisonment within a career from which the only escape was a distant pension.

Many people thrive on a lifetime commitment to one line of work. My correspondents had discovered too late that they couldn't sustain the commitment. I later met scores of resentful prisoners prepared to face the truth that medicine, as they practised it, was unlikely ever again to offer the challenge and excitement that had made them good at their job. It was a disturbing thought. They knew that bored doctors were dangerous doctors.

Since then medical 'career structures' have become even more rigid and our academic masters, in their commendable desire to raise standards and tidy things up, have behaved too often as if they were dealing with highly trained organisms and not with un-neat, quirky individuals.

I often wonder if some of those making decisions about postgraduate education are themselves refugees, taking on the job as an escape from a routine that was beginning to get them down. Trips to London or a foreign part, playing committee games, and a little pomp and ceremony are welcome breaks from the routine grind of hospital or general practice. Yet these escapists, with the best of intentions, imprison others within narrow careers.

A medical career should continually broaden an intelligent person's vision rather than restrict it. We need to re-examine the idea that practising medicine means a lifetime commitment to one specialty rather than to a series of tasks that serve our profession's common purpose. We now delegate many of medicine's technical manoeuvres to machines. What doctors need are not narrow specialist skills but the creative versatility needed to invent and programme the machines, a skill easily transferrable from one job to another.

Chekov, while still practising as a clinician, wrote:

*My medical colleagues sigh with envy when they meet me and talk about literature and say how sick and tired they are of medicine. The strange thing is that medicine has had a great influence on my literary work. It has widened the field of my observation and enriched my knowledge.*

We could free the resentful prisoners by promoting enrichment rather than disenchantment.

## Reservoir opening
Municipal ceremony that rides even higher in the Pooter

Pomposity League than Foundation stone laying (qv).

I am one of few outsiders to have witnessed this rare ceremony, revered by reservoir men in much the way bird watchers revere a sighting of a Short-billed Dowitcher.

The honour alighted upon me in the most casual of circumstance. On some municipal occasion to do with public health in Yorkshire, I was introduced to a local mayor resplendent in his full regalia. He was a jolly soul – his opening interdict was, "Now lad don't pull my chain cos I flush very easily" – and hearing I was born in Yorkshire, he expressed disappointment that I wasn't seeing my mother county at its best. "If you want a really good do," he said, "come back in June when I'm opening a reservoir. I'll get the clerk to send you an invite." And sure enough one week later the gilt-edged invitation flopped through my letterbox.

It's not an invitation you get every day of the week. I made a note in my diary and when people asked me to fix a date for anything I would riffle through the pages saying, "I know I can't manage the tenth of June because I'm going to the opening of a reservoir." The more I talked and thought about it, the more excited I became and speculated wildly about what might lie in store. How on earth did a mayor open a reservoir? I nurtured an impious hope but sadly, when the great day came, all he did was cut a tape.

Yet, in the speech that followed, he delivered himself of a sentence that remains imprinted on my cerebral cortex, as indelibly as Calais was on Queen Mary's left ventricle. With his chain gently agitated by the breeze, he announced: "There hasn't been much water to spare this year but I'm proud to say that we in the West Riding have been able to hold our own."

## Resignation
1. State of mind which helps younger doctors come to terms with the disruption caused by continual NHS reorganisation.
2. Action which helps older doctors do the same.

## Resilience
Enduring quality of the human organism.

My GP father advocated a gentle approach to treatment because, he claimed, practising medicine had a lot in common with gardening. You have to work really hard to kill anything.

When a power failure blacked out New York, its most terrified victims were those travelling in lifts which became marooned between floors. A couple of days after the black-out I interviewed a janitor who'd been one of a team that had to locate the immobilised lifts, establish the condition of the trapped passengers, then decide the order in which they would winch the lifts by hand to the nearest floor. After working for some six hours they reached their umpteenth marooned lift on the hundred and something floor and, having shouted reassurance, went into their routine.

"How many are you?"

"Six."

"Any torchlight?"

"No."

"Any children?"

"No."

"Any elderly?"

"No."

"Anyone pregnant?"

"Could be," said a woman's voice. "Ask me again in eight weeks."

Chirpiness in the face of adversity is not confined to the land of the stiff upper lip.

## Resisted dying

Squeezing the last drop of life from dying people. Achieved by continuing life-prolonging treatments even when patients have said they don't want them, or sedating people and depriving them of food and drink until they die 'naturally'.

In the opening decades of the 21st century, this was a fate difficult for old people to avoid in the general wards of NHS hospitals, but in November 2009 Alex Paton, a retired consultant physician, described in the *BMJ* how he helped his eighty-five-year old wife, Ann, to escape and receive true palliative care.

Over the years they had both given a deal of thought to the way they wanted to die, and in the months before Ann's death she had made her feelings clear to her family. Paton wrote:

*She wanted to die and we realised she meant it. She had a wretched summer, with several falls and difficulty getting about; she found it hard to read or embroider because of double vision; a keen plantswoman, she said there was no point living if she could no longer garden.*

Then one day she was admitted to hospital as an emergency after a heart attack and suffered a cardiac arrest. She had written an advanced directive stating she did not wish to be resuscitated. The hospital staff saw the directive but chose to ignore it. They inserted a pacemaker which did little to improve her condition and parked her in a depressing geriatric ward where she ran the danger of further unwanted treatment.

Alex Paton knew the safest place for his wife was at home. And, as a former hospital consultant, he knew how to get her there. Despite his clout, he still had difficulty persuading the doctors to let her go, but he and his family were unyieldingly persistent. Eventually, after signing a form confirming they were discharging her against medical advice, they were able to take her home.

The fight was worth it.

*During the last fortnight of her life, surrounded by our four children and their families, she was able to talk and laugh and share in the gossip till near the end. Professional support was impeccable: practice doctors came on request, and our own doctor appeared regularly on the doorstep "to see how you're getting on; relatives need support as well, you know". District nurses came every day to regulate the morphine and midazolam pump; in spite of a heavy caseload they seemed to have all the time in the world.*

Two weeks after returning home Ann died peacefully with her family around her.

Alex Paton believes, as did Ann, that we are entitled to die with dignity,

*Each of us should have the right, when life becomes intolerable, to choose a way out rather than suffer the interventionist nightmare often imposed by modern medicine. The decision (preferably in advance) must be left strictly to the individual and must never be influenced by friend or foe...*

*Of course, we appreciate the strength of feeling that separates us from those who believe that life should be preserved at all costs. We respect their views and hope that they tolerate ours. We are not trying to persuade them to join us: that way lies conflict and the tactics of fanatics like the antiabortionists in America.*

## Retirement party

A formal acknowledgement, in days when lives were shorter, that a GP's race was run and that he or she had reached the winning post.

In ancient times, say fifty years ago, when GPs engaged in bizarre activities such as staying on call for their own patients four or more nights a week, those who managed to survive seemed to relish the rubric of departure. I recently trawled through a collection of 1960s regional newspapers and the ritual was remarkably consistent across the country.

The old boy's patients – in those days there were just a few old girls – would organise a gathering in a local hall where, feeling guilty perhaps over the havoc they'd wreaked in his coronary arteries, they would invite him to take tea or coffee with them, eat cupcakes and maybe sip a glass of brown sherry before they handed him a cheque, gold watch, or carriage clock – occasionally all three – to carry across the threshold to oblivion.

The GP's speech of thanks, according to local reporters, followed a traditional pattern: an expression of humble thanks, an explanation of the joy derived from every second of a hard working life, and an admonition to the young fellows coming into the profession today who didn't seem to have the same qualities of self-sacrifice and dedication "that we had in our time."

My GP father took a more positive attitude to retirement. He saw it as a time to extract some retrospective pleasure from the hard slogging that preceded it. He claimed he'd go on living for a year in the house from which he practised and whenever the doorbell rang would appear wearing old clothes and affecting a gross tremor.

"Oh, I'd love to help you," he'd tell the patient on the doorstep, "but, as you can see, the old health has let me down. Still, there's a clever new doctor down the road. Let me give you a tip – a secret I can pass on now I'm no longer in the business. This new fellow's brain functions much better at night. So don't call him now. Wait till he's had an hour or two in bed. Then you'll get him at his best."

Sadly he never made the winning post. One winter's night, like many a GP who is cynical in word rather than deed, he insisted on doing his evening surgery with a crippling pain in his chest and, as it turned out, a large infarct in his myocardium. And that, as they say, was that.

## Risk

An assessment based more often on perception than on measurement.

One oddity of the current model of homo sapiens is a flawed perception of the risks associated with medicine. People, for instance, will worry about a risk with a drug that is one thousandth of that which they run every time they get into their cars, and will happily accept a scale of risk with surgery they would never countenance with a medicine.

This flawed perception has a political quality. The mathematician Sir Hermann Bondi described a Swedish experiment designed to study the Aurora Borealis by firing instrument-carrying rockets into it. When the rockets were spent, the burnt-out remnants were due to fall over an area of Lapland so sparsely populated that the mathematical risk of anyone being hit was minute. Even so, the Swedish government felt it should offer protection to those who lived there and, before the exercise started, lifted out the isolated reindeer herders by helicopter.

Sir Hermann calculated that the mathematical likelihood of anyone being hit by a piece of rocket was at least one hundredth that of a helicopter accident. But he also considered the political implications.

If someone had been hit – or just been given a nasty fright – by a rocket fragment, there would have been public outrage that the Interior Minister had done nothing to protect people for whom he was responsible.

Yet, if there had been a helicopter crash, people would have accepted a ministerial statement: "We deeply sympathise with the relatives of the victims of this tragedy. We used a well tried helicopter, flown by a well trained and experienced crew. We are appalled at what has happened but there is no other precaution we could have taken."

There would have been no outrage because the crash was clearly what the small-print on insurance policies describes as an Act of God.

Some think doctors are too ready to quote risks as a way of explanation. The case was well put in the *BMJ* by Peter Arnold, an Australian GP now retired.

When he had coronary bypass surgery twenty-three years ago the surgeon told him he had "a 70 per cent chance of living for ten years". But he couldn't tell him if he was one of the lucky seventy or or one of the less fortunate thirty. The truth was that the surgeon didn't know; the sad thing was that he didn't say so. Writing in the *BMJ*, Peter asks:

*Is it not time to give up our antediluvian pretence at omniscience and learn to tell our patients the truth: 'I don't know?' Is it not time that we conditioned ourselves, and our patients, to learn that life is a lottery, that we are all compelled to take chances, that no human action is risk-free and that we are, quite simply and honestly, unable to truthfully answer many of their questions.*

*No amount or detail of statistical theory nor of statistical understanding can tell the individual patient what will or will not happen to them. It is that which is their concern and none of us knows the answer.*

## RLF (Retrolental fibroplasia)

The original double-blind disease in which neither patient nor doctor could see what was happening. A defining moment in 20th century medicine that is now largely forgotten.

Most people remember that, in the 1960s, the drug thalidomide caused 8,000 children to be born deformed. Few recall that, ten years earlier, another treatment administered with uncritical enthusiasm had blinded some 12,000 babies.

In 1941 a Boston paediatrician, making a routine visit to a three month old baby, was shocked to discover that a grey membrane covered the back of the lenses in both her eyes. The condition, later named retrolental fibroplasia (RLF), was extremely rare before 1941, yet by 1950 had become the main cause of blindness in infants as it spread from the US to other affluent countries: Britain, France, Sweden, Holland and Australia.

By 1951 a few paediatricians had noticed that most cases occurred in hospitals using modern incubators and, in 1953, an English researcher showed that young animals exposed to high oxygen levels developed eye changes similar to RLF.

A group of American paediatricians, led by Professor William Silverman, set up a scientific study to determine if there was a link between RLF and oxygen and, after much argument over the ethics of depriving some babies of what was considered a life-saving level of oxygen, premature infants at eighteen hospitals were allocated at birth to a "routine oxygen" group or a "curtailed oxygen" group.

The trial lasted a year and showed conclusively that the routine group ran a much greater risk of RLF than the curtailed group. Hospitals reduced the oxygen level in incubators and the RLF epidemic came to an end. Yet during the trial Silverman and his colleagues were denounced for "human experimentation" and depriving the "curtailed" babies of life saving treatment.

Many people are still repelled by the idea of allocating patients randomly to treatment. Despite the evidence that guessing in medicine carries horrific risks, a well-intentioned guess by a kindly doctor is seen as less cold and unfeeling than a random allocation. To maim or kill with well-meaning guesswork is acceptable because it is not perceived as "human experimentation" but scientific trials, carried out under controlled conditions, still draw pejorative headlines.

## Road glee

Psychopathy induced by regular driving in congested traffic. Commoner than road rage but less well publicised.

The City of Reading is renowned for its notorious circular bypass which entraps visitors for an hour or so before hurling them like shot from a sling onto a route they never intended to travel. It is also known – and there could be a connection – for notoriously competitive motorists.

I was gifted both those snippets of information by a doctor who worked in a local A&E Department. He told me how one evening, while he was treating a casualty, he overheard a policeman in the next cubicle interviewing a pedestrian who'd been knocked down by a hit-and-run driver.

The policeman asked the victim if he'd seen the face of the driver of the car that struck him.

"No," came the reply, "but I'd remember his laugh anywhere."

## Rolling news

Also known as twenty-four-hour news. Reporting news before it happens.

Encourages politicians and journalists to spin yarns and irritate doctors.

On Monday October 28, 2002 BBC television news told us that the results of a poll to be published later in the week would show that hospital consultants had rejected a pay increase of 10 per cent.

On Wednesday the same source and *The Times* and *Guardian* reported that consultants would reject a rise of 15 per cent.

On Thursday, when the result of the poll was actually announced, television news programmes reported that hospital consultants had rejected a rise of 20 per cent, though by evening one commentator bumped this up to 24 per cent.

On Saturday we learned, but only if we read a discreet paragraph in the *Guardian*, that the actual offer was 7.5 per cent.

Ironically, one of the consultants' complaints had been about the political manipulation of NHS statistics. That fact never appeared in rolling news because it had actually happened. Predicting what might happen is real news; reporting what has happened is old news i.e. unrolling news.

## Rolling Stone Syndrome (RSS)

Common form of travel sickness. When its victims visit new places they look without seeing, listen without hearing, then roll home as uncontaminated by the experience as a highly polished snooker ball.

RSS discourages travellers from pausing to look around in wonder while encouraging them to hurry off to visit things called 'sights' and to stare at stuff called 'scenery'.

You can always identify a 'sight' because it's usually impossible to enjoy, indeed often impossible to see, because of a surrounding barrier of coaches and crowds of oddly clad travellers gazing at history through Japanese view finders or on the screens of mobile phones.

'Scenery' is stuff you see from the window of your car or coach. It's not a place that man has lived in, or struggled to tame, or even a place where you can pause and let your imagination roam; it's stuff you digitise into your camera or phone.

It is also something you can't afford to miss. A few years ago I pulled my car off an Alpine road into a lay-by enticingly labelled *Vista*. I climbed up a slope from the parking place and, as I stood on a rock, reluctant to move from surroundings with which for a moment I felt in near perfect harmony, another car pulled in alongside mine. A family got out, glanced cursorily around, and gazed confusedly at map and guide-book. Then the father climbed up the rocks towards me. "It's truly magnificent here," he said, "but I wonder could you tell us which way we face to see the famous view."

## Romantic fiction
Preferred style of 19th century medical biography.

One of the great Victorian romances was the tale of Dr John Snow and the Broad Street Pump. In 1854 a cholera epidemic devastated the Soho parish of St James. On its fringe lived John Snow, an anaesthetist at St George's Hospital. One evening he made a dramatic intervention at a parish meeting. In the words of his biographer, Sir Benjamin Ward Richardson:

*A stranger asked in modest speech for a brief hearing… He advised the removal of the pump handle… The vestry was incredulous but had the good sense to carry out the advice. The pump handle was removed and the plague was stayed.*

One minor flaw in the story is that it isn't true. Nor is the alternative version, still purveyed in medical schools, that Snow himself removed the handle from the pump, thus stopping people from drinking the water and halting the epidemic.

If you read what Snow, rather than his biographer, wrote, you discover that long before the immobilisation of the pump the locals had taken traditional preventive action.

*There is no doubt that the mortality was much diminished by the flight of the population… The attacks had so far diminished before the use of the water was stopped that it is impossible to decide whether the well still contained the cholera poison in an active state or whether, from some cause, the water had become free from it.*

His investigation was, in the parlance of today, a retrospective study. He mapped the houses occupied by cholera victims and found they were linked by their source of drinking water.

At the time of the Soho epidemic, the received truth was that cholera descended from a miasma, an invisible cloud of disease that hovered above afflicted communities. Snow's contemporaries ignored his evidence that the cause could be polluted water and when he died, four years after the epidemic, few doctors accepted his hypothesis. Only when the organism that causes cholera was identified thirty years later, did the medical establishment accept it was a waterborne disease.

Broad Street was later renamed Broadwick Street and today the site of the pump is marked by a red kerbstone outside a pub. In 1955, to mark the centenary of the publication of Snow's *Observations on Cholera,* a group of epidemiologists persuaded the owners of the pub to rename it the John Snow and for years a visitors book, kept behind the bar, accumulated signatures of international pilgrims who came to pay homage at the birth place of epidemiology.

The change of name was marked by a small ceremony. A clutch of respectful epidemiologists gathered on the pavement while their leader Austin Bradford Hill who, with Richard Doll, used Snow's technique to demonstrate the link between cigarettes and lung cancer, climbed a rickety ladder to unveil a new inn sign bearing the Great Man's picture.

The centenary was also marked by an exhibition at the London School of Hygiene which featured a fine portrait of Snow lent by his great nieces. They were strict teetotallers and not best pleased to hear about the pub. Bradford Hill tried to persuade them that you had to be a pretty important person to have a pub named after you but they ignored the epidemiologists and bequeathed the portrait to the Faculty of Anaesthetists. Their declared reason was that Snow made the use of chloroform during childbirth acceptable by administering it to Queen Victoria. Bradford Hill suspected there was another reason though, as a punctilious epidemiologist, he never claimed a direct causal connection.

## Royal colleges

Impressive institutions built above well-stocked cellars and born of a realisation that comes to male doctors of a certain age, as inevitably as the symptoms of prostatic obstruction, that playing academic games, discussing the philosophy of medicine with wise men such as themselves – and maybe a carefully selected handful of women – meeting with influential members of society, issuing declarations on the great moral and ethical dilemmas of our time, and proffering advice to government, is a pleasanter way of life than the daily grind of caring for troublesome patients.

## Runny nose

A physiological signal to others that you are in need of advice. When you suffer from a cold, the only person who won't, at the drop of a handkerchief, offer you their own infallible cure is a doctor.

Like all great national traditions the British Cold (qv) spawns traditions of its own. And the greatest of these is the British Cold Cure whose name is legion, with each nostrum inspiring enormous pride in those who use it.

Nearly fifty years ago I set out with a television film crew to interview David Tyrrell, head of the internationally renowned Common Cold Research Unit near Salisbury. While the crew adjusted lights and microphones before the interview, he told me that, by ironic chance, he suspected he was incubating a cold caught not at work but from a member of the choir in a local church where he played the organ.

When we finished and went for a cup of coffee, the cameraman and sound man, in turn, cornered the scientist, who knew more about common cold viruses than any person on earth, and urged him to use their own sure fire method of preventing a threatening cold from "coming out." As I remember it, one favoured Vitamin C and the other a complex ritual involving lemons, chives, cinnamon, and whiskey. My abiding memory is of the great man listening to their advice with the Christian stoicism for which he was renowned.

# S

## St Elsewhere's

A mythical Centre of Incompetence that doctors create to convince themselves of their own excellence.

It's extraordinary how many doctors define their success in terms of other people's failure.

Surgeons teaching new techniques they've invented will say, "Thanks to what we're going to do to this chap, we'll have him back at work in a week. If the poor unfortunate had gone to St Elsewhere's they'd have encased him in plaster for ten days."

The head of a department will tell a committee: "With this system, patients will be treated and back home within weeks of first being seen. At St Elsewhere's they would still be stuck on the waiting list."

It's not only doctors. I wonder how many of us could determine our identities without a fantasy Them – or even a real Them – whose ineptitude, stupidity, ignorance and sloth allow us to perceive ourselves as the bright, industrious persons we know ourselves to be; a Them whose capacity for evil makes us, if not wholly free from human frailty, at least persons of honest intent.

If you eavesdrop in a fast food eaterie you hear a lot about our common enemy: "Of course, They'd like us to think that They are very busy in Head Office"; "I see They've raised the price of petrol again"; "Did you see the dreadful rubbish They put on Channel Four last night?"

While fighting the good fight against disease and ignorance, some doctors identify enemies – for a hospital doctor it may be The Administrator, for a few GPs it may, sadly, be their patients – but the commonest enemy by far is the doctor at St Elsewhere's whose low clinical and ethical standards are our only measure of the excellence of our own.

Our patients, we know, are treated by wise, knowledgable, and kindly doctors, aware of their ethical responsibilities, conscious that each patient is not a mere collection of symptoms but an individual enmeshed in an interconnecting social network etc. etc.

Less fortunate patients are treated by Them.

## Sanctuary
What hospitals used to offer before they became Health Care Providers.

Dr Jonathan Paisley of Glenrothes claimed the following conversation took place at 2 a.m. through the intercom alongside the locked main door of a local community hospital.

"Hello, let me in. I need the toilet."

"I'm sorry this is a hospital."

"Well I'm a member, let me in."
"Sorry I can't let you use the toilet."
"In that case just throw me a newspaper."

## Saniflush

All-conquering concept of psychotherapy. Popular in California.

Bruce Sloane, a British expatriate psychiatrist working in Los Angeles, once explained to me why psychotherapy and cosmetic surgery were logical adjuncts to the American Dream. Both conformed to the Saniflush concept: people believing that they have it within them to achieve greatness – even become president – if only some therapist or guru can flush out the hang-ups that get in the way.

## Sarcasm

Medical tone of voice that occasionally earns its just reward.

By the time I was called up for national service in 1954, I'd shrugged off many of the attitudes I'd absorbed when working in teaching hospitals and had learned in general practice how to treat patients as equals. Then along came the army and re-introduced me to a world in which doctors were officers and patients were other ranks.

But social change was on its way. One morning I was apprenticed to an army doctor of the 'old school' doing routine medicals on a batch of conscripts. He prodded one fat-bellied recruit in the midriff and said: "You'll have to lose that. You look pregnant."

"I'm not surprised," came the response, "the way I've been fucked about this morning."

## Satanic possession.

If, as some claim, it is a disease, it is damned difficult to acquire.

I should know. I think I was nine, though I could have been ten, when I first tried to sell my soul to the devil. I'd assessed my prospects and resources and concluded that a deal with the devil was the only way I could acquire what I most wished from life – a piano accordion and the ability to play it.

I whispered my request up a chimney whenever I got the opportunity and hung about for weeks with my soul on offer, prepared even to sign the contract in blood provided it could be extracted painlessly. But Satan never put in an appearance.

By the time I was ten, or it could have been twelve, I was glad I hadn't settled for a piano accordion. By then I would have signed, even in painfully extracted blood, for the ability to run as fast as a boy called Allardyce. But try as I might to conjure up the devil he never appeared, not even for a laugh.

I suspect that, at the time, I wasn't so much under the influence of Goethe as of the cone-hatted magicians and mysterious orientals who wandered the pages of the Hotspur and the Wizard dealing with baddies in short sharp magical ways and transmogrifying weakling goodies into strong, athletic, accordion-playing heroes. They were the successors to the fairy godmothers who, six or seven years earlier, disguised themselves as witches and went round offering woodcutters three wishes which the silly old fools always went and wasted.

I remember round the age of six – or was it seven? – being irritated to the point of despair by the corporate lack of imagination in the woodcutting industry. I would need not three but only one wish because, quick as a flash and before the good fairy could renege on the deal, I would wish that all my future wishes would come true. Yet fairy godmothers, it seemed, never put anything on offer to precocious kids like me but wasted their magical powers on those old boneheads in the woodshed.

God knows I tried. I lay awake at nights waiting for a wish-offering creature to materialise; I took to walking in local woods hoping to find an elephant with a thorn in its foot or an ugly transmogrifiable toad in some form of distress. I visited junk shops and gave a surreptitious polish to every brass article I could find in the desperate hope of conjuring up a genie. But I conjured up nothing save frustration. I suspect it was when I realised I would never get anything out of the goodies that I decided to put my soul on offer to the arch baddie. No wonder I felt cheated when he too rejected me.

When I was fifteen, or it could have been sixteen, I called the whole thing off. I had discovered girls. They were easier to find than accordions and more pleasurable to squeeze.

## Scalpel power

Power that surgeons wield outside the operating theatre.

Early in her career, Katharine Hepburn made a series of films that even she considered were not so hot. They all got lousy reviews and Hollywood began to regard her as "box office poison."

The writer Cleveland Amory noticed, however, that the newspapers in Hartford, Connecticut, carried glowing notices of one of the films. When he met Hepburn's father, a Hartford urologist, he mentioned this heartwarming loyalty of local newspapers.

"Do you know what I do?" asked Dr Hepburn.

"No."

"I specialise in prostatectomies. I have already operated on half the newspaper publishers in this city and I confidently expect to operate on the other half."

## Scientific paper

Gobbets of ill-written, ill-digested information published in a scientific journal or read in laborious monotone at a scientific meeting. (See Data.)

Most people write them not because they're bursting to tell us something but for more solemn reasons: another line on a CV, another step towards a job or a research grant. When they finish a piece of research they don't ask, "How do we make this understandable" but "How many papers can we get out of this?"

In 1976 our profession missed a priceless opportunity when Dr J B Healy of Dublin wrote to the *Lancet* and, like another Irishman 250 years before him, submitted a modest proposal.

*It seems to me that we should for an experimental period of a year, declare a moratorium on the appending of authors' names and of the names of hospitals to articles in medical journals. If the dissemination of information is the reason why papers are submitted for publication, there will be no falling off in the numbers offered. … But if far less material is offered to the journals, we shall have unmasked ourselves.*

No editor was brave enough to conduct that experiment. Not even Richard Smith who, when editor of the *BMJ*, claimed, "… only 5 per cent of published papers reach minimum standards of scientific soundness and clinical relevance and in most journals the figure is less than 1 per cent."

Time was when doing research and 'writing it up' were part of the same process, equally deserving of time and thought. People who wrote in the hope of being read needed to be conscious of their audience and use language that would hold its attention; those who now write only to be published are free from this tiresome restraint. So the dominant prose style in scientific 'literature' is Decorated Municipal Gothic (qv), constructed from words and phrases that, like all clichés, make life easier for writers who haven't time to waste on thought. The prose is so unattractive that far from inviting readers it actually deters them. (See Prefabricated prose.)

Journals' tolerance of thoughtless prose encourages authors to write not only obscurely but too often. We live in a world that equates data with knowledge. Medicine may have moved from mystic certainty towards scientific uncertainty yet many of its practitioners still behave as if Galileo never lived. Wedded to the inductive approach of Francis Bacon, they choose to act like vacuum cleaners, sucking up vast quantities of data then dumping the contents into a journal.

Writing in the *New England Journal of Medicine*, Drummond Rennie, deputy editor of *JAMA*, summed up the whole sorry process in a single sentence.

*There seems to be no study too fragmented, no hypothesis too trivial, no literature citation too biased or too egotistical, no design too warped, no methodology too bungled, no presentation of results too inaccurate, too obscure, and too contradictory, no analysis too self serving, no argument too circular, no conclusions too trifling or too unjustified, and no grammar and syntax too offensive for a paper to end up in print.*

## Second phase syndromes
New conditions that appear in the wake of fashionable illnesses or drugs.

Viagra's spectacular success in enabling men to achieve erections encouraged women to demand drugs to improve other aspects of men's performance. Those they suggested included:

### Skyagra
A drug designed to stiffen a man's resolution to watch less televised sport.

**DIYagra**
Men taking this drug would be more likely to finish one DIY job before starting another.

**Triagra**
In a double-blind study, over 80 per cent of men who took the drug before starting a car journey would stop and ask for directions when they got lost. In a control group, the enquiry rate would be 0.4 percent.

**Buyagra**
When taking this drug 76 per cent of subjects would agree to spend money on household essentials.

## Self-improvement workshop
The only place to learn essential 'life skills'. More accurately defined as patronising talkshop.

Originated in the US in the 1980s when teachers who hadn't shed ideas they dreamed up as students in the days of hippiedom and flower power inflicted them on junior doctors. Later appeared in the UK as part of what the *BMJ's* primary care editor Domhnall Macauley described as the "happy clappy" side of general practice conducted by "cosy groups in woolly cardigans."

When the original progenitors of the 'life skill' workshops asked their victims to suggest suitable subjects for discussion, irreverent young doctors in California offered a list:

- Creative Suffering.
- Overcoming Peace of Mind.
- Guilt Without Sex.
- The Primal Shrug.
- Dealing with Post Self-Realisation Depression.
- Whine your way to Alienation.
- How to Overcome Self-Doubt Through Pretence and Ostentation.

## Send for the doctor
Ritual expression of the belief that every problem has a medical solution.

| Macbeth. | *Canst thou not minister to a mind diseas'd,* |
|---|---|
| | *Pluck from the memory a rooted sorrow,* |
| | *Raze out the written troubles of the brain,* |
| | *And with some sweet oblivious antidote* |
| | *Cleanse the stuff'd bosom of that perilous stuff* |
| | *Which weighs upon the heart?* |
| Doctor. | *Therein the patient must minister to himself.* |

## Send in the clowns
The NHS way to improve management.

The Institute of Health Care Management, after a diligent search for the ideal trainer to improve the skills of its 10,000 members, settled for a "freelance clown" called Bosco. For the modest sum of £200 per student, Bosco, complete with baggy trousers and a red nose, was happy to teach managers the traditional NHS skills of spinning plates, walking tightropes, and hurling trifle.

An enthusiastic member of the Institute, Andrew Corbett-Nolan, suggested to the equally hyphenated Kate Watson-Smyth of the *Independent* that the skills of the Big Top could be usefully extended to the medical profession.

*It is an exercise of the absurd, but there is also something to gain from it. In industry they have been doing this for years – sending people off to desert islands and abandoning them on Welsh mountains.*

The point of the seminars, he said, was to encourage people to approach a typical problem in a different way to find out how they behaved in a team.

*So it could be they must talk about two hospitals merging, and while one talks the others will spin plates and walk tightropes and, to show how it could all go wrong, they might throw a custard pie.*

Mr Corbett-Nolan would watch from the sidelines and decide whether anyone had "development issues".

Anyone who pointed out that the NHS already had too many freelance clowns would presumably be stripped of his tickling stick.

## Sensitive areas
Delicate subjects, often to do with sex or gender, that GPs learn to handle skilfully.

In the 1970s my brother-in-law Larry Morton was a GP in North London. One day his daughter Una, aged about ten, asked him out of the blue: "Daddy, what is a lesbian?" Larry was not just a good GP, he had also read most of the childcare gurus of that time. So he dealt with Una's question with skill and sensitivity. He sat her in a comfortable chair and gave her a simple, factual, unemotional answer to her question. Una, perched in the huge chair her feet barely touching the ground, listened intently, eyes wide open.

When Larry finished his explanation, he asked, "Do you understand what I have told you?"

Una nodded her head to signify 'Yes'.

"And have you any questions?"

Una shook her head to signify 'No'.

She was sent off to play and Larry did what many a GP does when he thinks he's been rather clever: he went to tell his wife about it. Only when he spoke to my sister did he discover that the reason Una had asked the question was that she was puzzled by the news that the family which had moved in next door were Weslyans.

## Serial killers.

Also known as character assassins.

In 1997 an epidemiological study published in the *BMJ* revealed that the most dangerous job in the United Kingdom was not bomb disposal expert, steeplejack, or racing driver but being a character in a soap opera.

Deaths in soap operas were almost three times more likely to be from violent causes than would be expected from a character's age and sex.

The research revealed that Brookside Close, Coronation Street, Albert Square, and Emmerdale were dangerous places to live. Characters tended to die young and from a variety of obscure and often violent causes, ranging from a mystery virus in *Brookside*, which killed three, to a plane crash in *Emmerdale*, which killed four.

The risk was not evenly spread. A character in *East Enders* was twice as likely to die during an episode than a similar character in *Coronation Street*. The researchers suggested that characters in these serials should be advised to wear good protective clothing (designed to withstand sharp implements, sudden impacts, and fire) and to receive regular counselling to blunt the psychological impact of living in an environment akin to a war zone.

## Sex Education
Subversive activity designed to encourage promiscuity, the spread of disease, and the destruction of civilisation as some would like to know it.

An anonymous doctor writing to the *Daily Telegraph* drew the world's attention to an under-publicised danger:

*Sex researchers are increasing women's expectations of sex. They are beginning to expect satisfaction. Soon, they may be demanding that their psychiatrists ensure that they have multi-orgasms, something neither their doctors, nor their husbands, may be able to fulfil.*

Less disturbing was the woman who called an American phone-in programme:

*These people claim that sex education in schools causes promiscuity. If you have the knowledge, they say, you use it. Heck, I took algebra. Yet I never do maths.*

## Sexism
Minefield for NHS bureaucrats who face not only their traditional enemies – grammar and syntax – but have to grapple with the notion of "correctness" without quite understanding what it means.

Dr Dick Ford, a GP in Bideford, wrote to the Secretary of State for Health:

*I was amazed to read your missive which refers to all doctors as he, and all nurses as she... I can assure you that not all doctors are male and certainly not all nurses are female.*

Back came an explanation from M A Garley (Sex undisclosed):

*I should explain that Section 6 of the Interpretation Act 1978 provides that any reference in legislation to the masculine includes the feminine, and similarly any reference to the feminine includes the masculine. Consequently all references in the Statutory Instrument to male or female include the other sex, and the regulations, of course, apply equally to all doctors and nurses. In this particular case, the regulations were drafted to refer to male doctors and female nurses solely to avoid any possible confusion and to make it absolutely clear when the reference was to the nurse and when to the doctor.*

We can console ourselves with the thought that unsexing is less dauntingly performed with a statutory instrument than with a surgical one.

## Sexual intercourse

Unseemly human activity that for most of the 20th century was considered unsuitable for discussion in polite medical society.

Martin Bax, paediatrician, novelist, and founder of the Arts magazine *Ambit* has written of his time as a student at Guy's Hospital, London, in the late 1950s.

*Some things we are taught and some we aren't. On family planning we get one lecture from a man who seems to purvey rubber goods, but any attempt, when we are doing our gynaecology and obstetrics, to find out more about the problem meets with an evasive answer from the consultant, who actually says to me: "You'll know more about things when you are married yourself."*

In those days undue reticence damaged people's health in many ways. The only public information on offer about sexually transmitted disease, for instance, was a list of *Venereal Disease clinics* posted inside public conveniences by the London County Council. This practice occasionally unveiled admirable aspects of the British character.

One evening a music hall performer, who earned his living as a siffleur, entered what was called the 'special department' at a London hospital, its unmarked entrance hidden discreetly down a dark forbidding alley. Still wearing the clothes he used in his act – white tie, tails, top hat and white gloves – he doffed his topper to the receptionist and announced in carefully modulated tones: "I've come in answer to your advertisement in the gentlemen's lavatory in Leicester Square."

Even at the turn of the century, some doctors – or at least BMA members – wished to protect themselves from discussion of 'that sort of thing'. Issues of the *BMJ* published in January 1999 carried a warning on the cover: *The ABC of Sexual Health contains sexually explicit material.*

## Shellacking

Technique of coating inaction with an Arcanian (qv) glaze in the hope of making it acceptable.

James Willis, when a GP in Alton, received a letter from Hampshire County Council Social Services:

*Please accept our assurance that having accepted this referral, we will ensure that it is allocated to the appropriate Care Manager, who will arrange to make an assessment at the earliest convenience. Whilst we would not want to delay this, I must point out that we are currently working to a pending list.*

A GP, Trefor Roscoe, received this note from a body calling itself Community Health in Sheffield (sic):

*Unfortunately owing to a crisis staffing situation the implementation time scale of this project has been dramatically increased.*

## Shibilance

Disorder of articulation. Sufferers can switch off sibilant sounds only by inserting an aspirate, making them sound as if they are talking through loose false teeth. (*Shome mishtake shurely.*)

I thought the condition was restricted to speech until an Abingdon GP Dr Frank Debney diagnosed a case in a caption in his local paper:

*The Saxton Road Playgroup is shown receiving a tree, one of the first offered by the Vale of White Horse District Council as part of their campaign to SHIT IN THE SHADE.*

## Shroud

Item of death-wear politicians accuse doctors and nurses of waving if they attribute unnecessary deaths to administrative decisions.

If the deaths can be attributed to clinical decisions the preferred phrase is "inexcusable failings."

## Side-effects

Trivial discomforts patients use as an excuse to stop taking drugs doctors know are good for them.

My abiding memory of the first press conference on the 'breakthrough' beta-blocker drugs is the uniformity of expression on the faces of the male journalists when a cardiologist told them that one of the new drug's 'minor side-effects' was impotence.

## Sigmund Freud

Self regarding story teller who, for a time, clouded the understanding of the human mind fostered by more perceptive writers such as Fyodor Dostoevsky and Gustave Flaubert. His writings, I'm reliably informed, are still a major cause of neurosis among psychiatrists.

Best remembered as devisor of the psychogame (qv) which during the first half of the 20th century enjoyed the same social cachet as *Times* crossword puzzling and 'serious' bridge. In its heyday it removed the drama from Oedipus and the fun from sex, and ensured that the versatile acrobats Ego and Id were good for an evening's bouncing on the conversational trampoline. It was especially popular in the United States where it was often the only way patients could get a doctor to listen to them.

In the 1970s I met a young woman who had worked as a receptionist for a Beverly Hills psychoanalyst. She soon discovered she'd enrolled as a player in a game she couldn't win. If she arrived at work early her boss told her she was showing signs of insecurity; if she was late the cause was underlying hostility; if she arrived on time she was accused of being obsessional. After six months, she left and found true happiness working for a cardiologist. Like most of us, I suspect, she preferred an employer more influenced by heart than mind.

She was not the first to discover that Freud's game enables his disciples to prove to themselves that they are always right. The same awareness of the nature of the game can dawn on patients – or, as some prefer, clients – such as the one described in a letter from a therapist to her GP, Dr Ron Manton.

*There has been a certain degree of ambivalence towards therapy, where Ms X has not fully engaged. She has latterly described our sessions as becoming 'aimless' with little forward momentum. This may be a further manifestation of her avoidance strategies with particular regard to examining deeper core beliefs and her level of inter-action with others.*

A non-analyst might call that rationalisation… not by the patient but by the therapist.

Just occasionally the game players get their comeuppance. Dr

Bruno Bettelheim, the child psychiatrist known for his psychoanalytic interpretation of nursery rhymes, was notoriously tyrannical towards his students. One day, when he saw a woman knitting during one of his lectures he turned to her and remarked acidly: "Do you know Miss Kupperwitz that what you are doing is a substitution for masturbation?"

Miss Kupperwitz glanced up from her needles. "Dr Bettelheim," she said, "when I knit, I knit."

## Silly or Sensible

An engaging way to divide the world into two groups. The writer Geoffrey Wheatcroft has suggested that we are all members of either the Silly party or the Sensible one.

It's easy to spot the divide in medicine. The Sensibles move gravely about their business making 'Important Decisions' on committees at the GMC, the BMA, and a Royal College or two, drafting protocols and frameworks, dining with the great and the good. In the presence of other Sensibles, they express concern about the behaviour of medical Sillies whom they consider irresponsible and in need of supervision by sensible persons such as themselves.

In the eyes of the Sensibles, the Sillies overindulge in irreverence, ill-considered humour, and unconstructive criticism. They lack judgement, their behaviour is often 'inappropriate', and they are prone to commit that most grievous of sins, 'overstepping the mark'. The Sillies are aware of these criticisms but, because of their source, regard them as accolades.

Sensibles admit that, although they cope with the big issues and take the grave decisions of which Sillies are incapable, the Sillies may have more fun. But they make that admission only to emphasise their gravitas (qv). As Sidney Smith said of his brother the bishop: "He has risen by his gravity and I have been sunk by my levity."

I once heard a medical grandee, a doyen of the Sensible party, try to patronise a notorious Silly.

"Still busy pursuing lost causes?" he asked.

The Silly was too weary to rise to the bait but managed a smile. He knew that his inquisitor, like all good Sensibles, pursued only causes that were already won.

## Silver tongue

Metaphorical award bestowed on folk who show a talent for saying what their listeners want to hear without revealing their own thoughts nor sacrificing their integrity.

Found more often in servants than in employers, in those who've been colonised than in the colonisers. Sixty years ago the silver tongue was endemic in peripheral communities in the British Isles where tourists were incomparably richer than the locals, such as the Scottish highlands and the south west of Ireland.

In the 1950s, two consultants from my teaching hospital, a surgeon and a pathologist, went on a fishing holiday in West Cork and soon discovered that Donal their gillie was so eager to please that he never contradicted them. A long family history of poverty had conditioned him to say nothing that might cost him his job.

After a few days, his smiling deference began to irritate the surgeon. I know it stretches belief that a St Thomas' Hospital surgeon could be irritated by somebody agreeing with him all the time but maybe he resented echoes of the workplace intruding on his holiday. He came to see Donal's attitude as a challenge and, one night in the bar, laid a hefty bet with the pathologist that, next day, he would get Donal to contradict him.

The following morning a Force Eight gale had blown in from the west and rain travelled horizontally across the fields. Donal, trying to find shelter, squatted in a corner of the hotel courtyard, swathed in a couple of overcoats and with a sack over his head. The surgeon strode over to him and, cupping his hand against the blast, bellowed in his ear: "There's not much wind this morning, is there Donal?"

And back came the silver tongued response: "Oh no, sir. You're quite right, sir. You're quite right. But what little there is 'tis very strong."

## Simple truth

That which comes from the mouths of children.

When I was a GP my five-year-old daughter attended a local school where each day began with the children telling their teacher what was happening in their worlds. One morning the discussion turned to the sort of jobs that daddies did. When it came to my daughter's turn, she said rather sadly: "We don't have a daddy. We have a doctor."

When the teacher told me the story I had to pretend to share her delight. I'd had my first insight into the effect my work as a GP was having on my family.

I soon learned that GPs whose children attend local schools are always at risk. One victim sent me this confession.

His young son, on his first day at a new school, let fly with a four letter word.

"That's a nasty word," said the teacher. "Goodness me, where on earth did you hear that?"

"My dad says it."

"Well don't you say it. You don't even know what it means."

"Oh yes I do. It means Mrs Enright has asked for a visit."

## Single parent
Paradoxical status awarded to someone who acts as a double parent.

## Sixth sense
The sense of self-importance. Highly developed in those who operate in medicine's High Places.

Those who work in Low Places are less at risk: daily contact with patients is a great leveller. Clinicians may occasionally succumb to flattery from sycophantic patients and begin to wonder whether a divine spark doesn't after all flicker somewhere about their person, but the evening they try on the divine robes for size will likely be followed by the morning after when a patient confidently diagnosed as having acute cholecystitis produces the mocking rash that heralds shingles.

Hence the ancient medical proverb: *The further a physician moveth from daily care of the sick, the greater groweth his sense of his own worth.*

Sadly, a few don't need to moveth at all: their sixth sense is congenital rather than a acquired. Here is a letter David Jobling, a GP in Knaresborough, received from a consultant.

*This gentleman did not attend for his appointment today. A DNA*

*(Did Not Attend) is certainly a risk factor for a large psychological element to a chronic pain. I would however advise you to guard against the mistake of relying on classical Cartesian mind body dualism when dealing with chronic pain problems.*

*It is now clear that the mind resides in the brain and the brain functions by being an adaptive network of nerves. This adaptation occurs not just in the brain, but throughout the nervous system extending to the tips of C fibre endings. This can not only affect nerve function, but also things like erythema and swelling around the site of injury, all under neural control. It is therefore very unclear where the mind ends and the body begins, or vice-versa.*

A mere detail, like not having seen the patient, is no barrier to pontification by those with a finely tuned sixth sense.

## Sleeping tablets

Decorative cards bearing uplifting messages that hoteliers place on the pillows of their 'guests'.

My first tablet was dispensed in a small hotel in upstate New York.

*Have a peaceful night secure in the knowledge*
*that we are here to care for you.*

The kindness of the thought was only marginally blunted when I turned over the card and found an advertisement for the security company that sponsored it.

The sleeping tablet habit is not confined to the US. A few month's later I found a printed card on my pillow at *The Compleat Angler* in Marlow:

*Another busy day passes into a quiet night*
*Bearing gifts of peaceful sleep and pleasant dreams.*
*Thus the comfort of night passes into the wonder of day*
*Bearing gifts of new people and special experiences.*

The verse wasn't bad enough to be funny nor good enough to denote satirical intent, so I spent a rather uneasy night.

More uplifting was the message on my pillow when a production company parked me in an hotel internationally renowned as an emporium of bad taste:

*From the mint on every pillow, to the sparkle in the bellman's smile,*
*to the quality of the hotel stationery,*
*the Helmsley Palace Hotel leaves no bedspread unturned*
*in its quest to become the best hotel in New York.*

Most uplifting of all was the card I found on my pillow on my first night in Tokyo:

*You are invited to take advantage of the chambermaid.*

## Small talk

Dangerous venture for doctors more accustomed to Big Talk with their patients.

The headmistress of a celebrated girls' school was vetting a newly fledged consultant paediatrician to see if he were a suitable person to supervise the health of her young ladies. The job would open the door to a treasure house of private practice so the young man was on his mettle and extremely nervous.

For a moment the conversation sagged and the doctor, desperate to revive it, spotted an elegant vase on the mantel.

"What an exquisite object that is," he said. "I'm sure you cherish it."

"Cherish is hardly the appropriate word," said the headmistress. "It contains my husband's ashes."

'I'm terribly sorry," stuttered the doctor, his cheeks aflush with embarrassment, all hope of the job now gone. "I hope… '

"However hard I try," continued the headmistress, "I just can't get him to use the ashtrays."

## Smile

Enigmatic facial expression. Occasionally a harbinger of laughter; more often an unconscious reflection of a mood that lies anywhere along the route from fear to delight.

An obstetrician at a meeting of the Royal Society of Medicine claimed that the source of the smile of the Mona Lisa was all too obvious to a member of his trade: it was that of a woman who'd just been told she was pregnant. A woman in the audience interrupted to say, equally persuasively, that it was the smile of a woman who'd just been told she was not pregnant.

One cherishable quality of the subconscious smile is that it is a genuine expression of emotion. That's why it is dangerous for non-actors to try consciously to 'turn it on'. Gordon Brown's facial antics after his image advisers told him to smile more on television hastened his Downing Street defenestration.

One of the most outrageous take-over bids of the 20th century was the attempted acquisition of National Smile Week by, of all people, dentists – most of whom know as much about inducing a smile as Ken Dodd knows about drilling teeth.

The idea of a National Dental Health Smile Week was an abomination. Can anyone seriously suggest that all that Sir Alan Sugar or John Redwood need to give them warmth is a few quids' worth of bridgework?

The only smile dentists can influence is the ersatz expression favoured by politicians and game show hosts, memorably defined by S J Perelman in his suggestion that the smile of the young Shirley Temple "could melt the glue out of a revolving bookcase".

## Smoothsayer

A 21$^{st}$ century soothsayer who practices the art of misleading without actually lying: saying something that is statistically correct but expressed in a way that makes listeners think it means something else.

An art born in the public relations industry but eagerly developed by politicians who cherry-pick statistics to make it sound as if they are proposing 'evidenced-based policy' when they are really offering 'policy-based evidence'.

A recent example is a statistical argument the Prime Minister, David Cameron, and the Health Secretary, Andrew Lansley, used to support their government's plans to 'reform' the NHS. They claimed that UK survival rates for cancer and heart disease were the worst in Europe. The claim was true; the pretence was that survival rates are what matter to patients. Those who know the difference would prefer to hear the mortality rates: the number of people who die each year of the disease and a truer measure of the standard of treatment.

Survival rates are affected by a number of things, particularly by how early you diagnose a disease. If you diagnose it early you don't necessarily extend someone's life, you may just lengthen the time they have a diagnosis. Despite the increased survival rate, the mortality rate can remain the same… and often does.

An easy way to understand the difference is to compare the survival and mortality rates for breast cancer in women in the USA and the UK. The UK screens women by mammography every three years starting at the age of fifty; the American Cancer

Society recommends that women be screened every year starting at the age of forty. In 2001, the five-year survival rate in the US was 89.1 per cent; in the UK it was 80.3 per cent. So a smoothsayer could hint that treatment results are 'worse" in the UK. Yet the mortality rates are much the same: 25.0 per 100,000 women in the US and 26.7 per 100,000 women in Britain.

A US health economist put it this way: "The same number of people are dying every year. We have just moved the time of diagnosis up and subjected people to five more years of side-effects and reduced quality of life."

For those who dislike being manipulated by smoothsayers, but have neither the skill nor inclination to unravel the intricacies, a bunch of experts waging war on statistical illiteracy has assessed the terms that appear in press releases, news reports, and political speeches.

Terms that are 'transparent' – i.e. mean what it says on the tin – are absolute risks (qv), mortality rates, and natural frequencies: those where meaning is clouded by equivocation and easily manipulated by smoothsayers, include relative risks, five year survival rates, and conditional probabilities.

## Smut
Anglo-Saxon words that provoke an acute allergic reaction in sensitive subjects, many of them doctors.

In 1958 when Eric Partridge wrote *Origins,* he replaced the central vowels of the two most familiar four-letter words with asterisks and wrote: "Outside medical and other learned papers, they cannot be printed in full."

Thirty years later both those Anglo-Saxon words appeared without asterisks in books and newspapers but authors in medical journals still used euphemistic verbs of Latin derivation such as defecate, micturate, and copulate.

Some claim that terse Saxon expressions have no place in 'learned writing' because they sound ugly. Yet 'folk' and 'luck' make much the same sound as 'fuck' and are not considered ugly. Maybe one day we will be able to restore the pithiest Anglo-Saxon words to respectability but there seems no reason why medical writers shouldn't make a start by supplanting words like 'eructate' and 'expectorate' with 'belch' and 'spit' and re-identify the passing of genteel flatus as an honest Anglo-Saxon fart.

Indeed, medical writers could be the first people to use the word 'fuck' to mean fuck. Most users don't. Making this point in *World Medicine,* Paul Vaughan used the example of a soldier on a charge who was asked to explain his behaviour.

"Well, sir, I went down the fucking pub, had a fucking pint or two and met this fucking bird, walked down the fucking lane, and then, er, well...'

'Yes?'

'Well, sir, intimacy took place.'

Vaughan's illustration provoked sack-loads of letters from outraged doctors. Typical was the comment from Dr J Doohan of Manchester:

*Paul Vaughan should have enough literary skill to be able to avoid the guttersnipes' language and you, as editor, should have enough manners not to be so vulgar as to print in your magazine such vagrants' language.*

In his memoir *Skip all that,* Robert Robinson offers the definitive description of that odd 'television first' when he was chairing the satire-and-chat show *BBC3* and Kenneth Tynan used the word 'fuck.'

When the novelist Mary McCarthy commented, "I suppose it's a historic moment," Robinson responded, "Then history's made very easily."

Some weeks later he was waylaid in a Chelsea street by an elderly woman in a ginger fur coat who turned out to be Lady Normanbrook, wife of the chairman of the BBC governors.

"You know that word Mr Tynan used?" she said.

"I'm afraid I do," said Robinson.

"Well, it doesn't form part of my vocabulary."

"I shouldn't have supposed so."

"But ever since I heard Mr Tynan say it, I use it all the time."

## Social engineering

Temptation doctors find difficult to resist. Hence the maddeningly enigmatic letter a consultant wrote to a Nottingham GP.

*I reviewed this seventy-year-old. He came for a chat about treatment of his impotence and at the moment has decided just to await events. He has one girlfriend who is keen on sex and another who is not. So I have pointed him in the optimal direction.*

Am I the only one who wonders which direction that is?

## Socialised medicine

Phrase US citizens use to denounce any healthcare system more equitable than their own.

If we are to believe the arguments they use when they argue about their own dysfunctional system, many Americans see Britain's NHS as a crypto-communist organisation that subjects patients to long waiting lists, out-of date medicine, low tech hospitals, and sets up "death panels" to decide which patients should be treated and which left to die.

As for NHS doctors, they are "lackeys who serve political masters", have "denied their ethical heritage", "debased the professional standards we hold so dear", "sold out to the Devil" and, engaged in unspecified "dangerous practises" denounced in tones that hint they could make you blind if you overindulged.

Yet if US citizens want to know what socialised medicine is really like they need to look not at the NHS but in their own backyard. For there they harbour one of the world's largest welfare states, which not only offers universal healthcare and educational opportunities but seeks to curb income inequality. They call it the Military.

Nicholas Kristof described in *The New York Times* how the US Military knits together citizens of all races and from diverse backgrounds, invests in their education and training, provides them with excellent health care and child care, and does so with minimal income gaps. "A senior general earns about ten times what a private makes, while, by my calculation, C.E.O.'s at major companies earn about 300 times as much as those cleaning their offices."

The armed services, Kristof points out, led the way in racial desegregation, "and even today do more to provide equal opportunity to working-class families – especially to blacks – than just about any social program."

The US Military is "a rare enclave of universal health care", looking after servicemen, servicewomen and veterans at a much lower cost than the US system as a whole. And it provides "superb" affordable daycare for the children of its employees. "While one of America's greatest failings is underinvestment in early childhood education (which seems to be one of the best ways to break cycles of poverty from replicating), the Military manages to provide superb child care."

As General Wesley Clark, former supreme commander of NATO forces in Europe, told Kiristof: "It's the purest application of socialism there is."

## Social Needs

Needs that those who know best choose to recognise. All other needs are social problems.

In the 1990s, when Britain lead the way in extending the vocabulary of deprivation, "marginalised" replaced "ignored" and Christine Tyrie, a consultant psychiatrist in Carlisle, described how those who struggled to help people in need of "care in the community" were no longer allowed to refer to "unmet needs." They were dealing instead with "preferred option shortfall."

A few years later the acceptable vocabulary was defined in a newsletter for people working in community social and health services in Northumberland:

> The word "need' has been used to mean two different things:
> 1. A way in which someone's life falls short of what they might reasonably hope for.
> 2. A requirement for a service, which has been accepted by the body responsible for providing it.
> Only the second of these should be called a "need". The first should be called "a problem".

Hence the progression: I have rights. You have needs. He has problems.

## Something for the weekend, sir?

Traditional phrase that 'Gentlemen's Hairdressers' murmured to departing customers in the years when the law forbade the public display of packets of condoms.

Half a century later the Dublin government modified the phrase when it sought to cope with the arrival of the best known post-war product of the city of Cork (apart from Roy Keane), the impotence-treating pill Viagra. After grave deliberation government officials decided to limit the number of tablets allowed on state-funded prescriptions to four per month. Like a discreet and deferential hairdresser, the state murmured: "Just one for the weekend, sir."

The official reason for this restriction was is to prevent men from "abusing" the drug, presumably by having too many erections. Juliet Bressan, a Dublin GP, was quick to ask, "What if having sex only four times a month is dysfunctional for women?" But answer came there none. I doubt the question entered the consciousness of the unworldly folk who determined men's monthly ration.

Dr Bressan was not done. Viagra was later touted as a way to enhance sexual desire in women. If it were licensed for this, she asked, would the state be prepared to cough up?

*Bearing in mind the moral panic which accompanied the reluctance to allow gay men, single men, and non-impotent men to use state subsidised Viagra, I think we can look forward to the health-budgeting civil servants sitting down once more to agonise about the NHS funding of female multiple orgasms. Or not.*

## Spa therapy

Masochistic ritual devised at 18th century resorts where the overfed and under-exercised 'took the cure' and lost their money at the tables.

In truth, the 'cure' was a penitential offering to expiate the gambling. Many who came to the spas were less interested in repairing their debilitated "nervous systems" than in enjoying the company, the gaming, and the gossip. Their approach was that of the Duchess of Bedford, recorded in the *Percy Anecdotes*.

*Her Grace, after inquiring of many of her friends in the rooms what brought them there, and being generally answered for a nervous complaint, was asked in her turn, what brought her to Buxton. "I came only for pleasure," answered the duchess, "for, thank God, I was born before nerves came into fashion."*

British spa towns were slow to acknowledge the real reason for the popularity of the 'cure' and, when they closed their gaming tables, the water lost much of its therapeutic potency.

The burghers of French and German spa towns were less foolish. When I visited Baden Baden in the 1970s, I discovered that the municipal government plundered the casino takings even more voraciously than the doctors, hoteliers, and shopkeepers plundered the pockets of those seeking a cure for their 'neuro-vegetative organic disturbances'. All this prosperity derived from water that sprang from the ground and which, because it came from the Friedrichswelle, I decided to call Fred.

Fred wasn't just for drinking. An impressive therapeutic menu, available under the German equivalent of the NHS, included:

- Wildbad thermal bubble bath.
- Grosse Gesellschaftsbad thermal steam and hot-air movement community bath, which sounded like fun.
- Fango mud pack sluiced off with lashings of Fred.
- Thermal Movement Bath: pretentious name for a swimming bath filled to the brim with steaming Fred. Underwater massage recommended for 'low blood pressure and poor circulation' was delivered with a high power jet of pure Fred.
- An exciting room where devices could squirt Fred at or into any part of your anatomy.

When it came to drinking, those who preferred harder stuff seemed to favour Henry – Nürtinger Heinrichsquelle – "indicated for liver, bile, stomach and intestines" and, like Fred, available either bottled or on draught.

The handout from the Kurdirektor left few conditions un-embraced.

*The baths and treatments help and heal in cures of rheumatism, arthrosis, neurotis, neuralgia, paralysis consequent on brain and spinal disease; sport injuries; damage resulting from bodily wear and tear; conditions of exhaustion accompanied by neuro-vegetative organic disturbance, especially circulatory disorders, work, war and civilisation injuries, general old age symptoms; chronic catarrh of the pharynx and trachea. bronchial catarrh and bronchial ectasia; and chronic women's disorders.*

Fred was no ordinary fellow.

## Speed

Once the most prized of surgical skills. In the days before anaesthetics, patients heavily dosed with rum or opium had to be held down or strapped to the operating table. A speedy surgeon shortened the torture they had to endure and created the legend of the Surgeon as Hero.

One hero, whose reputation as a speedster spread from his native Scotland to Europe and North America, was Robert Liston. His operating speed was such that one observer wrote, "the gleam of his knife was followed so instantaneously by the sounds of sawing as to make the two actions appear almost simultaneous." Others described how, to free both hands during an operation, he would clasp the bloody knife between his teeth.

Born in 1794, a son of the manse, Liston studied medicine in Edinburgh and was a surgeon at the Royal Infirmary before moving South to become professor of surgery at University College Hospital, London.

There he built his reputation as the fastest surgeon in town and his operating sessions attracted packed galleries of students and their friends. An impressive man, six foot two tall, Liston would stride across the blood-stained floor of the operating theatre in Wellington boots and bottle-green operating coat calling to the students who stood in the galleries, pocket watches in hand, "Time me, gentlemen, time me." His speed sometimes had 'side effects.' Once, when he amputated a patient's leg in his routine time of two and a half minutes, his flashing knife also removed the poor man's testicles.

The operation that won him his place in medical folklore was another leg amputation. He managed it in under his usual two and a half minutes but sadly the patient died later from surgical gangrene, as patients often did in the days before antiseptics and asepsis. During the operation Liston inadvertently amputated the fingers of his young assistant, who also died of gangrene, and slashed through the coat tails of a distinguished surgical spectator who, terrified that the knife had pierced his vitals, dropped dead from fright. So, as modern surgeons point out, with a relish that borders on pride, Liston performed the only operation in surgical history to have a 300 per cent mortality.

Soon after the legendary triple, the arrival of anaesthesia from America gave surgeons more time to operate and eventually the high speed skills of men like Liston became redundant. Ironically, he performed the first operation in Europe to be done under anaesthesia. On 21 December 1846, disregarding the time advantages conferred by the new technique, he amputated a leg in his usual two and a half minutes before growling: "This Yankee dodge beats mesmerism hollow."

## Spice doctors
Those who add seasoning to routine exchanges with colleagues.

A GP friend of the Steve Jenkins, consultant cardiologist at St Thomas' Hospital, London, wrote to him about a patient: *If this man has mitral stenosis, I'm the Queen of France.*

After examining the patient, Dr Jenkins wrote back: *Dear Mother, he has. Your loving son, The Dauphin.*

## Spin doctors
Specialists most in demand in the NHS internal market.

> In January 2000, after wide publicity given to a woman whose cancer became inoperable while her treatment was repeatedly cancelled, the prime minister Tony Blair, announced on a television programme – where else? – that UK spending on health would rise to the European average over the next five years. The *BBC* television programme *Panorama* called it the most important statement in the history of the NHS, with profound implications for public sector spending.
> Later Downing Street explained that Mr Blair's "pledge" was in fact "an aspiration". By March of that year, the Treasury had downgraded it to "a long term challenge".

> The press handout in which the London Ambulance Service announced it was withdrawing hospital transport for blind patients and amputees carried the headline: *Planned Improvements for Patient Transport Services.*

The best definition of a spin doctor to come my way was written by an appellant to a Welsh disability tribunal who claimed that her GP had referred her to "a rumourtologist".

## Spontaneous tissue generation
A characteristic of foods that leave you with more on your plate when you've finished than there was before you started.

The prime example is an artichoke but I encounter the same phenomenon when I eat mussels or prawns or have a go at a fully articulated lobster.

## Sport
(Obsolete.)

Inconsequential activities once called games.

(Obsolete.)

1950s dream of underprivileged youth seeking health through joy on Duke of Edinburgh playing fields.

(Current.)

Aggressive, humourless, track-suited activities that fill the back pages of tabloid newspapers and the front pages of television schedules.

Sixty years ago, when walking my dog, I used to watch nine-year-old schoolboys playing football in Battersea park. One boy would stand in each goal, blowing on his fingers and shouting: "Please, sir, can I come out now sir?" while the other twenty chased the ball around the field in a joyful pack like a boxful of clockwork toys that had been wound up and poured onto the pitch.

Two years ago I walked past the the same pitch. The boys were the same size but were clearly engaged in sterner activity. There were few smiles, no free-for-all chases after the ball, and track-suited adults standing on the touchline shouted the aggressive clichés of our time: "Get stuck in", "Make your presence felt", "Put yourself about".

The nine-year-olds knew what was expected of them, as they kicked and tripped and rolled on the ground feigning injury. To my jaundiced old eyes they seemed to be having a lot less fun than their grandfathers had on the same patch of grass.

I've since heard that on the public tennis courts where, when I played, the game included rituals unknown at Wimbledon, such as the regular counting of the balls, a fracas broke out last summer and the police had to be called when a fight broke out over a disputed line call. But then Sport isn't meant to be fun. I mean, it's all about winning, isn't it Gary?

Yet it seems only yesterday that Danny Blanchflower, one of the great footballers of his day, wrote:

*The great fallacy is that the game is first and last about winning. It's nothing of the kind. The game is about glory. It's about doing things in style, with a flourish; about going out to beat the other lot, not waiting for them to die of boredom.*

I indulge this grouch not because I hanker for times past, though I do, nor because my attitude to sport is unashamedly middle-class, though it is. I indulge it because I object to people justifying this celebration of aggression by claiming it is healthy when I'm damn sure it isn't.

Sport's misappropriation of the notion of health is crystallised in the tale of the jogger who dropped dead while at his exercise. His companion looked down with pride at his friend and said: "What a way to go. In the peak of condition."

## Stable relationship

Harmonious association more easily achieved by horses than by humans. In horses it is based on geographic approximation. In humans it is occasionally based on love but is more reliable if based on greed.

George Mikes used to tell a story about his fellow Hungarian the playwright Ferenc Molnar, best remembered as the author of *Liliom;* the play that provided the book for *Carousel.* When Molnar was middle-aged and wealthy, he made a trip to America but left his young mistress behind in Budapest. When he returned, the scandal mongers eagerly offered him details of her infidelity while he was away. Molnar would listen to their tales unmoved, then shrug his shoulders and say: "With them she sleeps only for love. But for money, she sleeps only with me."

## Stethoscope

Assumed by outsiders to be an aid to auscultation. Recognised by doctors as an aid to meditation.

Newly qualified doctors soon discover that if they place the business end of a stethoscope over an inert portion of a patient and use the other ends to plug their ears, they create the perfect ambience for contemplating not just trivial problems such as 'What is the matter with this patient?' but more serious ones such as 'What is her name?, or 'What crisp, reassuring, non-discussion provoking phrase will get me out of here in time to watch the football on television?'.

The beauty of this clinical manoeuvre is that the very act that enables you to struggle with your own problems gives your patients the impression you are thinking deeply about theirs. As a result, you can make decisions free from the pressure of time. The longer you take, the more your patient is impressed by your thoroughness.

Sophisticates improve this empowering quality by bunging the earpieces with cotton wool to eliminate distracting sounds that may intrude if they inadvertently place the business end over the heart or other noisy organ. Soundproofed stethoscopes are particularly useful for dealing with talkative patients whom a doctor can halt in full flow by applying the instrument to their chests and telling them to breathe deeply.

Over the years, doctors have found many uses for the stethoscope – as a tourniquet, a paperweight, a hook for retrieving packets that have fallen behind chests of drawers, and an effective binder for boxes with loose lids. I knew a senior doctor who used an old stethoscope to keep his trousers up and a junior who, when faced with a personal credit crisis, used his to siphon petrol from cars left overnight in the residents' car park.

All in all the stethoscope has proved, in the right hands, to be a useful, versatile and safe instrument, provided doctors are not unduly influenced by anything they hear through it.

## Stroke prevention
Ban on the use of hyphens imposed by the *British Medical Journal (BMJ)* in a bid, claimed the editor, to save hours of discussion. When implemented consumed more hours than it saved.

The writer Keith Waterhouse regarded hyphens as a necessary evil and regretted that the choice lay between 'second-hand-car salesman', which he thought fussy, and 'second-hand car salesman', which suggested that the salesman was second hand. Sir Ernest Gowers had already suggested that a fried fish merchant is not quite the same thing as a fried-fish merchant.

Dr Jeff Aronson pointed out that the *BMJ's* ban had led it into headlining a news item, *Vaccine tailor made to treat cancer.* "Poor chap," said Dr Aronson.

And Dr Dominic Horne complained the ban had caused the journal to publish a misleading headline. *Five yearly checks for over 40s will save 650 lives a year* suggested that the over forties would be checked five times a year rather than once every five years.

## Student

Person of any age who relishes subversion.

The American physician Richard L Day defined a student as, "Someone who thinks otherwise" and suggested it was dangerous to treat this healthy state of mind.

Doctors who have the stamina to remain students for most of their lives come to be known as 'troublemakers'. They ask rude and awkward questions, criticise received truth, and their abrasive qualities disrupt the smooth running of official machinery. They have occasional moments of triumph when they reveal to the conformists that their emperor is wearing no clothes but they also serve a useful day-to-day purpose by keeping authority on the defensive, which is the only safe place for it in a democracy.

Doctors were once rather good at troublemaking but the tradition seems to have gone into a decline. It's time more doctors won the accolade J B Priestley awarded to Margaret McMillan when he described her as one of "those beastly agitators who are always bringing up awkward subjects and making decent people feel uncomfortable."

## Success

Prize that managers strive energetically to win. More difficult concept for clinicians for whom success is inevitably followed by failure.

Doctors who practice, as opposed to those who preach, can find themselves out of tune with the managerial ethos that dominates 21$^{st}$ century culture. One reason, I suspect, is that it harps so much on success as if that were the ultimate human achievement. Yet doctors practice a craft in which the ultimate 'outcome', no matter how clever they may be along the way, is a patient's death. And much of the art of medicine – well, the sort of medicine I want practiced on me – is concerned with trying to help people survive the short spell they have on this earth in some sort of harmony with the world around them.

George Orwell suggested that, seen from within, every life is a succession of failures. Experience has taught me that failure doesn't matter. A lesson I learned in clinical medicine – and now apply to less worthy activities – is that life can still be rewarding if you strive for perfection while knowing you're unlikely to achieve it. Maturity dawns when failure becomes a worthy objective. You can fail only if you try to do something; the surest route to success is doing nothing.

I hope Valhalla has a special hall for those whom success-chasers call 'losers': a European navigator, maybe, who got to America ten years before Columbus but liked it so much he didn't bother to come home to boast of his success.

Valhalla would need a much bigger hall for those who *know* they are successful: the 17th century intellectuals, for instance, who said of Galileo, "He's a decent enough chap but he's got this fixation about Copernicus. Insists the earth moves round the sun when he just needs to stick his head out the window to see he's wrong."

## Suffering
Traditionally regarded by hospitals as the only route to joy.

An antique truth handed down from generation unto generation and exemplified in a memorandum from Mrs Edwards, Assistant Domestic Manager to Sisters and Heads of Department at the old Oldchurch Hospital in Romford: *As from 12 November the issue of pre-packs will now contain hard toilet rolls, due to excessive use of soft.*

## Superstition
The irrational beliefs of other people. Our own irrational beliefs we call Faith.

One evening when the world and I were young, by which I mean the early 1970s, I found myself dining in a gazebo in the middle of a tropical garden on the island of Bali. The head of the local WHO unit had taken me to dine at the home of a missionary, a tall, lean and, it proved, erudite man: a Jesuit priest who had come to Bali from Argentina. In a film he would be played by Gregory Peck.

The WHO doctor had explained in the jeep that the priest's interpretation of his mission had less to do with converting the Balinese to Christianity than with perfecting a breed of long-bodied pig, perfect for local conditions and a cheap source of rich protein.

It was a magical evening. The canopy of the gazebo was supported by four slim stilts and there were no side walls. The only curtains were streams of rain that fell vertically from the sky onto the lawn outside. In the vaults of the canopy above us, fireflies flickered back and forth, as grateful as we were for the shelter.

The food was delicious and the conversation wandered widely, from energetic exploration of what we had learned from English literature to what well-intentioned intruders from affluent societies could do for impoverished ones. The subjects were serious but the talk was never solemn. We laughed a lot and I noticed that the most radical and subversive ideas, and the wittiest observations, came from our Jesuit host.

It was my first visit to the island and late in the evening, and because the meal was not alcohol-free, I launched into an energetic declaration of my love for the Balinese: their gentleness, their music, their dancing, their painting, and the innate aesthetic sense that all of them seemed to possess.

"Ah yes," sighed my host, echoing my admiration. "But you have to remember, doctor, that they are very superstitious people… oh dear me, very superstitious people."

And, as he repeated the phrase, he blessed himself, his right hand travelling in a broad sweep from brow to breast to shoulder to shoulder.

I doubt he was aware of the gesture. But I was.

## Surgical spirit

Jaunty attitude that male surgeons once adopted – and maybe still adopt – towards colleagues and students who have the misfortune to be women.

In his book *Trust me I'm a Doctor,* Phil Hammond offers a woman's description of what happened in 1995, when she was a student and assisted a surgeon in the operating theatre:

*First he asked me if I was from the Home Counties. When I said yes, he started calling me Tinkerbelle and said I looked the sort of girl who'd had a horse between my legs. Then he asked me if I'd lost my virginity up against the wall of a horse-box while my mother was outside watching a gymkhana. The registrar and the other theatre staff started laughing too. It was like being in a monkey house. At the end, he asked me if I minded him being sexist in theatre – "Women like to know what men want." Then he made a hole in the gall-bladder and said, "Look what you've made me do."*

## Sweet reason

Seasoning used to disguise the bitterness of revenge.

I discovered its value at my medical school soon after World War Two when a group of students decided to take revenge on an administrator they thought had dealt with them unjustly.

One hot summer day they scoured the North Downs near the hospital's country branch and captured three basking adders. They brought them back to town in a basket, and set them free in the tiny apartment where the administrator lived alone. A pretty routine medical student prank you may think but they sweetened their revenge with a note they left on his desk: *Dear Mr X, we have left four snakes in your room.*

Fifty years later, a well respected San Francisco physician arrived at the Customer Relations counter in the basement of a department store. She was carrying an electric toaster.

"Do you remember persuading me to have this repaired instead of getting a new one in exchange?" she asked.

"I do indeed," said the blue-rinsed 'customer counsellor',

"Perhaps you could remind me how I need to operate it. I've brought along two slices of bread."

"Certainly," said Ms Blue Rinse. She plugged in the toaster, inserted the bread, and pushed down the lever.

Every light in the basement went out.

# T

## Talk Therapy

20th century activity popular with Californians and would-be Californians with time to fill between cosmetic surgery and colonic lavage.

Now eagerly embraced by the new rich, the new idle, and the not so rich but easily exploited. The menu is generous, varied – and expensive.

*To say 'Hello' rightly is to be aware of the other person as a phenomenon, to 'happen' to him or her and be ready for him or her to 'happen' to you! This course will provide a theoretical base, through the concepts of Transactional Analysis, to help you to reflect upon your attitudes and beliefs in order to be more open and natural – in Transactional Analysis terms to be more authentic, autonomous and spontaneous.*

University of Lancaster Summer School prospectus.

*What the aesthetic drama has done for deities like Dionysus, Brahma or Jehovah and the representative characters like Hamlet, Macbeth or Oedipus, the psychodrama can do for every man.*

J L Moreno' in *Sociometry.*

*The last session was a demonstration of primal therapy. For the spectator this is less interesting than a wrestling match, and lasts longer.*

Bulletin of the British Psychological Society.

*Those who feel they need psychotherapy tend to be the very people who are most easily exploited; the weak, the insecure, the nervous, the lonely, the inadequate and the depressed, whose desperation so often is such that they are willing to do and pay anything for some improvement of their condition.*

Foster Enquiry into the Practice and
Effects of Scientology.

## Targets

Ridiculous goals set by compulsive modernisers.

In 2009 a GP surgery in Preston, Lancashire, was docked £375 from its income because it had had no complaints from patients.

The NHS rewards GP surgeries for hitting targets, one of which is demonstrating how they deal with complaints. The Preston surgery lost out because, having had no complaints, it couldn't demonstrate how it dealt with them. A spokesman for the local NHS trust said it had to follow guidelines.

## Teamwork
Concept of interdependence instilled in doctors early in their tutelage.

I learned its value as an undergraduate in post-war Cambridge. One of the great sporting events of 1947 was the first post-war rugby tour of the mighty Wallabies. On the day they were to play the university at Grange Road, the Professor of Anatomy insisted, under threat of dire penalty, that every student should attend a lecture carelessly timed to start twenty minutes before the match. Everyone dutifully signed in but five minutes into the lecture one of the male students fainted. Later calculations revealed that it took twenty-seven of his colleagues to carry him out. I was number twenty-six.

## Teflon skills
Rules GPs have evolved to protect themselves from impromptu consultations.

- Never use the front door of a hotel which harbours lonely old people as permanent residents. Always approach via the kitchen and the back stairs. Ingenuous fools who walk through the residents' lounge deserve what they get.
- Never take your car onto a caravan site. Leave it down the road and approach on foot trying to look like a rent collector.
- If nobbled in the street, try a pre-emptive strike before the patient speaks. "How nice to see you looking so well, Mrs Cadwallader. Haven't seen you looking healthier for years. Must dash."
- If entrapped, don't neglect the Classical Deterrent originally designed for cocktail parties but effective in any public place. "Just drop your trousers and we'll have a look."

## Telephone advice
Dangerous activity for young GPs, especially after dark.

When I retired from general practice, my first life enhancing discovery was that the telephone beside my bed was no longer an enemy that threatened me by night but a friend that could serve up cheerful conversation during the day.

The worst feature of a night call was its instigation: the insistent ringing that penetrated my sleep while I tried desperately to dream it away. Just as the droning of German bombers during my childhood meant the siren would soon sound and I would have to get out of bed and head for the air-raid shelter, so the ringing of the bedside telephone meant I would have to get up and visit a patient, even if I were asked only for advice. I'd learned that, if I didn't go, I'd lie awake for much longer than it would take to make a visit, wondering if I'd done the right thing. I envied those who mastered the skill of giving advice without actually waking up.

One of my medical school contemporaries told me how, when he was a young GP, his senior partner insisted that he "always turn out for babies." On his first night on call, he obeyed instructions when the mother of a nine-month-old baby telephoned at two in the morning because she was worried by her baby's "snuffles."

He examined the child carefully, explained to the mother that her daughter had a mild upper respiratory infection, was not in danger and needed to be nursed and cosseted. If she were still worried in the morning she should give him a ring.

The mother nodded. "I thought you'd say that, doctor. I didn't really want you to come. When my other daughter had the same trouble, Dr X (the senior partner whose advice he'd followed) told me over the phone that all would be well till he came in the morning." Then she added: "Of course he would be more experienced than you, wouldn't he?"

In those days the process was called 'learning by apprenticeship': learning, that is, not about night calls but how to unload irksome tasks on to your juniors, one of medicine's great Hypocritic traditions.

Today, of course, it's a lesson few need to learn. Most GPs – but not all – unload 'out of hours' calls onto strangers whom they never meet.

## Testiculator
One who waves his arms about while talking balls - *Cambridge University Medical School slang.*

## Themarket
Ancient God to Whom some believe all of human life must be subservient.

Belief in His supreme power was revived in the final decades of the 20<sup>th</sup> century by two powerful sects, the Thatcherites and the Reaganites, and later adopted by the neotribe of Blairites.

Themarket was hailed, among other things, as the saviour of health services on which His mystic power would confer efficiency – but only by people who were aged under sixty or had lost their memory.

The Oxford historian Charles Webster, explained in a lecture to the Royal College of Physicians (see Market traders):

*Experience (of health services during the inter-war period) had demonstrated that the market system was a failure. Even according to narrow criteria of efficiency gains, the achievements of the early NHS were of an altogether higher order than anything claimed for the current wave of experimentation with market systems. The forms of administration and management introduced by Bevan were not an irresponsible and wasteful experiment in socialism but the logical conclusion of an evolutionary development which had been underway for more than a decade. It is therefore the early NHS, not the chimeras of the marketeers, which represents the realisation of Britain's native genius in the field of health care.*

## The patient
Mythical creature who exists only in the minds of those who claim to represent it, and of doctors who use it as a collective noun for people they've never met.

Don't get me wrong. I don't mean a patient, or patients generally, all of whom are fellow members of the human race. I mean The patient, depersonalised by the definite article so often used to homogenise groups that are heterogeneous to fault: The public, The people, The listener, The viewer, and so on.

One summer evening in 2004, I returned from my GP's crowded waiting room and, in masochistic mood, logged on to the *BMJ* website. I should have known better. The first thing I encountered was a string of 'rapid responses' from an ill-assorted bunch urging us to listen to "The patient's voice", by which of course they meant their own.

Not for the first time the definite article got under my cuticles. The GP's waiting room from which I'd just returned had, I suspect, harboured as many different voices as different faces. Indeed I don't suspect, I know. One of the few truths I've learned from experience is that The patient's voice is legion. And when it comes to interpreting what our voices are saying I would put greater trust in the GP who was running 45 minutes late because of the care with which he listened to our stories than in any of the *BMJ* responders who presumed to speak on our behalf – not even the Fourth Earl Baldwin of Bewdley, formerly Viscount Corvedale, educated at Eton and Trinity, Cambridge, whose only occupations declared in *Who's Who* were membership of the House of Lords and former Chairman of the British Acupuncture Accreditation Board.

Doubtless all the responders were motivated by the very best of intentions but, at my time of life when I am more patient than doctor, I get irritated by people in High Places such as the Department of Health, the House of Lords, and the groves of academe who presume to speak in patronising tones on behalf of me and my friends in low places.

Most of us are quite capable of speaking and thinking for ourselves, thank you. Just as most of us – and, over the past few years I have made a lot friends in waiting rooms and hospital wards – seem able to find doctors who are prepared to listen to us and help us make our decisions.

## Time lapse

An easy way to outwit dogmatic doctors.

Johannes Brahms, like many a composer, enjoyed his food. One day, when feeling the Viennese equivalent of the English 'a touch under the weather', he had the misfortune to consult a mean-spirited doctor who ordered him to start immediately on a strict diet.

"But this evening I am dining with Strauss," said Brahms, "and we shall have chicken paprika."

"Out of the question," said the doctor.

"Very well," said Brahms. "Please consider that I did not come to consult you until tomorrow."

## Tonsils and adenoids

Lumps of lymphoid tissue whose only purpose is to provide for the private education of the children of ear, nose, and throat surgeons.

## Tool

Multipurpose implement commended to NHS workers when no money is available.

> *High quality and cost-effectiveness are two sides of the same coin. Both are needed. The Government is providing new tools to ensure they are achieved.*
> Department of Health consultation document.

> *The indications are that there are serious shortcomings in perception, understanding and managerial capacity which will need to be tackled if the NHS is to move forward in its use of standards as a strategic development tool.*
> Clearly Competent: The Strategic Use of Occupational Standards in the NHS.

> *It is recognised by the Trust that establishing an open and blame free culture and environment is crucial in underpinning the entire risk management process as a policy of openness and honesty will allow the Trust to learn from mistakes when they occur and utilise them as a proactive management tool.*
> Management Policy Statement. Mid Yorkshire NHS Trust.

## Top doctor

Any doctor a journalist finds at home and willing to give a 'quote' close to a deadline.

## Touch of

Passing acquaintance the English claim to have with a disease so they can use it as an excuse without being seen to make a fuss.

'A touch of flu' or 'A touch of the old trouble' are acceptable reasons for a break in regular attendance at saloon bar or golf club, or non-appearance at a reunion dinner.

The phrase is also a useful conversational segue. A

correspondent to the erstwhile *Lancet* column, *In England Now,* claimed the only thing he learned when he served in the RAMC was that he could sustain any conversation in the mess with just four remarks: 'Pity', 'Really?', 'You don't say', and 'A touch of arthritis'.

## Toy soldier

An army doctor – a person whom regular soldiers used to describe as "always an officer, sometimes a gentleman."

In the days of national service, conscripted doctors could savour the delights of a peacetime army. Within a week of my call up, my garrison was on ceremonial parade. It was impressive: bayonets fixed, flags flying, bands playing, and lots of people stamping their feet and shouting. I was safely anonymous in the middle ranks but, thanks to some quirk of military protocol, one of the four officers standing in front of the parade was a national service doctor from the local military hospital. The three proper officers had crisply pressed uniforms, mirror-like toe-caps on their shoes, and had rammed the peaks of their caps down onto their noses. The doctor wore a rumpled battledress and suede shoes, and his RAMC cap perched uneasily on a mound of frizzy hair. Then, as the general who had come to inspect us ascended his podium, and the RSM bellowed a loud incoherent command, the doctor looked impatiently at his watch and strolled casually off the parade.

Next morning when wheeled in front of an apoplectic commanding officer, he explained he was already seven minutes late for his clinic and didn't want to keep his patients waiting.

He wasn't playing a game. Most conscripts had been drafted soon after qualifying and were keen as mustard on practising their medical skills. Many of the 'regular' doctors, who'd spent most of their professional lives looking after healthy young men, acknowledged their medical limitations and admitted they'd joined the RAMC to get away from the drudgery of clinical practice.

The CO of one hospital, a kindly soft voiced Dubliner, told me: "I expect my junior officers to get on with the medicine. I specialise in good living." He'd joined the Indian Army medical service in the 1930s and, when he boarded his troopship at

Southampton, his only baggage was two polo saddles.

His humour was a useful antidote to the earnestness of the conscripts but some of his regular colleagues had dangerous pretensions. When John Seale, one of my national service contemporaries, was hidden behind screens examining a patient, he overheard a regular army surgeon say to a colleague: "I hope they call me in on that case. I haven't been inside a chest for years."

## Traditional British diet
Stirring patriotic phrase used by food manufacturers seeking to defend the eating habits they promote from the likes of Jamie Oliver.

Evokes an image of Essex and Elizabeth exchanging wicked glances over platefuls of baked beans, sausages, and fatty chips, and hints that the glory that blazed at Agincourt, Blenheim, and Waterloo was won by yeomen with knapsacks stuffed with packets of crisps, chocolate bars, Turkey Twizzlers, and bottles of brown sauce.

## Training
Instant solution for NHS problems. Not to be confused with education.

Some people seem incapable of developing the empathy and understanding you need as a doctor yet folk in High Places would have us believe that this defect can be corrected by 'training' in Communication or Empathy.

Imagine Mark Elder having a quiet word with the leader of his band. "I don't want to worry you, Charlie, but the old Halle sounds a bit scratchy on the fiddles these days. What we need are a dozen well-trained fiddlers. Nip down the pub like a good boy and pick a few likely lads. We'll send them on a violin training course and before you can say Simon Rattle we'll be back at the top of the charts."

If this training business is all it's cracked up to be, why waste it on doctors? Let's train half a dozen Leonardo da Vincis, four Isaac Newtons, a couple of Shakespeares, and a brace of Beethovens. Then we can all lie back and watch them build the new Jerusalem.

Kenneth Calman, when the government's Chief Medical

Officer, told me in an interview: "To be trained is to have arrived; to be educated is to continue to travel."

## Transcultural medicine
Intractable problem facing doctors trained south of Watford who have to work north of the Wash.

> Conversation, reported in the Lancet, between a newly recruited houseman and a patient's husband in a Leeds hospital.
> "And is she eating 'owt?" asked the husband.
> "Oh no," said young doctor. "She has all her meals in the ward."

> When Dr Gillon Ferguson was a registrar in Dundee, he heard a houseman, trying to sort out the beds in an overcrowded ward, ask a typical Dundee 'Wifie': "And who are you?"
> He got the reply: "Fine. Hoo's Yersel?"

## Trivial illness
An illness suffered by someone else.

## Trust
Paradoxical title given to NHS management units that inspire little confidence in their employees.

## Two-way dialogue
Tautology employed to give 'innovative' spin to ancient ideas.

According to the news sheet published by the Royal College of General Practitioners, an Oxfordshire practice received a *communication award* for *an innovative project designed to establish a two-way dialogue between the surgery and their patients.*

What's innovative about that? If they'd managed to establish a one-way dialogue or even a two-way monologue that would have been something.

# U

## Unconditioned reflex

Subconscious physiological response that produces an instantaneous reaction to a stimulus with no time for conscious thought.

When an advertising salesman asked the surgeon/novelist John Rowan Wilson what was the meaning of Mons Veneris, he instantly replied "Fanny Hill." John then looked puzzled and asked out loud, "Where on earth did that come from?"

Oliver St John Gogarty, Irish poet, ENT surgeon, and Buck Mulligan in Joyce's *Ulysses*, walked into a pub and saw a friend wearing an eye patch. Without pause for thought, he said: "Drink to me with thine only eye."

Frank Muir and Denis Norden often made me contemplate the physiology of repartee. Did their minds flash tangentially in search of ideas? Or did they have accelerated retrieval of lines they wrote years before. Whatever the answer, the result was impressive.
During a recording of *My Word,* I asked Frank, without warning, what historical incident he would like to have witnessed. With bare a pause he replied: " I'd like to have been present at the destruction of the cities of the plain. I've always wanted to know what went on in Gomorrah."

I was dining with people I didn't know too well when my host 'outed' me as a doctor. The first to strike was the woman on my left. Her husband was about to have coronary angiography. Dye, she gathered, would be injected through a tube into his coronary arteries and she assumed he'd be left with a puncture wound in his chest where the cardiologist inserted the tube. So why, she asked, would he have to lie flat on his back after the procedure with a pressure pad over his groin?

While my mind was elsewhere I heard my voice explain that these days the safest way to a man's heart is through his groin.

## Uncooperative patient

One who is impervious to simple straightforward explanation.

Such as the seventy-three-year-old woman described in a letter from a surgeon to Dr R S Smith, a GP in Helston.

*I explained that surgery carries a four per cent risk of stroke, and that after surgery her risk of stroke is about one and a half per cent per year. This will give her a five year stroke risk of about ten per cent. I have explained that best medical treatment carries about an eleven per cent risk of stroke in the next year and about seven per cent risk of stroke every year after that. This would give her a five year stroke risk of about forty per cent.*

*I have also advised her of the nature of carotid surgery and the recovery expected. I am afraid she seemed a little bewildered and taken aback by my explanations.*

## Undertaker

Onetime stalwart of the community.

When I left general practice in the mid-1960s an undertaker was one of a cadre of non-commissioned officers that sustained local communities: verger, school caretaker, park keeper, Bobby on the beat, and the AA motor cyclist who directed traffic at weekends. GPs knew them all but knew the undertakers best because they met them more often in, as it were, the way of business.

Yesterday, when rain stopped play at the Test Match and I switched channels, I saw a young man in a smart suit being introduced, to my dismay, as a funeral director's marketing manager. He was quick to explain he was no mere coffin maker nor coffin carrier but a highly skilled bereavement therapist.

Goodness gracious me. When I became a GP in 1953, undertaking – I beg its pardon, funeral directing – was largely a part-time business. Our undertaker, like most others, was a local builder. If you lived near one of his sites you would occasionally hear the foreman blow three blasts on a whistle and see the cheery chaps who were effing and blinding their way through the day put aside their tools and line up to be driven away on a sand-spattered lorry. Thirty minutes later they would reappear in smart morning suits with eyes downcast and faces frozen in solemnity as they walked as pall-bearers alongside a hearse or as marshals of a sombre procession.

By the 1950s most hearses were what the local paper called "motorised" but important figures in the community – bookies, county councillors, and what would now be called celebrity criminals – often chose to be ferried to eternity in a stately carriage drawn by a pair of black horses with plumes on their heads.

Within half an hour of the interment the pall bearers would be back on the building site in muddy boots and ragged trousers, shouting cheerful obscenities at one another and whistling at any young woman who dared pass by.

Intrigued by the sighting of the bereavement therapist, I trawled the internet and discovered that the University of Bath, established in 1966, offers a Foundation Degree in Funeral Services. The three year course includes the study of grief and bereavement, ritual and ceremony, developing professional competence, green issues, children and death, historical and sociological aspects of funerals, the running of a contemporary funeral business, and, inevitably, health and safety.

No mention there of brick laying or pick swinging. Oh where is the life that once we lived, or thought we lived or hoped we lived? Mechanised, modernised and now academicised beyond recognition.

## Unexpected question

Valuable diagnostic tool for clinicians and journalists. Sometimes elicits an unexpected, and revealing, answer.

An unexpected question is alleged to have provoked one of the Great Medical Moments of the 20th century.

Nixon's historic visit to China in 1972 set off a fashion. Not only governments but national institutions hurried to visit what was then a largely unknown country. Medical organisations were quick off the mark and the British Medical Association was one of the early visitors. The Irish Medical Association was further down the queue and by the time its turn came, the Chinese had established a standard tour: a bit of traditional medicine, a bit of acupuncture, a walk on the the wall and, as a grand finale, an interview with Chairman Mao.

Throughout the tour one of the Irish delegates, still referred to as Dr O'Nonymus, tried hard to devise a question that might elicit from Mao something more rewarding than a diplomatic platitude.

When the final day came the delegates sat in a polite semi-circle before the Chairman. Each in turn commented on the fruitfulness of the visit, the generosity of the hosts, a future of better understanding, opportunities for cooperation, and so on and so on... until it came to O'Non's turn. Instead of making a comment he posed his carefully prepared question. "What does the Chairman think would have happened in the world if, instead of J F Kennedy, Kruschev had been assassinated?"

The question, translated by the interpreter, was considered by Mao for a long, long time – no doubt inscrutably. Then back, via the interpreter, came the answer. "The chairman says that only one thing is certain. Onassis would never have married Mrs Kruschev."

In Ireland O'Non has now become a legend which means, when translated, that no one knows for sure that he existed. But that's of little consequence in a land where good stories exist not to be verified but to be told.

## Unfortunate symbolism
Something for which the NHS has an unhappy talent.

On July 5th 1948, the 'appointed day' on which the NHS was born, I was visiting my parents in a Yorkshire colliery village. (A local councillor once explained to the BBC that it wasn't twinned with anywhere but it did have a suicide pact with Grimethorpe.)

My father was the local GP and very much part of the community; one of my childhood memories of the 1930s Depression is of helping him load his car with the medicaments he said his patients needed – not bottles of medicine but tureens of stew. (See Care.) He was also one of a tiny group in the local BMA who actually applauded the coming of the NHS.

So maybe we shouldn't have been surprised when, on the morning of July 5th 1948, the colliery band assembled outside our house and celebrated the birth of the NHS with rousing variations of 'If You Knew Souza Like I Knew Souza'. It was the sort of serenade they gave us every Christmas morning and, when they'd blown themselves out, my dad and I, as we did each Christmas, carried out trays of beer and whisky.

Nick Timmins later described the event in his masterly biography of the welfare state *The Five Giants* and in 1998, as part of the celebrations of the NHS's 50th anniversary, the local Trust decided to re-enact the scene. But it had a problem. After the miners' strike, Mrs Thatcher's apparatchiks not only closed and sealed the pit but abolished the colliery band and took away its uniforms. Undaunted, the Trust's publicity whizzers hired a band from elsewhere. They also planned to hold the ceremony not outside our old house but in front of a new health centre they were eager to publicise.

The result was a happening more symbolic than they intended. In 1998 the South Yorkshire mining villages had the highest rate of unemployment in the country and the folk who'd been around in 1948 were among the nation's most deprived. How better to celebrate this achievement than by importing outside musicians to play the wrong music in the wrong place. When they invited me to take part I found business elsewhere... but my dad would have enjoyed it.

## Unjust dessert
A dish GPs grow used to consuming.

An elderly woman who lived alone and appeared to have few friends was admitted to a London hospital. Her GP, knowing she would be lonely and fearing she might be disorientated, went to visit her. He described in a medical journal how, because there was no space in the car park, he left his car in the road on a double yellow line with a polite note on the windscreen explaining the circumstances and ending: *Forgive us our trespasses*.

The old woman didn't recognise him and refused to see him and, when he returned to his car, he found a parking ticket on which the warden had scrawled: *Lead us not into temptation*.

## Unlicensed surgery

Routine surgical operation performed by an untrained person.

It is something of a national scandal that this includes the commonest operation performed in Britain every day: the surgical removal of trichotic filaments from the facial epidermis. Every morning men perform it without benefit of protocol or training, using a surgical blade honed, if we are to believe the advertisements, to the highest degree of sharpness known to man.

My investigations reveal that these dangerous surgical instruments are freely available in High Street shops where vulnerable teenagers can buy them across the counter and set about using them with no appropriate training, not even a book of instructions. And many bear the scars to prove it.

We're used to the Department of Health being dilatory in such matters but I'm astonished that the issue hasn't been taken up by the Royal College of Surgeons, founded as it was by barbers seeking to protect their trade.

Let's face it, we're not talking just about untrained surgeons but unnecessary surgery. Bernard Shaw described how at the age of five he watched his father shaving and asked him why he was doing it. "He looked at me in silence for a full minute before throwing the razor out the window and saying 'Why the hell do I?' He never did again."

It's odd that no journalist has had the courage to challenge this form of self-mutilation for here surely is a scandal worthy of a Panorama investigation, a proliferation of victim support groups, or even, dare I say it, an Esther Rantzen Special.

## Unnatural selection

Unfair discrimination by antivivisectionists and animal welfare organisations who never campaign on behalf of creatures whose slaughter is measured not in tens per hour, or in thousands per year, but in millions per second?

Sixty years ago, I wrote a revue lyric that expressed my concern. Here, to give you the flavour, are a couple of stanzas. If nothing else, they reveal what little effect the passage of time has on human barminess.

*Why are we so cruel to bacteria?*
*Let me ask you, by the way of introduction,*
*Why it doesn't seem to shock us*
*That we kill the staphylococcus*
*By inhibiting its powers of reproduction.*
*Why should we think bacteria*
*In any way inferior*
*Because they're small and singularly plain?*
*And are we sure a bite*
*From a hungry leucocyte*
*Doesn't cause unnecessary pain?*

*Why are we so cruel to bacteria*
*When kindness always helps to clear the air?*
*Perhaps the salmonella*
*Is a friendly little fella*
*Who is longing for a little loving care.*
*Each small bacterium*
*Has a loving dad and mum*
*And a virus*
*Should inspire us*
*Every one.*
*Yet the poor old spirochete*
*Who only wants to live and eat*
*Is murdered 'cos he complicates our fun.*

## Unprecedented
Adjective used by hospital administrators to describe emergency admissions every January.

## Upper lip rigidity
A Briton's first line of defence against disease or discomfort.

Allegedly sustained by a diet rich in moral fibre and usually associated with a stiffening of the backbone. Lack of moral fibre in the diet of foreigners causes a streak of yellowish discolouration of the skin overlying the spine.

Discussing the British admiration of a stiff upper lip, the American journalist Lynn Payer quotes a report that suggested British psychiatrists tend to regard people who are quiet and withdrawn as normal but prescribe tranquillisers for those who seem unsuitably overactive.

More direct evidence came when Ms Payer saw an English woman tell a television interviewer how she'd given birth to twins on an Italian train. The woman's main concern had been that she might wake the other passengers.

## Venereal revenge

A vindictive form of retribution reported by Samuel Pepys.

The avenger was Robert Carnegie, Earl of Southesk; his victim the Duke of York, later to become James II.

On Monday 6 April 1665 Pepys recorded how, when the Earl discovered his wife was having an affair with the Duke, he bade her to continue the liaison. Pepys writes:

[He then] *went to the foulest whore he could find, that he might get the pox; and did, and did give his wife it on purpose, that she (and he persuaded and threatened her that she should) might give it the Duke of York; which she did, and he did give it the Duchesse; and since, all her children are thus sickly and infirm – which is the most pernicious and foul piece of revenge that ever I heard of. And he at this day owns it with great glory, and looks upon the Duke of York and the world with great content in the ampleness of his revenge.*

The incident Pepys records is substantiated by two of his contemporaries who also described it: Gilbert Burnet, theologian, historian and Bishop of Salisbury; and the Comte de Gramont whose *Mémoires*, though regarded by many as jewel of French literature, were written for him by an Englishman, Anthony Hamilton.

Other adulterers allegedly subjected to this form of retribution featured regularly in courtly gossip in succeeding centuries. And, in the 1980s, a 'reliable source' – a doctor whom Richard Gordon, British medicine's national treasure, met in a London pub – swore it was wreaked on a British cabinet minister in the 1960s.

## Verbal Autoimmunity
Syntactical condition induced by medical surroundings. Words become allergic to their own meaning.

> I first became aware of the condition while lying on a trolley in the A&E department at Royal Surrey Hospital in Guildford. A passing ambulance driver said to his mate: "I'd give my right arm to be able to play the guitar."

> Grammatical advice that the journalist Tim Albert found in an article purporting to help medical writers: *Data is always in the plural.*

> Proud boast I saw in the window of an old fashioned chemist's shop in a South Coast town: *We dispense with precision.*

> An anxious man to his Torquay GP: "I'm very worried about our marriage. If my wife's agoraphobia gets any worse I fear she may walk out."

## Verbal incontinence
Congenital affliction endemic in the South of Ireland.

A beguiling quality of Irish anecdotage is the love affair the people conduct with words, not just with their meaning but with their fabric and their sound. 'Tis said that in England you can say what you like as long as you do the right thing, while in Ireland you can do what you like as long as you say the right thing. Add to that passion for words a manic depressive national personality and you create a society in which, in the words of Mahaffy, the inevitable will never happen but the unexpected often occurs.

> Joyce Delaney, author and psychiatrist, told me that when her father, who was Dublin GP, visited her in Birmingham, he saw his first televised party political broadcast. He switched on in the middle and watched in silence for several minutes. Then he turned to his daughter and said: "If that man knew anything more, he'd be confused."

At the annual meeting of the Irish Medical Association, I heard a country GP give a long, complicated, yet highly entertaining, account of some political happening. "Excuse me interrupting, Joe," said the chairman, "but we're pushed for time. Could you just give us the gist."

The speaker waxed indignant. "It's all gist," he said.

## Versatility

Essential quality – I beg its pardon, 'core requirement' – in general practice. Not always appreciated by outsiders.

At the turn of the century, when a cranky politician questioned the social usefulness of general practice, I invited GPs to send me case histories to rebut the accusation. Thanks to their response, I acquired evidence of the pivotal role GPs played in late 20$^{th}$ century Britain. Here are just two of many doctors who served their communities well.

In Luton, Dr Paddy O'Donnell rendered valuable service to a stranger who turned up at his surgery. The stranger, a policeman, had been accused of sexual harassment by a woman PC who claimed he'd boasted noisily in her presence about his sexual attributes including his decorated penis.

He wanted a certificate stating that his penis was unpierced. The good doctor examined him and certified with due solemnity that the vital organ was unadorned. The policeman, said Dr O'Donnell, paid his £7.50 gratefully but left rather hurriedly. With the stroke of a pen the good doctor had stilled what could have been disruption in the ranks of Luton's finest.

Martin Kent of Westcliff-on Sea was asked to visit an elderly woman who'd had her haemorrhoids injected the previous week. The reason for the call, recorded in the visit book, was *Cannot go to toilet*.

Soon after he arrived at the woman's home, Dr Kent discovered the cause of her symptoms. Her lavatory seat was broken and the council wouldn't fix it. With the unruffled skill of a professional, he reduced the dislocation of the seat, tightened the loose bolts, and left the patient, in his own word, "contented".

## Vetting

Rigorous screening of applicants for sensitive NHS posts.

Like most politically dangerous jobs best delegated to 'private providers' who can do it on the cheap and be blamed if anything goes wrong.

A few years ago a series of tragedies spurred government officials to search for ways of checking the suitability of women who offer themselves as children's nannies. Hardly had the search begun when a friend who runs a nanny agency received a leaflet from a couple of experts who offered "a fast professional and confidential service" which could reveal "what a person is really like and whether she is genuine... an essential part of the vetting procedure in securing the best nanny."

Their "outline analysis", they claimed, would provide "insight into integrity, emotional balance, maturity and reliability"; their more expensive "in-depth analysis" would reveal the quality of the nanny's adaptability, attitude, application, and intellect.

The beauty of their technique was that the analysers did not have to see the candidate, only a specimen of her handwriting. Both persons offering the service – outline analysis £40, in-depth analysis £90 – were members of the British Academy of Graphology.

If Insight Graphology – yes, that's what it's called – can be used to still the fears of working mothers, what a gift it will be to hospital managers in search of 'private providers' to screen applicants for jobs in their hospitals' most sensitive areas.

## Village cricket

Traditional sport of rural GPs. Presence on village green gives the appearance of availability while deterring interruption.

Dr W.G. Grace never left the crease no matter how grave the summons. Even umpires found it difficult to dislodge him. Once when he was leaving his house carrying a cricket bag an anxious young woman accosted him. "I think my twins have got measles," she said. "Can you come?"

"Not just now," replied the doctor. "But contact me at the ground if their temperatures reach 206 for two."

## Virtual medicine
Imagery with which minds untutored in science interpret illness and its treatment.

Dr Tom Madden encountered two characteristic examples in his South London surgery.

"I said to myself: 'What's that snapped in my inside, and it went all round my belly like a needle and then settled in the shoulder'."

The sister of an elderly man who was admitted to hospital in a confused state described one of the investigations he'd endured, a telescopic exploration of his lower bowel via the rectum: "The doctor used this instrument to blow all the dust off his brains and he's back to his old self again."

Michael Winstanley gave me an example he encountered when he was a Manchester GP.

When an old woman died the widower dutifully handed back all her medicines to the doctor. Every bottle was empty and when the doctor asked what had happened to the left-overs, the old man replied: "Oh, I supped 'em. I thought 'appen they might find a weak spot somewhere."

Another GP friend offered this experience.

"I had to do a rectal examination on a nice old woman. She lay patiently on her side on the couch and as I crossed the room with gloved and anointed finger held aloft, she asked: 'Is it all right if I keep my teeth in, doctor?'"

## Visitors
Persons who come to plague the sick in hospital and sit uncomfortably at their bedsides waiting for some blessed signal that it's time to leave.

It is, however, possible to break with tradition. One of the many things I've learned as an octogenarian is the role my contemporaries want me to play when I visit their sickbeds, not as a doctor but as a friend.

The *New Yorker* columnist and critic, Alexander Woollcott defined it in the instruction he gave to a visitor during his final illness in 1943:

*I have no need of your God-damned sympathy. I only wish to be entertained by some of your grosser reminiscences.*

## Visual aid
Any illustration that gets in the way of understanding. (See Communication aid.)

*Thank you for publishing the photographs of my collection of kidney stones. The photo on your cover shows what I had told you was a kidney stone in the shape of Margaret Thatcher, the former Prime Minister of England. I was mistaken. It was not a photo of a kidney stone. It was a photo of Margaret Thatcher.*
Letter to *Annals of Improbable Research*.

## Vital Statistics
National guidelines for plastic surgeons.

In France the ideal bust measurement is 33 inches, in America 39 inches. Breasts reduced by surgeons in France would be treasured in America. As a result, in the United States, breast augmentation is performed twice as often as breast reduction. In France reduction is almost four times more common than augmentation.

Asked why face lifts are less common in France than in the United States, a Parisian surgeon explained: "In France, to age is to enter a social category that has its place."

## Vocation
Mystical influence that guides people towards a medical career.

The problem with my own vocation was less mystical than fiscal. When I finally decided I wanted to become a doctor, I was exempted the pre-clinical years thanks to my Cambridge degree in Natural Sciences but the only way I could fund three years living in London while doing the clinical course was to keep up my part time jobs as stage-hand at a West End theatre, occasional scriptwriter for the BBC Variety Department, and petrol pump attendant in Streatham.

Rumour had it that St.Thomas' was the most likely of the London hospitals to countenance odd-ball students so that's where I applied. Before my interview I carefully constructed an opening gambit in the bar of The Two Sawyers, the pub across the road from the hospital. So, when ushered to a chair in the Dean's office, I pre-empted any discussion of my profound desire to save suffering humanity by asking: "Could this hospital countenance the idea of a part-time medical student?"

To which Allen Crockford, secretary to the Dean, replied "Is there any other kind?"

After that, the conversation was too low-flying to include notions like vocation. Allen Crockford saw no reason why I should give up my part-time jobs while I 'walked the wards'. (He didn't use the phrase but, even in 1949, others still did.) He offered me a place on the understanding I would write the St Thomas' Christmas Show which before the war had earned the same reputation as the Cambridge Footlights Revue.

Times have of course changed. As has the nature of vocation. Recently a GP told me about the evening he helped out at a Careers Night in a local school. His first customer was a shy sixth former accompanied by a forceful mother.

"So you're thinking about becoming a doctor," he said to the boy.

"Yes."

"Which branch of medicine do you think you might be interested in?"

"Private," said his mother

## Voice of the Profession

Portentous tones adopted by medical politicians who regard themselves as 'leaders of the profession'."

Not to be confused with the 'voice of the doctor' which patients, if they're lucky, hear in consulting rooms or at their bedsides: a softer, less certain and more sceptical tone than that which fills the air at political summits.

If doctors as a profession wish to foster the respect that most of them still command as individuals, the best way to do so is to avoid the seven deadly clinical sins defined by Richard Asher: obscurity, cruelty, bad manners, over-specialisation, spanophilia (love of the rare), stupidity, and sloth.

And, whisper it gently, some would say those sins are more often committed at the summit than at the foot of the mountain.

## Vox humana
The voice of patients speaking truth unto their doctors.

Tom Madden heard most of these in his South London practice. The rest were sent to me by other GPs.

> "I'm glad I've got somebody to console my troubles to."
> "When I retired they gave me a nice clock to see my time pass away."
> "My boyfriend is a bit of a suet pudding, more filling than satisfying."
> "My husband wears a protective but sometimes he forgets himself."
> "It's not me but the wife who's incompatible."
> "Tragic really. They'll be no use to him again… not as feet."
> Resident in old people's home: "We're like battery hens here… I like to keep a little free range."
> GP talking to woman in retirement home: "Why don't you sit outside in the sunshine on one of the benches?"
> "Oh, I wouldn't risk it. I don't want to be a poppy show. There's only one here who does. They call her the News of the World."

Last week as I sat, as a patient, in my GP's waiting room I heard a woman articulate the central paradox of general practice. She turned to her neighbour and said: "I feel much better, now that the doctor's found out there's really something wrong with me."

## Waiting room

Medicine's purgatory: a region where tormented souls linger unhappily for a time before being admitted to the healing presence.

James C Ruddie, writing in *Hoolet*, a serious but unsolemn magazine much loved by sceptical Scottish GPs, captured the ambience.

*We are soothed by piped music in an atmosphere heavily saturated with exotic germs and viruses. Despite a standard of living superior to that of all people who have ever existed, most of us cannot come to terms with the realities of life and express our unhappiness through illness.*

*"Chernobyl," the man sitting next to me says. "Chernobyl. That's what did for us. We're all knackered... and these bloody doctors? They're all useless. It's all parrot talk and probing and pretending with them. Mark my words, son."*

*I mark his words...*

*A Neanderthal rises, goes to reception and shouts "Do you know I've been sitting here for three quarters of an hour. What do those bastards do in there anyway?"*

*"Crosswords," replies the receptionist.*

*Nonplussed, he returns to his seat.*

A man, having waited overlong in the outpatients of a Dublin hospital, rose to his feet and announced to the congregation of fellow sufferers: "I think I'll go home and die a natural death."

## Waiting to happen

Where accidents linger for a time before being set free.

A man had fallen off a hospital trolley and broken his hip. At lunch time a television news reader interrogated one of the hospital's surgeons who was determined to give a mundane explanation. Irritated, the news reader sought to add urgency: "Wouldn't you say, doctor, that this was an accident waiting to happen?"

The surgeon, God bless him, replied: "Er... No."

Later the news reader wound up the bulletin: "And on this programme a member of the medical staff denied that this was an accident waiting to happen," thus giving the incident a roundness of zen-like perfection. It was as if the Revd Ian Paisley had walked out of a negotiation and said: "It's all over bar the shouting."

## Weathercock

Medical politician with a well honed sense of which way the wind is blowing... and of the most rewarding direction in which to face.

A weathercock gifted with reasonable intelligence and a constipated imagination finds it easy to give an impression of mediocrity, the quality so revered by the British establishment: "not too clevar by half... decent chap or gel... maybe a bit of a plodder but..." and here the trumpets sound, "... a safe pair of hands."

Winifred Holtby described the dominant characteristic in her novel *South Riding* when she wrote of the chairman of a County Council:

*Never in his life had he uttered an unexpected sentiment, and what he said could be noted down before he spoke it almost as easily as after it.*

Because weathercocks pose no threat to the craftily ambitious, a few are allowed to bumble away for so long that they end up in the old persons' annexe to the Palace of Westminster (see Peerage) where they can nod their lives away in consensual conversation.

## Welsh Rarebit

Versatile victual employed by 18th century accoucheurs in the Principality.

Francis Grose describes the practice in his *Classical Dictionary of the Vulgar Tongue*.

*The Welch (sic) are said to be so remarkably fond of cheese that, in cases of difficulty, their midwives apply a piece of toasted cheese to the janua vitae to attract and entice the young Taffy who, on smelling it, makes most vigorous efforts to come forth.*

## Who do you think you are?

Phrase that epitomises snap judgements that some people, not all of them doctors, make of other people's worth.

Carys Margaret Bannister won an international reputation while at the University of Manchester and was only the second woman to become a consultant neurosurgeon in the UK. In 2010 her obituary recorded how an exasperated milk man, unimpressed by her excuse that she hadn't paid him because she kept being called into work, asked, "What are you then? A bloody brain surgeon?"

An outstanding feature of the Edinburgh Festival in 1977 was the inspired playing of the London Symphony Orchestra under Claudio Abbado. One evening, just ten minutes before one of the concerts was due to begin, I saw Abbado, chauffeured by his wife Gabriella, being driven up the alley to the artists' entrance of the Usher Hall. Their path was blocked by a large Edinburgh policeman and Abbado, with an impish grin, nipped from the car and sprinted through the stage door leaving Gabriella to cope with the law. I couldn't hear what was being said but she clearly wasn't winning so I went over to intervene.

"Excuse me," said I, pointing to the crowds converging on the Usher Hall. "Do you know that this woman's husband is the reason all these people are flocking here this evening?" "That's as maybe, sir," said the policeman politely. "But he's not going to get his car up this lane without an official pass. And I would say just the same if he were Billy Connolly."

At least Abbado had his wife to act as buffer. One week before, Daniel Barenboim, after giving a stunning recital in the Usher Hall, arrived in the Pompadour Restaurant in the Caledonian Hotel to join Clifford Curzon for dinner. As he hurried across the room, still in white tie and tails, an angry diner grabbed him by the elbow and demanded: "Am I ever going to get the sauce for my fish?" "I will attend to it immediately, sir," said Barenboim. He flicked his fingers at a waiter and pointed at the angry diner. When he saw the waiter respond he bowed to the customer before joining Curzon at his table, thereby winning immediate entry to my register of nature's gentlemen.

One evening, Alan Coren, when editor of *Punch*, motored too sportingly along the Mall. A large policeman stepped into the road, waved him to a halt, then walked slowly round to the driver's window. "Now, now, sir," he said. "What have we here? Some sort of humorist, are we?"

## Whore's throat

Sometimes known as Clergyman's Throat.

Occupational malady.

A GP who acts as a medical agony aunt for a group of newspapers received a letter that began:

*Dear Doctor, I wonder could you tell me what you would prescribe for a whores throat. My throat has been whores for so long I can't even sing in the church quire…"*

## Why be unreasonable?

Question to which the only reasonable answer is "Why not?".

I've just attended a medical committee meeting at which two lively, if unorthodox, ideas were rejected largely because their implementation would not have suited the personal ambition of the chairman.

It's not an unusual experience. Over the years I've noticed that members of committees that wield real power can get so involved with the mechanics of committeemanship that they lose touch with the purpose for which they were originally convened. Maybe the honourable course is not to join them but to accept Sir Barnett Cocks's definition that "a committee is a *cul de sac* down which ideas are lured and quietly strangled" and devote your energy to trying to curb committee power.

I'm also ill at ease with the assumption made by most medical committees that progress will come through consensus. (Once, when I suggested that a GMC committee should settle a contentious issue by taking a vote, the chairman accused me of breaking the "unwritten rules". How's that for Catch 22?)

Consensus is a commendable way to stabilise established positions but is no way to seek ideas. As Bernard Shaw wrote in *Man and Superman*:

*The reasonable man adapts himself to the world; the unreasonable one persists in trying to adapt the world to himself. Therefore all progress depends on the unreasonable man.*

Perhaps the answer is to create enough committees to keep the games players occupied, reward them with honours rather than power, and feed them enough paperwork to keep them out of the hair of unreasonable people whose ideas may lead us to greener pastures.

## Will Rogers effect

Presentational change achieved by moving the goal posts when reporting research data.

Sometimes used to improve the look of clinical trial results, particularly those sponsored by pharmaceutical companies.

Named after the observation by the American humorist Will Rogers that, if the least intelligent ten per cent of Californians were to move to Ohio, it would significantly increase the level of intelligence in both States.

## Wilsonism

Any trick of the trade that is guaranteed to work. Name coined by Antony Jay, author of *Yes Minister* and other delicacies, for the practical wrinkles known to insiders in every profession.

When Jay, fresh out of Cambridge, tried his hand at teaching, he spent his first morning in a classroom of rowdy boys who ignored his shouted commands to "Shut up." During the break, a gnarled old teacher took him aside and told him it was no use shouting general exhortations. He should include a name in his command and shout: "Shut up, Wilson." It wouldn't matter if there were no Wilson in the class, everyone would quieten down and look round to see who was being admonished. Jay tried the phrase and found it worked.

He later discovered that similar wrinkles exist in every trade, rarely written down but passed by word of mouth from generation to generation. One of medicine's most valuable Wilsonisms was passed to me by Richard Leech: actor, doctor, and grandson of a distinguished Dublin physician, Richard Leeper.

Leeper's gift to his grandson went something like this: "Never give medicine to a dying man. Always give him brandy, for everyone knows that brandy never harmed anyone. Give the patient medicine and someone will say: 'God forgive me if I wrong him, but the doctor's draught was the last thing the poor man took'."

Grandfather Leeper must have received that advice round about 1880 and no one knows how many generations before that had passed it on. It could well have been devised in ancient Greece by one of those who used the pseudonym Hippocrates (qv) because that quality of learning has an imperishable validity.

## Wishful science

Phrase coined by the Nobel Laureate Irving Langmuir to describe cases in which enthusiastic scientists grow blind to the way in which subjective judgement and wishful thinking are leading them astray.

On 16 December 1961 the *Lancet* published a letter from Dr William McBride, a thirty-two-year-old Australian gynaecologist working in Sydney. It suggested that thalidomide, a sleeping pill women took during pregnancy, could be responsible for their babies being born with deformed limbs. When further research confirmed McBride's findings he won international acclaim and, during the years of litigation that followed, his international celebrity turned him into a national hero. He was the 1962 Australian of the Year and named as one of the one hundred most influential Australians of the 20th century. His fame enabled him to get resources for his own research centre, *Foundation 41*, at the Women's Hospital in Sydney.

Twenty years later, McBride issued a warning about another drug given to pregnant women. He and two junior associates at *Foundation 41* published a paper describing how eight rabbits were born with deformed limbs after their mothers received the drug. When one of the associates, Phil Vardy, read the published paper, he saw that the data in it were not those he had recorded. It was a traumatic moment. Vardy, confined to a wheelchair after breaking his back in a motorcycle accident, hero-worshipped his boss. His proudest day, he said, was the day McBride offered him a job. He talked to the other author, Jill French, but, when they confronted McBride, he refused to admit to fraud, just muttered phrases like, "Look, I'm very disappointed in this", and "I'm sure you're mistaken."

Within a week Vardy and French were fired. They wrote to the *Australian Journal of Biological Sciences* which had published the paper, but the journal didn't print their letter. Vardy found it impossible to get another job locally and when he eventually found one in Tasmania, the separation from his wife contributed to the foundering of his marriage.

McBride's fraud remained concealed for another five years. Then by chance Vardy met Norman Swan, an Aberdeen graduate who had worked as a paediatrician in the UK before emigrating to Australia and becoming a journalist. Swan, the first person Vardy had met who took his story seriously, used a handwriting expert to confirm McBride had altered the data. But Vardy was reluctant to publicise the story. He didn't want to topple an idol he had once revered, nor damage the reputation of Australian science.

Swan spent months trying to persuade him that staying silent did more damage to Australian science than speaking out. Only when Swan was sure that, if needed, Vardy would testify in court did he go on ahead with a programme now regarded as a milestone in Australian broadcasting.

In the programme's aftermath some newspapers defended "the lion of Australian medicine" with stories hinting that Vardy was after money, but once journalists tempered their immediate disbelief, they started to ask awkward questions. Eventually *Foundation 41* set up an internal inquiry headed by a former chief justice which, after a long hearing, found McBride guilty of fraud. He had to resign from the Board but, after "a decent interval", rejoined it. Later the New South Wales Medical Tribunal, after a protracted hearing, found him guilty of scientific fraud.

Swan, named Australian Radio Producer of the Year, received Australia's top prize for Science Journalism and a string of other awards. Vardy turned his back on the past, helped to establish sailing for the disabled in Australia, and laid the groundwork for his country's success in the Paralympics. McBride eventually admitted he had changed some data "in the long term interests of humanity".

## Women of a certain age

Patronising euphemism for women of uncertain age. A definitive example was Barbara Walters, the *grande dame* of American television, who was not only coy about her age but liked everyone else to be coy about it too.

One of the guests on her chat show was a sprightly ninety-year-old man, the mayor of an Irish city. After wheedling his age from him and encouraging the round of applause with which audiences congratulate old folk for surviving, Ms Walters asked him coyly what age he thought she was.

"Madam," said the dignified old boy, "in my country that is a question that is never asked and if asked would never be answered."

Then emulating the patronising smile of his hostess, he added: "But I'll tell you this. Whatever age you are, you certainly don't look it."

## Word Blindness

Visual defect that occurs when doctors grow so used to a cliché they become blind to its meaning.

I first encountered the condition as a medical student working the night shift in Casualty.

An ambulance delivered a patient with something nasty going on in his abdomen. I can't remember what it was but I've never forgotten what the surgical registrar said. "We must admit this chap for the students to see. He shows the typical picture and we don't see that very often."

"Is it is a rare condition then?" I asked.

"Oh no. Very common. But it's rare to see a typical presentation like this."

In my innocence I wondered why such a bright young man used 'typical' as a synonym for 'untypical'. Now I realise that medical usage had blinded him to the word's true meaning. This form of blindness affects doctors not just when they speak but when they write.

*Europeans living on diets of Buddhist monks have low blood cholesterol level – MRC News.*

A surgeon at St Richard's Hospital Chichester wrote to Tim Fooks, a GP in Pulborough: *This lady was reviewed in fracture clinic today. Her fourth finger of her right hand came off remarkably lightly after her dislocation.*

John Parrish, a GP in Kingston upon Thames, was relieved to read the headline: *Oral sex poses higher risk than thought,* implying, as it does, that just thinking about sex remains relatively safe.

## Worry
Infectious sense of unease.

Doctors are allowed to be anxious, tense, concerned, or perturbed; to agonise, brood, fret, lose sleep, torment themselves, or suffer the willies or the heebie-jeebies. But they must never show signs of worry in the presence of patients because it is dangerously infectious.

A month or so after I qualified, while doing a holiday locum in my father's practice, I was called to see a miner who'd taken to his bed with vague abdominal symptoms. I can see him now: thin-face, high-forehead, watching anxiously while I examined and re-examined him, did lots of investigations, but detected nothing abnormal. I was so worried about him that I took to visiting him every day and watched him daily grow more ill. I couldn't see that the more I worried about him, the more he worried about himself.

In desperation I called in my father for a second opinion and my brain still retains the image of him bursting into the patient's bedroom radiating good cheer.

"Now George, what the hell have you being doing to my son?" he said. "You should be ashamed of yourself, worrying him out of his wits."

Then he sat on the side of the bed engaging in cheery conversation with my patient who, for the first time since I'd seen him, allowed that drawn face to melt into a smile. My father then examined him as thoroughly as I had, chatting away merrily as he did so, and extracting the news that George was having problems with a foreman who seemed to have it in for him. When he'd finished his examination, he prescribed the treatment.

"You'd best get out of bed," he said. "Lying there is doing you no good. I think you've let this business at the pit get to your stomach but you need to be up and about. I'll give you a note to Ernie Bicknell to help you get on a different shift. In the meantime stop putting the fear of God into well-meaning young doctors."

As we left the room I turned and saw that the thin worried face that I'd visited daily had fattened into an expansive grin.

### Xenophobic oath

Affirmation of a medical truth acknowledged in every civilised country. Students, teachers, and clinicians are encouraged to swear by Apollo, or any other fashionable deity: "Our medicine is the best in the world."

I once asked a meeting of some 300 British GPs if anyone could name a French medical journal. No one could. And when a British anaesthetist told the European Society of Anaesthesiologists that, "These figures show the incidence is the same in England as it is in Europe", he seemed genuinely puzzled when the audience burst into laughter.

Sometimes the attitudes are fashioned by cultural differences. French doctors tend to be more concerned with the intellectual process than with its outcome. Hence that nasty French habit – at least in British eyes – of taking the temperature *a derriere*. Rectal temperatures are indeed more accurate than oral temperatures but while British doctors claim such precision is unnecessary, French doctors revere the intellectual quality of accuracy and attribute the British attitude to Puritanism.

The Atlantic borders of medical culture were neatly defined at a meeting of the American College of Cardiology, when the chairman hinted to his local audience that the European data that Britain's Professor Peter Sleight would present came from a rather primitive corner of the planet. Peter responded with the traditional eccentricity expected of an Oxford professor. He ostentatiously removed his shoes and socks, walked across the platform to the lectern and introduced himself as a visiting European "barefoot doctor".

## Xmas
Season when doctors enter into the festive spirit.

My father was a GP in a Yorkshire village and one of his seasonal duties twas to dress up as Father Christmas, make a surprise entrance at the Mixed Infant's school, and hand out the presents. Like many a GP he'd grown used to putting on a performance and entered his Christmas role with gusto.

Every year after doing his stuff he would arrive home in a state of high exhilaration and repeat the performance long after I and my sister had reached the age of Santa rejection. Then one year he crept into the house distinctly under-exhilarated. We later learned that, after he handed one Mixed Infant her present, she said: "Thank you very much, doctor."

"Ho, ho, ho," he said in theatrical basso profundo, "I'm not a doctor. I'm Santa Claus."

To which the girl responded: "Then why are you wearing the doctor's shoes?"

When I was a GP, one thing that never ceased to amaze me at Christmas twas the procession of patients bringing presents to my door. The value of the present always related inversely to the service I'd rendered; the nearer I'd come to actually killing someone, the more flamboyant the acknowledgement. That shouldn't have surprised me because there's nothing like making a mistake to render a GP dedicatedly attentive. As we desperately try to repair the damage we've done,we grow lavish with our time and our concern, and the punters interpret our hyperactivity as an expression of loving care.

Many of the presents were bottles wine and spirits and it was a sobering moment – if you know what I mean – when I realised that that my clinical incompetence kept my family in booze for about six months every year.

## Yorkshire relish

Delight provoked in those who live in the Ridings by the antics of those who don't. According to Simon Henry, author of *Tourist's Guide to the British*, a smile on the face of a Yorkshireman is a sign only of impending breaking wind.

In the 1970s, the *Yorkshire Post* ran a series of stories chronicling the progress of a party of twenty visiting Japanese chicken sexers who were visiting the county to share their skills with local poultry keepers. A West Riding GP claims that one morning, as he crossed the bridge at his local railway station, he saw one of the porters gazing down on the visitors bunched on a platform below.
As the GP approached, the porter turned and said: "They may be bloody clever these Japanese but they don't know the right platform for Sowerby Bridge."

A patient came to my friend John Oldroyd's surgery in Batley with a travel insurance application form that had to be countersigned by the traveller's doctor. When John glanced down the form he saw that under the heading, *Person to Notify in Case of Accident,* his patient had written: *Anybody in sight.*

# Z

## Zeal

Essential yet dangerous component of medical practice.

In an ideal world, radical treatment would be given only by conservative doctors, and conservative treatment only by radical ones. That would ensure that the doctor's attitude always worked in the patient's favour.

## Zen for the older person

How to walk the path of wisdom with one who knows.

> *Do not walk behind me, for I may not lead.*
> *Do not walk ahead of me, for I may not follow.*
> *Do not walk beside me, for I may not like it.*
> *Just leave me the hell alone.*

## Zero

Useful number for doctors who like to get their own way. Dangerous one for politicians who like to do the same.

One London public health doctor was proud of the way he made use of the fact that zero is a number. If under pressure at a council meeting, and fighting for a cause in which he believed, he would claim he had the support of local doctors, having discussed his proposal with a number of them.

Politicians should beware of boasting, as Mrs Thatcher did, that "our national investment in research is second to none", lest a numerate listener translate that as "less than zero".

Postscript.

Notes, acknowledgements, and references are posted on the website www.barefacedoctor.com.

This book started as a form of therapy after the sudden deaths of my wife Catherine and my younger daughter Lucy; it has ended as a celebration of times I shared with three generations of my family... and of the fortunate life I've been granted, despite doing precious little to deserve it.

My continuing good fortune led me, when my spirit was at its lowest, to the island of Menorca and the magical Biniarroca hotel where its creators, Lindsay Mullen and Sheelagh Ratliff, their ethereal garden and their skilled and genial staff offer not just peaceful refuge but the civilised ambience in which this book flourished.

Loxhill, October 2012